Antibodies in Radiodiagnosis and Therapy

Editor

Michael R. Zalutsky, Ph.D.
Associate Professor
Departments of Radiology and Pathology
Duke University Medical Center
Durham, North Carolina

CRC Press, Inc.
Boca Raton, Florida

Library of Congress Cataloging-in-Publication Data

Antibodies in radiodiagnosis and therapy / editor. Michael R.
Zalutsky.
p. cm.
Includes bibliographies and index.
ISBN 0-8493-6303-9
1. Antibodies, Monoclonal--Therapeutic use. 2. Antiblodies,
Monoclonal--Diagnostic use. 3. Cancer--Diagnosis. 4. Cancer-
-Radiotherapy. 5. Radioimmunoimaging. 6. Radioimmunotherapy.
I. Zalutsky, Michael R., 1949- .
[DNLM: 1. Antibodies, Monoclonal--diagnostic use. 2. Antibodies,
Monoclonal--therapeutic use. 3. Neoplasms--radionuclide imaging.
4. Neoplasms--therapy. QZ 266 A629]
RC271.M65A58 1988
616.07'57--dc19
DNLM/DLC 88-7659
for Library of Congress CIP

Direct all inquiries to CRC Press, Inc., 2000 Corporate Blvd., N.W., Boca Raton, Florida, 33431.

International Standard Book Number 0-8493-6303-9

Library of Congress Card Number 88-7659
Printed in the United States

PREFACE

The contents of this book are focused on the development of radiolabeled monoclonal antibodies for use in the diagnosis and treatment of cancer. This area of research has attracted the interest of scientists from a wide variety of disciplines, reflecting the multidisciplinary nature of the challenge. Realization of the full potential of labeled antibodies for increasing the selectivity of cancer-cell identification and destruction will require continued efforts by researchers in tumor-cell biology, immunology, pharmacology, radiopharmaceutical and protein chemistry, as well as in clinical medicine.

The purpose of this book is to provide a basic background of the various aspects of labeled monoclonal antibody development for investigators in these diverse fields. Although it is difficult to avoid omitting the latest innovations, particularly in a rapidly proliferating area of research such as this, methodological problems in areas such as antibody production, characterization, and radiolabeling have been discussed in detail. However, the long-term value of this volume lies in the authors' attempts not only to evaluate the limitations of currently available technologies and approaches, but also to speculate upon future directions of research.

The editor gratefully acknowledges the efforts of all the contributors, many of whom have presented previously unpublished results.

THE EDITOR

Michael R. Zalutsky, Ph.D., is Associate Professor of Radiology and Assistant Professor of Pathology at Duke University Medical Center in Durham, North Carolina.

Dr. Zalutsky graduated in 1970 from Clark University, Worcester, Massachusetts, with a B.A. degree in chemistry and received his Ph.D. in chemistry from Washington University, St. Louis, in 1974. Prior to joining the Duke faculty, he held appointments at Argonne National Laboratory, the University of Chicago, and Harvard University.

Dr. Zalutsky has published more than 75 research papers and reviews. His current research interests include radiolabeled monoclonal antibody developments, the chemistry of astatine, and the therapeutic use of radionuclides.

CONTRIBUTORS

William D. Bloomer, M.D.
Professor and Chairman
Department of Radiation Oncology
University of Pittsburgh School of Medicine and
Joint Radiation Oncology Center
Pittsburgh, Pennsylvania

Jorge A. Carrasquillo, M.D.
Medical Investigator
Department of Nuclear Medicine
National Institutes of Health
Bethesda, Maryland

Ann M. Carroll, Ph.D.
Research Associate
Institute for Cancer Research
Fox Chase Cancer Center
Philadelphia, Pennsylvania

Janet F. Eary, M.D.
Assistant Professor of Nuclear Medicine
Division of Nuclear Medicine, Department of Radiology
University of Washington
Seattle, Washington

William C. Eckelman, Ph.D.
Vice President
Diagnostic Research and Development
Squibb Institute for Medical Research
New Brunswick, New Jersey

Eliot Friedman, M.D.
Clinical Fellow in Medicine
Department of Medicine
Dana-Farber Cancer Institute
Harvard Medical School
Boston, Massachusetts

Brian M. Gallagher, Ph.D.
Manager
Immunopharmaceutical Research and Development
E.I. duPont de Nemours, Co., Inc.
North Billerica, Massachusetts

Mark I. Greene, M.D., Ph.D.
Head, Immunobiology Division
Department of Pathology and Laboratory Medicine
University of Pennsylvania School of Medicine
Philadelphia, Pennsylvania

Daniel F. Hayes, M.D.
Instructor in Medicine
Department of Medicine
Dana-Farber Cancer Institute
Harvard Medical School
Boston, Massachusetts

Shalom Kalnicki, M.D.
Assistant Professor
Department of Radiation Oncology
University of Pittsburgh School of Medicine and
Joint Radiation Oncology Center
Pittsburgh, Pennsylvania

William D. Kaplan, M.D.
Associate Professor
Department of Radiology
Division of Nuclear Medicine
Harvard Medical School
Boston, Massachusetts

Raj Kishore, Ph.D.
Reviewing Chemist
Food and Drug Administration
Rockville, Maryland

Kenneth A. Krohn, Ph.D.
Professor
Department of Radiology
Division of Nuclear Medicine
University of Washington
Seattle, Washington

Donald W. Kufe, M.D.
Associate Professor
Department of Medicine
Dana-Farber Cancer Institute
Harvard Medical School
Boston, Massachusetts

Su Metcalfe, Ph.D.
Senior Research Associate
Department of Surgery
Clinical School
University of Cambridge
Cambridge, England

Wil B. Nelp, M.D.
Professor of Medicine and Radiology
Division of Nuclear Medicine
University of Washington
Seattle, Washington

C. H. Paik, Ph.D.
Research Professor
Department of Nuclear Medicine
George Washington University Medical Center
Washington, D.C.

Howard Sands, Ph.D.
Supervisor
Pharmacology Group
Immunopharmaceutical Research and Development
E.I. duPont de Nemours, Co., Inc.
North Billerica, Massachusetts

John N. Weinstein
Laboratory for Mathematical Biology
National Cancer Institute
National Institutes of Health
Bethesda, Maryland

TABLE OF CONTENTS

Chapter 1

INTRODUCTION: THE CURRENT STATUS OF TUMOR IMAGING

William D. Kaplan

TABLE OF CONTENTS

I. INTRODUCTION

What is it that clinicians expect when they send their patients for "a radionuclide tumor scan"? What are the advantages and the limitations of current techniques, and what can be expected from the monoclonal antibody approach to tumor imaging?

We will try to put these questions in perspective by use of specific clinical examples and, hopefully, at the same time clarify which techniques are available and accepted.

First, it must be appreciated that current imaging technology really only allows the definition of macroscopic tumors. That is, if the tumor site identified by radionuclide imaging were to be surgically isolated and resected, the lesion would most likely be able to be seen with the naked eye. Albeit, the focus may be only a few millimeters in size, but in terms of the number of cell divisions that the malignant tissue has undergone, we are far from being able to detect truly microscopic disease. With this caveat in mind, what are the major indications for sending a patient for a tumor scan?

II. INDICATIONS FOR TUMOR IMAGING

There are three major indications for tumor imaging: (a) detecting the presence of tumor, (b) localizing the sites of disease, and (c) following the effects of therapy.

A. Tumor Detection

With respect to the first indication, certainly tumor detection is a major concern of medical practice today. This concern applies, in particular, to those individuals at risk for developing a malignant process, for instance the long-term smoker with a high probability of developing lung cancer who shows a change in his chest X-ray. In general, it applies to any patient with a constellation of clinical signs and symptoms which raise the suspicion of an occult malignancy.

B. Tumor Localization

In assessing the extent of the tumor, it is imperative that all sites of metastases be identified so that the most appropriate therapy can be directed at irradicating disease; detecting the full extent of the malignancy will have a major influence on the type of therapy prescribed. For example, if the disease is localized, a surgical approach, with or without concomitant radiation therapy, may be all that is necessary for a cure. On the other hand, if the disease is widely disseminated, as defined by radionuclide imaging techniques, local control will be impractical and systemic therapy will be in order.

C. Tumor Follow-up

The follow-up of the patient's course with radionuclide studies is as important as the staging applications of tumor imaging. These follow-up tumor imaging sessions allow the clinician to:

1. Assess the effects of the administered therapy
2. Predict early treatment failures as well as new sites of disease
3. Reinforce a sense of patient well being in those individuals fortunate enough to enjoy tumor response and an associated negative scan result following therapy

III. INDIRECT APPROACHES OF RADIONUCLIDE TUMOR IMAGING

The approaches of radionuclide tumor imaging most widely utilized today take advantage of the growth characteristics of neoplastic cells. As these tumor cells grow and divide, there

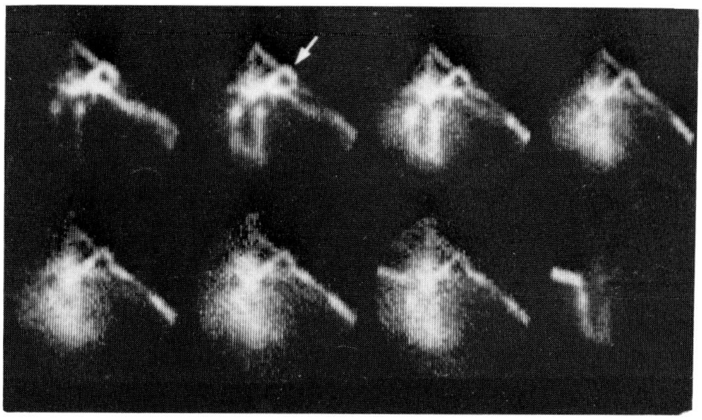

FIGURE 1. Anterior views of thorax (left to right, top to bottom) seen on eight sequential 1 sec images obtained following left arm injection of radionuclide (Frames 1 to 6) and right arm injection (Frames 7 and 8). Following left sided injection collateral filling of venous channels (arrow) in upper thorax are seen secondary to obstruction of left innominate vein. Right sided injection shows normal filling (Frame 8) of vena cava and heart with no evidence of collaterals. Patient was suspected of having vena cava (central vein) occlusion; however, radionuclide dynamic flow study showed peripheral obstruction.

occur resultant regional changes in vascularity and secondary effects on adjacent normal tissues. These changes in the local tissue environment combine to alter both regional organ anatomy and physiology. It is these indirect changes which produce an index of tumor presence on the radionuclide images. Examples of such alterations would be the increased bone seeking tracer uptake in the spine of a patient with skeletal tumor or the focal absence of radiocolloid uptake in phagocytic cells of a liver replaced by hepatic tumor. Some of these indirect approaches to tumor visualization will now be examined more critically.

A. Dynamic Studies

It is not uncommon for tumors to produce gross alterations in the regional vascular system; these changes can be readily evaluated by a dynamic tracer flow study. For instance, in patients with chest lesions, such as a primary lung cancer or a lymphomatous mediastinal mass, there is frequently some compression of the veins which return blood to the heart.[1] These patients may show signs ranging from slight distension of the superficial veins of the upper body to a full blown obstructive syndrome.

During the injection of any Technetium 99m labeled radiopharmaceutical, rapid sequence image collection (one picture every second) will allow definition of these vascular abnormalities.[2] The study is physiologic since only small volumes of injected material are administered, usually on the order of less than 1 mℓ, and the tracer can be delivered at relatively slow flow rates as opposed to the "bolus" injections needed to achieve X-ray contrast information (Figure 1).

B. Static Studies

Perhaps the two most common "indirect" static radionuclide studies for the detection of malignant disease are bone and liver-spleen scans. These tracer examinations take advantage of known chemical and physiologic principles to achieve the desired effect. Unfortunately for the patient, both of these studies are generally utilized for the evaluation of metastatic tumors, i.e., those that have spread from the original site of primary tumor growth to become disseminated throughout either the skeletal or hepatic system. Although this constellation

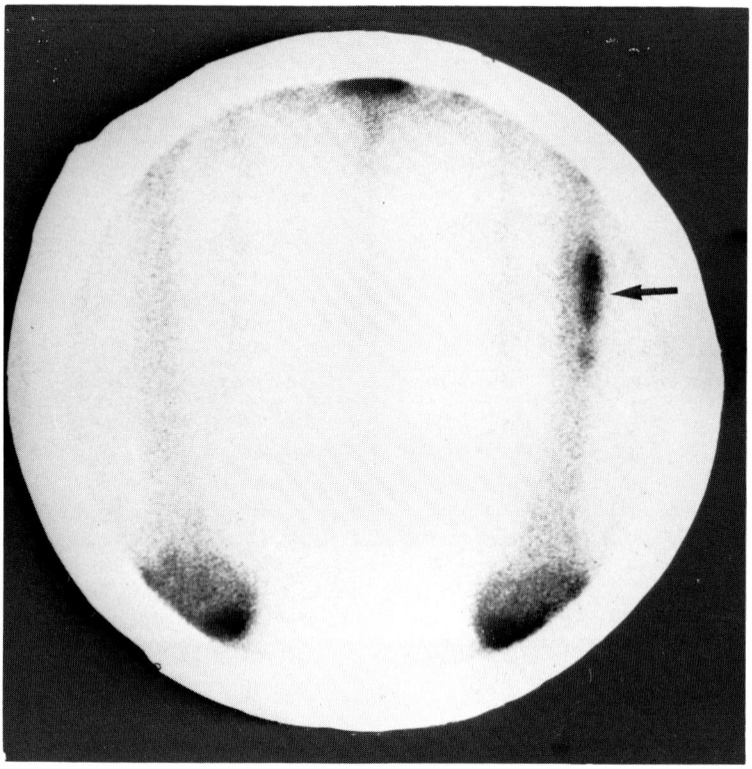

A

FIGURE 2. (A) Anterior view of femora in patient with carcinoma of the breast complaining of left leg pain. Note linear region of increased activity (arrow) localized to the cortical midshaft of left femur. (B) A left lateral X-ray of midshaft of left femur shows extensive lytic involvement (arrows) of bone due to metastatic tumor.

of clinical dissemination generally carries a poor prognosis in terms of cure, palliative procedures available at this stage of disease can offer some relief of symptoms.

1. Chemical Adsorption — Bone Imaging

The commonly used bone-scanning agents employ some form of phosphonate which has been labeled with Technetium-99m. After intravenous administration, this radiopharmaceutical quickly associates with the bony matrix of the skeleton. The precise mechanism of this association remains undefined; however, localization is thought to be primarily a function of adsorption of the phosphonate compound in association with the calcium hydroxyapatite crystalline lattice of the bone.[3] What is important is that the "concentration" of the radiopharmaceutical, as it is recorded on film, is directly related to the degree of regional bone activity. This activity reflects a combination of (a) bone blood flow, (b) bone turnover, and (c) metabolic activity of osteoblasts, those cells primarily involved with laying down new bone — particularly in the presence of skeletal metastases (Figure 2 a and b).

It is important to remember, however, that the increased bone uptake seen on the image is not necessarily indicative of skeletal metastasis. Changes in the skeletal system as reflected on bone scans can be due to any cause of bone turnover; therefore, trauma, infection, and degenerative disease may all be responsible for the abnormal scan findings. It is important to correlate the scintigraphic abnormalities with those seen on plain X-ray. The general rule of thumb is that a bone scan abnormality, which cannot be substantiated by plain X-ray as

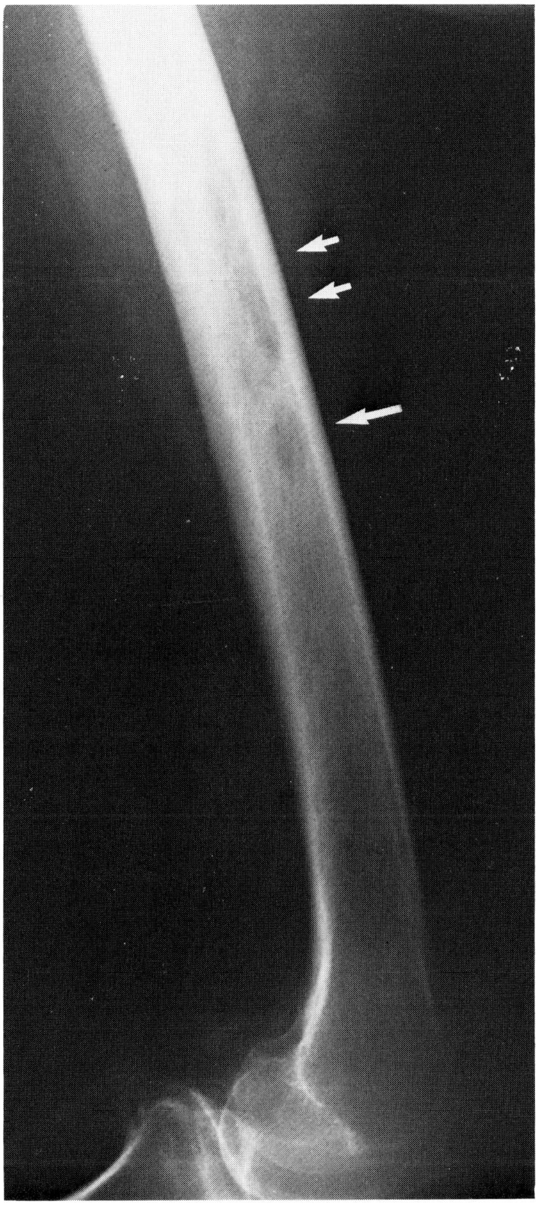

FIGURE 2B

having a benign etiology, should be considered to be metastatic in etiology until proven otherwise.

A key point in this exercise, however, is that although the bone scan is not specific, it is exquisitely sensitive; in approximately 20% of patients, the bone scan will detect a metastatic focus months to even years prior to plain X-ray change.[4] Earlier detectability is the basis for the utility of this test in evaluating the cancer patient.

2. Phagocytosis — Liver Scan

By injecting Technetium-99m labeled colloidal particles of 500 nm in diameter into the venous system, the distribution of the body's reticuloendothelial (RE) system can be outlined.

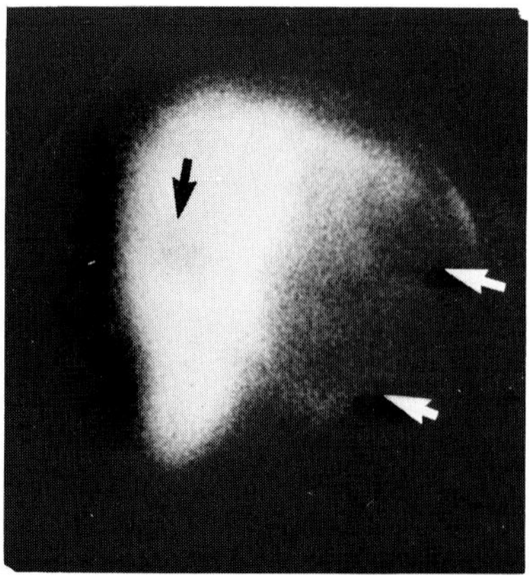

FIGURE 3. Anterior view of liver following intravenous administration of Tc-99m sulfur colloid. Patient with recently diagnosed breast cancer and elevation in serum liver function tests. Radiocolloid scan shows large intrahepatic focal abnormalities replacing functioning reticuloendothelial cells in both right (black arrow) and left lobes (white arrows) of liver, compatible with multiple metastatic lesions.

Most of the RE cells which line sinusoids are located within the liver. Consequently, on the radiocolloid liver scan, one can appreciate subtle alterations in regional hepatic blood flow (as is sometimes seen with early microscopic tumor infiltration from breast cancer or small cell carcinoma of the lung) or focal anatomic derangements from replaced RE cells, such as the larger macroscopic metastasis from colon cancer.

As with the bone scan, these findings are nonspecific, since a variety of disease processes can cause alterations in RE phagocytosis. For instance, hepatitis, whether due to an infectious etiology or induced by chronic alcohol abuse, will cause changes in intrahepatic blood flow; this is manifested on the radiocolloid liver-spleen scan as a heterogeneous pattern of radiocolloid distribution. Similarly, focal alterations in the liver may be due not only to metastasis (Figure 3), but to benign entities such as simple cysts or an intrahepatic abscess.[5,6] It is not uncommon that a second radiologic study, such as an ultrasound or a computerized tomographic liver scan, is needed to further evaluate the derangement seen on the initial radiocolloid scan in order to differentiate a benign from a malignant etiology.

Although these scintigraphic findings are nonspecific, the test is very sensitive; an abnormal pattern of radiocolloid distribution is usually synonomous with a pathologic process.

3. Phagocytosis — Lymphoscintigraphy

An interesting aside on the radiocolloid portrayal of phagocytic organ systems is the use of an ultra-small particle (50 nm in diameter) to image the lymphatics. The most common application of this technique is in the evaluation of the internal mammary lymph node chain, those lymphatics located just a few centimeters lateral and deep to the sternum.[7] These lymph nodes are at risk for harboring microscopic tumor in patients with breast cancer, particularly those patients in whom the primary lesion is located in the medial aspect of the breast. Standard radiologic techniques, i.e., chest X-ray and even computerized tomographic (CT) scanning of the thorax are unable to detect tumor cells within these lymph nodes until the nodes approach a size of 7 to 10 mm in diameter; at this point in time, patients usually have clinically overt evidence of disseminated disease.

By utilizing the physiologic principle of lymph node phagocytosis, and the subsequent alterations secondary to tumor deposits, we can readily define the earliest manifestations of breast cancer spread to the internal mammary chain. The pattern of abnormal radiocolloid

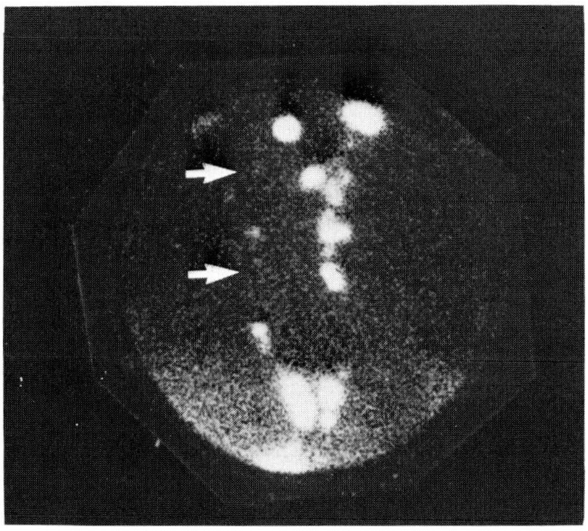

FIGURE 4. Anterior view of thorax in a patient with 3 cm lesion in medial aspect of right breast. Patient was injected bilaterally with radiocolloid. Note poor filling of patient's right internal mammary chain (arrows) when compared with normal appearing left lymphatics.

uptake is one which could be predicted based on experience interpreting the abnormal liver-spleen scan. There is an overall decrease in nodal uptake of radiocolloid as well as a "patchy appearance" of the lymph nodes. This is opposed to the normal lymphatic chain which shows a homogenous and uniform pattern of radiocolloid uptake (Figure 4).

Other major lymphatic groups with which clinical experiences have evolved include the internal and external iliac and para-aortic nodes which commonly drain tumors arising in the genito-urinary systems[8] and the cutaneous lymphatic pathways of the trunk which are evaluated in patients with truncal malignant melanoma.[9]

IV. DIRECT APPROACHES OF RADIONUCLIDE TUMOR IMAGING

The techniques just outlined centered around defining sites of disease by recognizing the secondary effects of tumor within an organ system. Of major importance, however, is the definition of the actual sites of tumor cells per se; for that task, a number of proposals have been put forth.

A. Radiolabeled Chemotherapeutic Agents

In the development of new tumor localizing agents, the absolute amount of radionuclide uptake is key, but the uptake of tracer within the tumor *relative* to adjacent tissue may have an even greater bearing on the clinical utility of the agent.

For example, Grove et al.,[10] in comparing Gallium-67 tumor scanning to the results obtained using the established antitumor agent bleomycin labeled with either Cobalt-57 or Indium-111, indicated that although the absolute tumor uptake of these three agents was about equal, the rapid urinary clearance of the Cobalt-57 labeled entity resulted in the highest tumor to non-tumor ratios. Thus, in their study, Cobalt-57 bleomycin appeared to be the superior tumor scanning agent.

Although work continues on the approach of radiolabeling known cancer drugs, no major, clinically useful breakthroughs have occurred to date. It may well be that as a result of labeling, drug kinetics are altered sufficiently to compromise tumor avidity.

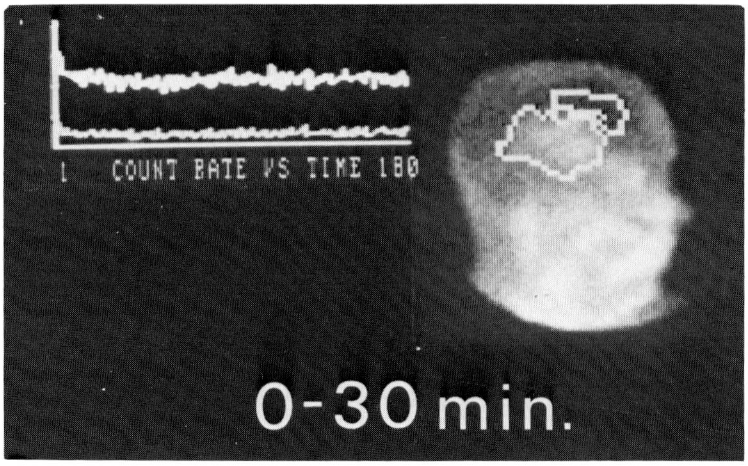

FIGURE 5. Right lateral Thallium-201 view of the head with resultant time-activity curves at one frame per 10 sec representing regions-of-interest drawn over the brain tumor (upper curve) and adjacent normal brain tissue (lower curve). Note rapid and persistent uptake of radiothallium within tumor focus.

B. Simple Ionic Substances

1. Thallous Chloride (Tl-201)

Thallous chloride has been shown to have clinical efficacy as a tumor scanning agent.[11] This gamma emitting radionuclide, commonly employed for myocardial perfusion studies, is thought to sequester in tissue as a potassium analogue. The exact mechanism of action for tumor uptake is unknown, but it may have some relationship to the maintenance of an intact sodium-potassium ATPase membrane pump.

Recent experiences in our laboratory have offered us an opportunity to study a group of patients referred for evaluation of gliomas, a type of primary brain tumor.[12] The major clinical question to be answered was whether or not a positive therapeutic effect could be documented by radionuclide scan in a group of patients in whom there was marked clinical improvement, yet a persistent and unchanged abnormality on a CT scan of the brain.

Thallium was shown to be an active metabolic marker of viable tumor cells (Figure 5). In those patients who were doing well clinically (in spite of the fact that a CT scan showed an abnormality) the thallium scan was normal. On the other hand, in those patients who demonstrated clinical tumor recurrence, the thallium scan was abnormal. At postmortem examination, correlation with the pathologic specimens showed that thallium uptake was restricted to areas of active tumor growth and did not reflect adjacent regions of edema, necrosis, or fibrosis.

2. Gallium 67 Citrate

Gallium 67 (Ga-67) as the citrate is probably the most widely used radiotracer for direct tumor imaging. Localization within malignant cells is felt to be related to the chemical similarity of Ga-67 (an inorganic cation of Group IIIB) to iron. There is documented binding of gallium to circulating transferrin and the presence of transferrin receptor sites on the surface of tumor cells can, to some extent, explain gallium uptake within a malignant focus. The intracellular site of radiogallium concentration appears to be cytoplasmic; electron microscopic studies suggest this localization to be within lysosomes.

Ga-67 has been shown to be very avid for a number of tumors. Those malignancies commonly imaged with this radiotracer include primary liver cell tumor (hepatoma), malignant melanoma, sarcoma, lymphoma, and primary carcinoma of the lung (Figure 6).

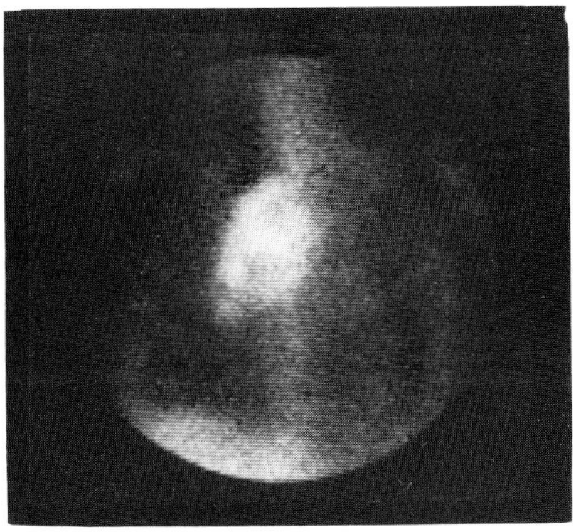

FIGURE 6. Anterior view of thorax in a patient being staged for chemotherapy protocol with small cell carcinoma of lung. Gallium scan shows markedly avid and abnormal uptake within known anterior thoracic primary lung cancer.

An example of the clinical utility of radiogallium is the frequent problem of evaluating the treated lymphoma patient.[13] It is not uncommon that such patients will manifest a residual mass in the previously treated area. The question of clinical interest is whether the mass represents persistent disease or inactive tumor and fibrosis. Since radiogallium does not sequester in nonviable, fibrotic, or necrotic tissue, a negative gallium scan in such a treated patient carries a high likelihood of indicating inactive disease. Persistent, abnormal gallium uptake in a site of prior tumor, on the other hand, is compatible with residual neoplasm and appropriate therapeutic steps to irradicate this nidus of disease must be taken.

A potential interpretive problem arising from the use of radiogallium as a direct tumor scanning agent is the nonspecificity of tracer accumulation. Areas of inflammatory change or abscess formation can also sequester gallium. However, it is usually possible to differentiate between a benign and malignant etiology based on clinical history and physical examination.

C. Metabolite Imaging

Positron emitting radionuclides, of biologically important elements such as oxygen, nitrogen, and carbon, have been actively incorporated into analogues of some of the common metabolites found in man. This labeling technique, coupled with the use of a positron emission tomographic (PET) camera, allows one to scintigraphically document pathways of metabolic activity previously unrecorded in vivo.

For example, definition of regional cerebral glucose metabolism in man has been achieved by using Fluorine-18 labeled 2-deoxy d-glucose, the latter competing for glucose transport at the cell membrane.[14] Once inside the cell, the deoxyglucose competes with glucose for phosphorylation. When this has occurred, it becomes trapped within the cell, no longer available to be further metabolized.

In looking at the correlation between glucose utilization and the grade of primary brain tumors, DiChiro et al.[15] found that the higher the grade of tumor, the greater the glucose utilization. Glucose utilization was also decreased in the surrounding, tumor-associated edema and in regions of brain tissue adjacent to tumor cells. In a clinical setting, when a cerebral mass is identified on CT scan, a Fluorine-18 2-deoxy d-glucose scan is performed; if tracer uptake is seen within the mass, this indicates dividing tumor tissue and the necessity for instituting therapy.

D. Receptor Imaging

Receptors, thought of as high-binding affinity proteins of finite capacity, are now accepted as important factors in pharmacology and for explaining the action of both endogenous biochemicals and therapeutic pharmaceuticals. Since receptors appear to be involved in a bewildering variety of biological systems, "receptor-ligand" interactions are an attractive approach to radiopharmaceutical development. Receptor systems and the diseases for which changes in receptor biochemistry have been suggested include estrogens and progesterones for breast cancer and androgens for prostate cancer.[16]

An example of the use of the receptor approach for tumor imaging and therapy is that described by Kimmig et al.[17] who used Iodine-131 labeled meta iodobenzylguanidine (MIBG) for the definition of neuroblastoma. MIBG is an analogue of the neuron blocking agent guanethidine and, therefore, sequesters in the ontogenetically related tumor, neuroblastoma. Kimmig showed that following the injection of labeled MIBG, greater than 30% of the injected dose of radioactive iodine localized within the neoplasm. The radiation dose to the tumor sites approached 2,000 rads when MIBG was labeled with 80 mCi of radioactive iodine. Therapeutic responses have been achieved by this approach.

E. Immunologic Imaging

Monoclonal antibodies have heralded a revolution in radiopharmaceutical strategy. Recent advances in biotechnology, particularly recombinant genetics, cell cloning, new radiolabeling techniques, and the characterization of cell receptors and antigens, have raised new hope for achieving the long-cherished goal of employing site-specific radiopharmaceuticals for medical diagnosis and therapy.[18]

The advantages of this biotechnology center around the ability to generate gram quantities of very pure and monospecific antibodies to a particular tumor-associated antigen. There are a number of practical considerations, however, which have been responsible for the slower than expected progress in this area of tumor imaging.

Optimally the antibodies utilized should show no cross-reactivity with antigens associated with either normal tissues or those expressed on the cell surface of other unrelated tumors. When cross-reactivity does occur, nonspecific uptake can lead to potential diagnostic problems.[19]

Variability in antigen expression can also lead to imaging difficulties. It has been shown, for instance, that some cell surface antigens are expressed in only specific phases of the cell cycle.[20] If the cell surface antigen is expressed only during the synthesis or S phase of cell growth, but at the time of external imaging, most of the tumor cells are in the G_0 or G_1 phase and a false negative scan can be the result.

A third problem centers around the potential for circulating serum antigens.[21] If the cell surface antigens are shed into the circulation, this can allow blood pool complexing of injected radiolabeled antibodies which results in (a) a decrease in the amount of radiolabeled antibody available for identification of tumor sites and (b) significant background in tumor images due to activity in the vascular space.

In spite of these considerations, clinical work with radiolabeled anti-tumor antibodies has made remarkable progress in the last few years and the use of these agents in the diagnosis and therapy of malignant disease has been suggested by some as representing an area that will become "a genuinely decisive technology".[22]

V. SUMMARY

Lentle et al.[23] have recently offered a thoughtful perspective on the future. "As tumor scintigraphy is refined during the next decades we will be driven by our oncologist colleagues to detect even smaller tumor-cell masses. We submit that there is no realistic technology that can be anticipated in the near future which might allow us to achieve scintigraphic techniques to meet these morphological constraints of cancer medicine. These unrealistic goals however are capable of being replaced by realistic and relevant goals: we should exploit the power of nuclear medicine to reflect some of the pathophysiological characteristics of a tumor. We need to know the invasiveness of the cancer, its anaplasticity, or whatever other characteristics are necessary to understand if a given tumor is likely to have metastized . . . Conceivably, monoclonal antibodies, if measured in quantitative terms proportional to a tumor mass, may reflect its degree of cellular differentiation or anaplasticity''. That is, monoclonal antibodies may offer us an exciting method of examining the behavior of tumors as well as recording their presence.

ACKNOWLEDGMENTS

The author thanks Deborah Hanson and John Buckley for their artistic and photographic contributions and Arlene Haury for her help in the preparation of the manuscript.

REFERENCES

1. **Kanji, A. M., Chao, J. H., Liebner, E. J., Lobo, P., and Thakrar, M. B.,** Extrinsic compression of superior vena cava: an analysis of 41 patients, *Int. J. Radiat. Oncol. Biol. Phys.*, 6, 213, 1980.
2. **Miyamae, T.,** Interpretation of 99mTc superior vena cavograms and results of studies in 92 patients, *Radiology*, 108, 339, 1973.
3. **Davis, M. A. and Jones, A. G.,** Comparison of 99mTc-labelled phosphate and phosphonate agents for skeletal imaging, *Semin. Nucl. Med.*, 6, 19, 1976.
4. **Brady, L. W. and Croll, M. N.,** The role of bone scanning in the cancer patient, *Skel. Radiol.*, 3, 217, 1979.
5. **Waxman, A. D.,** Scintigraphic evaluation of diffuse hepatic disease, *Semin. Nucl. Med.*, 12, 75, 1982.
6. **Drum, D. E.,** Current status of radiocolloid hepatic scintiphotography for space-occupying disease, *Semin. Nucl. Med.*, 12, 64, 1982.
7. **Ege, G. N.,** Internal mammary lymphoscintigraphy. The rationale, technique, interpretation and clinical application: a review based on 848 cases, *Radiology*, 118, 101, 1976.
8. **Kaplan, W. D.,** Iliopelivic lymphoscintigraphy, *Semin. Nucl. Med.*, 13, 42, 1983.
9. **Bennett, L. R. and Lago, G.,** Cutaneous lymphoscintigraphy in malignant melanoma, *Semin. Nucl. Med.*, 13, 1, 1983.
10. **Grove, R. B., Reba, R. C., Eckelman, W. C., and Goodyear, M.,** Clinical evaluation of radiolabeled bleomycin for tumor detection, *J. Nucl. Med.*, 15, 386, 1974.
11. **Tonami, N. and Hisada, K.,** Clinical experience of tumor imaging with ^{201}Tl chloride, *Clin. Nucl. Med.*, 2, 75, 1977.
12. **Kaplan, W. D., Takvorian, R. W., Morris, J. H., Rumbaugh, C. L., Connolly, B., and Atkins, H. L.,** Tl-201 brain scans: a comparative study with pathologic correlation, *J. Nucl. Med.*, 28, 47, 1987.
13. **Anderson, K. C., Leonard, R. C. F., Canellos, G. P., Skarin, A. T., and Kaplan, W. D.,** High dose gallium imaging in lymphoma, *Am. J. Med.*, 75, 327, 1983.
14. **Beaney, R. P.,** Positron emission tomography in the study of human tumors, *Semin. Nucl. Med.*, 14, 324, 1984.
15. **DiChiro, G., DeLaPaz, R. L., Brooks, R. A., Sokoloff, L., Kornblith, P. L., Smith, B. H., Patronas, N. J., Kufta, C. V., Kessler, R. M., Johnston, G. S., Manning, R. G., and Wolf, A. P.,** Glucose utilization of cerebral gliomas measured by (^{18}F) fluorodeoxyglucose and positron emission tomography, *Neurology*, 32, 1323, 1982.
16. **Kilbourn, M. R. and Zalutsky, M. R.,** Research and clinical potential of receptor based radiopharmaceuticals, *J. Nucl. Med.*, 26, 655, 1985.
17. **Kimmig, B., Brandeis, W. E., Eisenhut, M., Bubeck, B., Hermann, H. J., and zum Winkel, K.,** Scintigraphy of neuroblastoma with I-131 meta-iodobenzylguanidine, *J. Nucl. Med.*, 25, 773, 1984.
18. **Keenan, A. M., Harbert, J. C., and Larson, S. M.,** Monoclonal antibodies in nuclear medicine, *J. Nucl. Med.*, 26, 531, 1985.

19. **Hayes, D. F., Zalutsky, M. R., Kaplan, W. D., Noska, M., Thor, A., Colcher, D., and Kufe, D. W.,** Pharmacokinetics of radiolabeled monoclonal antibody B6.2 in patients with metastatic breast cancer, *Cancer Res.*, 46, 3157, 1986.
20. **Kufe, D. W., Nadler, L., Sargent, L., Shapiro, H., Hand, P., Austin, F., Colcher, D., and Schlom, J.,** Biological behavior of human breast carcinoma-associated antigens expressed during cellular proliferation, *Cancer Res.*, 43, 851, 1983.
21. **Goldenberg, D. M., Kim, E. E., Bennett, S. J., Nelson, M. O., and Deland, F. H.,** Carcinoembryonic antigen radioimmunodetection in the evaluation of colorectal cancer and in the detection of occult neoplasms, *Gastroenterology*, 84, 524, 1983.
22. **Larson, S. M.,** Radiolabelled monoclonal anti-tumor antibodies in diagnosis and therapy, *J. Nucl. Med.*, 26, 538, 1985.
23. **Lentle, B. C., Scott, J. R., Schmidt, R. P., Hooper, H. R., and Catz, Z.,** Clinical value of direct tumor scintigraphy: a new hypothesis, *J. Nucl. Med.*, 26, 1215, 1985.

Chapter 2

TUMOR CELL BIOLOGY: TUMOR SPECIFIC AND ASSOCIATED ANTIGEN

Ann M. Carroll and Mark I. Greene

TABLE OF CONTENTS

I. INTRODUCTION

A. Historical Background

The notion of tumor-specific antigen (TSA) expression and the awareness of its implications for immunotherapeutic approaches to cancer date back to Paul Ehrlich.[1] A series of observations from studies of transplanted animal tumors supported this notion, but these early experiments were conducted prior to the development of inbred animal strains and the awareness that disparate major histocompatibility (MHC) alloantigen expression could itself induce transplantation rejection.[1] Subsequent establishment of syngeneic, genetically inbred strains of mice provided the basis for meaningful tumor transplantation studies, which showed that tumor-specific immunity could, in fact, be elicited.[2] Initial evidence for tumor-specific transplantation antigens (TSTA) was provided by Gross, who showed that murine, chemically induced sarcomas did not form progressively growing tumors when inoculated intradermally.[3] Mice immunized in this manner rejected subsequent subcutaneous transplants of the same tumor, whereas tumors progressed in nonimmunized mice. Foley[4] and Prehn and Main[5] showed that a variety of chemically induced sarcomas expressed unique tumor antigens. Both cross-reactive and noncross-reactive TSTA were later shown for viral-,[6,7] radiation-,[8] and ultraviolet[9] light-induced rodent tumors.

These early descriptions of TSTA resulted in many attempts to develop specific antibodies which could be passively administered to cancer patients for therapy and diagnostic imaging.[10,11] Results of the initial attempts in both animal models and clinical trials were disappointing, due principally to two major obstacles. The first obstable was the limitation of conventional methodology for generation of large quantities of homogeneous, well-defined specific antibodies. The second obstacle was a limited understanding of the nature of tumor-associated antigens, and a lack of evidence for their widespread existence in spontaneous animal and human cancers.[12,13] Putative unique TSTA identified by conventional animal antisera to human tumor tissue have not stood up to follow-up analyses. Most were discovered to delineate quantitative rather than qualitative differences between normal and tumor tissue antigen expression.[14]

The first of these obstacles was overcome a decade ago by Kohler and Milstein's hybridoma technique for the generation of monoclonal antibodies.[15] The second obstacle remains; indeed, analyses with antigen-specific monoclonals have confirmed doubts that many proposed TSTA are actually the result of altered or aberrant normal antigen expression.[16] The current availability of specific monoclonal antibodies, clonal cell lines, and sophisticated biochemical and molecular biological techniques should provide better understanding of the nature and generality of tumor antigens. This review will discuss the current status of tumor-associated antigens and address the following questions:

- Do true TSTA exist?
- How widespread are they and for what tumor types?
- Do any present reasonable candidates as targets for clinical monoclonal antibody applications?
- Can tumor-associated antigens which are not tumor specific, but are narrowly restricted within the patient, also be used for these approaches?
- What role does the status of the normal or compromised host immune system play in the generation and maintenance of antigenic tumors?

B. Tumor Antigens Defined

A tumor antigen is an antigen expressed as a consequence of a malignant transformation event. The term TSA implies unique expression of antigen by a particular tumor or a particular tumor type and not by any normal nonmalignant tissue. In this sense, a true TSA would be expected to elicit an active host immune response, barring some compromise of the host immune system. Concurrent immune suppression and tumor generation has been shown for at least one tumor system[9] and is indicated in other models.[16,18] TSA expression might be a direct effect of the transformation event, which induces new genetic expression. Ideally for tumor immunologists, TSA expression would be an integral part of the malignant phenotype, i.e., all tumor cells would be antigen positive, and loss of antigen expression would also result in loss of the transformed phenotype; some oncogene associated TSA fulfill this condition (see Section II.A). For many TSA, expression is an indirect consequence of transformation effects, such as alterations in either processing enzymes, or exposure on the cell surface. Indirect TSA expression may occur concurrent with transformation, or could result secondarily from genetic instability of malignant cells during tumor progression.

The generality of TSA expression in human cancers remains uncertain. Carcinogen-induced rodent tumors often express unique tumor antigens, the biochemical character of which is becoming better understood, but spontaneous animal tumors show less evidence for TSA.[13] The etiology of most human cancers is uncertain, although particular viruses and chemical carcinogens are clearly involved in the genesis of certain tumor types. It is uncertain whether human cancers are more similar to carcinogen-induced rodent tumors or spontaneous rodent tumors arising in inbred strains raised under standard food and housing conditions. For obvious reasons, detailed direct studies of human cancer etiology are limited. However, the continued development of more sophisticated tools, such as molecular biological techniques and monoclonal antibody technology, should contribute much insight to the analyses of these basic questions of etiology, TSA expression and tumor immunological host responses. Experimental animal models, particularly in the area of oncogenes, are providing new, exciting, and detailed information about the multiple generative molecular events of carcinogenesis. Probes for identifying human oncogenes are now available. Clinical studies with specific monoclonal antibodies and other reagents are being utilized for systematically characterizing antigen expression on human cancers and studying malignancy-associated alterations in host immune parameters.

In the meantime, must an antigen meet the most stringent definitions for TSA to be considered as a target antigen for clinical trials involving in vivo antibody administration? Although detailed knowledge of the nature of antigen expression in the host is essential, antibodies to antigens which may be classified more loosely as tumor-associated rather than tumor-specific may indeed be useful. Some preliminary clinical trials using antibodies to well-defined antigens which are highly, although not completely, restricted to tumor tissue have shown documented success, as will be discussed.

This review is written to provide an understanding of both the current status of tumor antigens and the direction which current studies of tumor antigen expression and host immune status are taking. This review first addresses specific examples of clinical and animal research which indicate the existence of tumor-specific or very highly restricted antigens. The next section outlines current research efforts and approaches to the study of human normal tissue differentiation antigens which may provide a basis for selective, cautious use of less restricted monoclonals. Classification of particular antigens into these categories is for convenience and is not absolute; B cell idiotypic antigen as discussed in Section III.C, for example, is both a normal differentiation antigen and tumor-specific, due to the clonal nature of its expression. In the final section, we will consider the complexity of the available data and relevant host-tumor interaction factors and how this information will influence the future direction of tumor antigen research.

II. TUMOR-SPECIFIC ANTIGENS (TSA)

A. Oncogene-Encoded Tumor-Specific Antigens (TSA)

1. Introduction

In recent years, the principal focus of cancer biology has been the molecular biological analysis of oncogene transformation. By this model of transformation, specific oncogenes derive from "normally innocuous cellular DNA sequences whose inappropriate action during oncogenesis confers a novel transforming potency on the altered gene".[19] Oncogenesis can generally be related to the effects of either cellular (c-onc) or viral (v-onc) oncogenes. With c-onc, activation of pre-existing cellular sequences called proto-oncogenes is initiated by DNA modifying agents such as chemical carcinogens. With v-onc, cellular infection occurs via retroviruses which have previously acquired cellular sequences with transforming potential. A variety of related c- and v-oncogenes have been described,[20] but the extent of specific oncogene activation in clinical human cancer is uncertain.[21] Specific oncogenetic transformation poses a potentially important opportunity for tumor immunologists. Can identifiable gene products be utilized as target tumor antigens whose expression is essential to the transformation phenotype? And, are any of these antigens expressed on the cell surface, accessible to an in vivo administered antibody?

A variety of oncogenes have been shown to encode for cellular growth factors[22,23] or factor receptors, resulting in autostimulation of transformed cells which may both synthesize and respond to factors, or factor-independent stimulation via aberrant receptor structures.[24] The latter would provide the ideal tumor antigen, both essential for, and specific to, the transformed phenotype. Three oncogene-encoded cell-surface receptors have been described: erb-B, neu, and fms. The gene product of the cellular homolog of the v-erb-B oncogene of the avian erythroblastosis virus (AEV) was identified as a component of the receptor for epidermal growth factor (EGF).[25] Comparison of the EGF receptor and the v-erb-B oncogene product suggested that v-erb-B selectively encodes a tyrosine kinase activity-associated transmembrane portion of the receptor, but does not code for the external EGF binding domain. Lack of surface expression renders this oncogene product nonimmunogenic in intact cells, and, thus, normally inaccessible to a transfused antibody.

2. Neu Oncogene

An erb-B related receptor encoded by the rat oncogene neu, however, is exposed on the transformed cell membrane and does elicit specific antibody production in mice.[26,27] Neu oncogene expression is associated with rat neuronal tumors arising following transplacental administration of the carcinogen ethylnitrosourea (ENU). Injection of ENU into pregnant BDIX rats on day 15 of gestation results in the occurrence of neuro/glioblastomas in offspring. DNA prepared from these tumor-derived cell lines uniformly transforms murine NIH-3T3 fibroblasts by the "gene transfer" transfection technique[28] in which calcium phosphate precipitated DNA is acquired by cells during in vitro coculture.[19] The gene conferring this property, derived from four independently activated neuro/glioblastomas and characterized by specific restriction enzyme sensitivity patterns, was designated neu.[28] These results are exciting to tumor immunologists in that they show common expression of a transformation-associated antigen in tumors separately derived through the induction of a common chemical carcinogen, suggesting that antigen expression may be an integral component of the transformation phenotype.

Initial evidence for neu-oncogene transformation-associated expression of a novel surface component was provided by Padhy et al.,[26] who found specific antibody activity in sera of nude mice bearing NIH-3T3 tumors. These NIH-3T3 tumors were secondary transfectants; NIH cells were originally transfected with rat neuroblastoma DNA, and transformed cells were selected and used as a source of DNA for a subsequent round of transfection. These secondary foci contained virtually no foreign genetic material other than the transforming oncogenic sequence. When injected into young mice, they induced fibrosarcomas. Padhy showed that sera of these sarcoma-bearing mice could specifically precipitate a 185 kdalton polypeptide (p185) from radiolabeled lysates of rat neuroblastoma cells and primary and secondary NIH-3T3 transfectants. The protein was not precipitated from a variety of other transformed cells or NIH-3T3 fibroblasts. Based on these findings, Drebin et al.[27] immunized C3H/HeJ mice with a neu transfected NIH-3T3 cell line, B104-1-1, and fused spleen cells of these mice with NS-1 myeloma cells in an attempt to produce monoclonals to the p185 (and any other transformation-specific) surface structure(s). Initial screening for hybridoma supernatants that bound B104-1-1 was accomplished by indirect immunofluorescence and fluorescence activated cell sorter (FACS) analysis. Hybridoma supernatants positive for B104-1-1 were screened for specific binding using nontransformed NIH-3T3 cells and NIH-3T3 cells transformed by a distinct oncogene of Harvey sarcoma virus proviral DNA (cell line XHT-1-1a). Five of 3000 hybridomas screened showed this pattern of specificity, and one monoclonal antibody, an IgG2a designated 7.16.4., also specifically precipitated the p185 phosphoprotein from metabolically (^{35}S-cysteine) radiolabeled lysates of B104-1-1 cells. FACS analysis of 7.16.4. binding to an extensive panel of murine cells, including those which were nontransformed (NIH-3T3), transformed by independently derived neu-containing rat tumors (primary transfectants B52,B80,B103,B104) or transformed by a variety of unrelated viruses or carcinogens, showed p185 expression to be specifically associated with neu-mediated transformation (Table 1). Quantitative levels of 7.16.4. binding to neu-transformed cell lines varied, with high 7.16.4. immunofluorescence staining correlating with greater quantitative immunoprecipitation of p185 from radiolabeled lysates. Cytological compartmentalization analysis showed p185 to be distributed diffusely on the extracellular face of the plasma membrane of paraformaldehyde-fixed B104-1-1 cells. Functional studies of the effects of anti-p185 monoclonals on neu-transformed cells provided further evidence that p185 is required for maintenance of the transformation phenotype. Treatment of B104-1-1 with 7.16.4. resulted in rapid and reversible loss of surface p185 and reversion to a nontransformed phenotype, as determined by loss of anchorage-independent growth.[29] Administration of small quantities of purified 7.16.4. to B104-1-1-bearing rodents caused tumor regression (in nude mice and syngeneic BDIX rats) and even cures of preestablished tumor in nude mice; treated rats showed no side effects.[30] Based on these studies, Drebin et al.[29] postulated that neu-encoded p185 may be the prototype of a distinct family of tumor antigens whose cell surface expression is essential for the malignant behavior of the cancer cell. Studies of Schecter et al.[31] indicated nucleic acid sequence homology, but nonidentity between the neu gene and v-erb-B gene and its cellular homolog encoding the 170 kdalton epidermal growth factor receptor, strengthening evidence for a direct role of p185 in transformation. Nucleotide sequence analysis of a neu complimentary DNA clone, isolated from a NIH-3T3 neu transformed cell line, indicated a transmembrane protein product with extensive homology to the EGF receptor and evidence for a tyrosine kinase domain.[32] These results suggest that the neu gene encodes for an as yet unidentified growth factor receptor. A human cellular gene homologous to neu also has been recently identified.[33] This gene, c-erb-B-2, a v-erb-B related gene, is amplified and overexpressed in a human salivary adenocarcinoma and a gastric cancer cell line.

3. SM-FeSV fms Oncogene

Another oncogene encoding a cell surface expressed protein is v-fms, the transforming gene of the McDonough strain of the feline sarcoma virus (SM-FeSV). SM-FeSV induces fibrosarcomas in cats and transforms a variety of mammalian cells in culture.[34] The v-fms oncogene was originally acquired from normal cat DNA by recombination with proto-oncogene c-fms sequences.[35] V-fms encodes a set of related glycoproteins designated gp180,

Table 1
EXPRESSION OF p185 ON MURINE TUMOR CELL LINES

Cell line	Description	Immunofluorescence
NIH 3T3	Contact-inhibited mouse fibroblast	–
B104-2	1° Transfectant of B 104 rat neuroblastoma DNA	+
B104-1-1	2° Transfectant of B104 DNA	+ + + +
B104-1-2	2° Transfectant of B014 DNA	+
B103-1	1° Transfectant of B103 rat neuroblastoma DNA	+ + +
B103-5	1° Transfectant of B103 DNA	+ +
B103-1-1	2° Transfectant of B103 DNA	+ +
B103-1-2	2° Transfectant of B103 DNA	+
B50-1	1° Transfectant of B50 rat neuroblastoma DNA	+
B50-6a-2	2° Transfectant of B50 DNA	+ + + +
B50-6a-3	2° Transfectant of B50 DNA	+ +
B82-1	1° Transfectant of B82 rat neuroblastoma DNA	+
B82-3	1° Transfectant of B82 DNA	+ + +
B82-3-2	2° Transfectant of B82 DNA	+
XHT-1-1a	2° Transfectant of v-HA-ras proviral DNA	–
RSV 3T3	RSV-transformed NIH 3T3	–
MSV 3T3	Moloney sarcoma virus-transformed NIH 3T3	–
HaSV 3T3	Harvey sarcoma virus-transformed NIH 3T3	–
PyD2	Polyoma virus-transformed mouse fibroblast	–
PyBR	Polyoma virus-transformed mouse fibroblast	–
SVD2	SV40-transformed mouse fibroblast	–
S1509a	3-Methylcholanthrene-transformed mouse fibroblast	–
YAC	Mo MuLV-induced lymphoma	–
SP2	Mineral oil-induced plasma-cytoma	–

Note: Cell lines were prepared for FACS analysis on a Coulter Epics V Cell Sorter using saturating amounts of monoclonal antibody 7.16.4. Immunofluorescence was quantitated by subtracting the median fluorescence channel of populations stained with fluorescein isothiocyanate (FITC)-conjugated rabbit anti-mouse immunoglobulin alone (negative control) from the median fluorescence channel of populations stained with monoclonal antibody 7.16.4 followed by FITC-conjugated rabbit anti-mouse (positive staining). The resulting net fluorescence was expressed according to the following scale: –, less than two channels; +, 5 to 10 channels; + +, 11 to 15 channels; + + +, 16 to 20 channels; + + + +, >20 channels. 1° and 2° indicate primary or secondary transfectant created by passing the onogene through one or two sequential cycles of DNA transfection in NIH 3T3 mouse fibroblasts. MoMuLV stands for Moloney murine leukemia virus.

gp140, and gp120. Anderson et al.[36] prepared rat monoclonals to syngeneic FeSV transformed rat cells, and selected for antibodies that specifically immunoprecipitated v-fms encoded proteins. By subcellular fractionation analysis, and by immunofluorescence staining of permeabilized, v-fms transformed rat and mink cells, they showed that most v-fms products were organelle or membrane-associated, with the possibility of some surface membrane association. Dual-antibody immunofluorescence was used to show that the distribution of v-fms protein was coincidental with that of internal membrane-associated intermediate filament[37] and that a minor population of v-fms encoded antigens (gp140) could also be detected on lactoperoxidase iodinated cell surface membrane. Manger et al.[38] confirmed the surface localization of gp140 by surface labeling and immunoprecipitation and by immunofluorescence analyses with conventional rat antisera. These sera were obtained from weanling (Wistar-Furth × Fischer) F_1 rats which received injections of SM-FeSV transformed Fischer rat embryo cells and developed tumors at the injection site. Often tumors regressed, and sera of regressor rats were reported to have higher titer anti-v-fms activity. Binding of rat anti-fms sera to the surface of SM-FeSV transformed mink cells was studied by an immunofluorescence technique using viable, nonpermeabilized cells. The anti-fms antisera showed clear membrane staining in a fine, punctate pattern. Normal rat sera did not stain transformed mink cells, and uninfected mink cells were not stained by rat anti-fms antisera. Double label immunofluorescence studies indicated association of the v-fms protein with clathrin-coated pit structures characteristic of certain receptors (e.g., receptors for epidermal growth factor, transferrin, and insulin) which internalize bound ligand.[39] Clathrin association of gp140 led Manger et al.[38] to propose that this oncogene-encoded protein functions as an analogue for a growth factor receptor. This hypothesis was strongly supported by nucleotide sequence data of v-fms, which showed unexpected homology with other tyrosine-kinase encoding oncogenes, and predicted an internal membrane-spanning sequence.[40] Specific nucleotide deletion mutation studies of v-fms by Roussel et al.[41] and microsomal proteolytic digestion studies by Rettenmier et al.[42] showed that v-fms surface membrane expression is correlated with the transformed phenotype, and that membrane v-fms glycoprotein topology resembles that of other known cell surface receptors. Tyrosine kinase activity of the v-fms product was also shown.[43]

The c-fms proto-oncogene product, a 170 kdalton glycoprotein with associated tyrosine kinase activity, has similar tissue distribution and biochemical properties to the mononuclear phagocyte (and mononuclear phagocyte precursor) receptor for the macrophage growth factor colony-stimulating factor (CSF-1).[44] These similarities, and the ability of rabbit anti-v-fms antisera to precipitate both the feline c-fms product and the 165 kdalton putative mouse CSF-1 receptor, indicate a relationship and possible identity of these molecules.[45] A human gene homolog for fms has not yet been reported, although human homologs for other retroviral oncogenes, such as murine Moloney sarcoma virus[46] and simian sarcoma virus,[47] have been detected and chromosome mapped.

B. Tumor-Associated Aberrant Glycosylation

1. Introduction

Tumor-associated antigen expression may also result from oncogenetically induced changes in the synthesis and activity of glycosylation enzymes, resulting in modified surface carbohydrate composition. In a recent screening of monoclonals from different laboratories, 97 of 325 antibodies to differentiation and oncogenetic transformation antigens identified carbohydrate determinants.[48] These antibodies recognize oligosaccharide sequences of both proteins and lipids. Many of these antigens may not be truly tumor specific, but rather structures which are expressed normally in lesser quantities during specific developmental stages or in a cryptic, nonimmunogenic manner. Currently, aberrant membrane glycolipid and glycoprotein determinants are being studied by two approaches, the combination of which may permit the rational design of highly restricted, if not completely "specific", anti-tumor antibodies. These approaches are

1. Detailed chemical analysis of homogeneous extracted tumor cell (and control nontumor cell) glycolipid fractions

2. Characterization of the target determinants detected by monoclonal antibodies generated to whole cells, membrane fractions, or isolated characterized glycolipid fractions.

A recent review of tumor-associated carbohydrates indicates two basic processes are responsible: precursor accumulation (due to transformation-associated suppression of glycosyl transferase activities) and neosynthesis (attributed to activation, derepression, or altered substrate specificity of glycosylation enzymes).[49] Some tumors show diverse combinations of unusual precursor structures and novel, or retrogenetically expressed, glycolipids, with particular carbohydrate epitopes characteristic of certain tumor types. In addition, surface expression of glycolipids is controlled not only by the balance of enzyme-controlled synthesis and degradation, but may also be greatly influenced by surface organization of membrane components.[49] Surface organization is determined by the state of cluster, its dependence on membrane antigen concentration, the state of coexistence with other glycolipids and proteins (e.g., masking of antigenicity), and membrane ceramide composition, which affects steric antigenic stability and orientation.[50]

2. Precursor Accumulation

Precursor accumulation is attributed to blocked synthesis of normal glycosylated surface structures and consequent surface expression of the altered, unfinished structure. Early studies of in vitro virus-transformed cultured fibroblasts showed a pattern of transformation-associated incomplete synthesis of higher glycolipids[51-53] due to a block of one or more glycosyl transferases.[52-54] Murine and rat cells, transformed by chemical carcinogens, showed similar glycolipid alterations. Chemical glycolipid analyses of normal and malignant human tissues indicate that the transformation of human cells also is often accompanied by precursor accumulation.[55] Blood group antigens, which are the major human allogeneic antigens, (i.e., inherited and expressed in different forms from individual to individual, for example, ABH antigens of red blood cells) are expressed in a variety of tissue types, notably epithelial cells. Incomplete synthesis of carbohydrate blood group antigens may result in accumulation of surface precursor structures.[56] Incomplete synthesis of the ABH antigens, for example, may result in accumulation of a structure designated Ii,[56,57] shown to be associated with glycoproteins of epithelial secretory type cancers.[58,59]

By the monoclonal approach, two groups have described a novel glycolipid precursor structure of human melanoma. This neuroectodermal differentiation antigen, a GD3 disialoganglioside identified by Nudelman et al.[60] and Pukel et al.,[61] results from precursor glycolipid accumulation. This antigen was used as a target structure in a clinical trial for antibody treatment of melanoma patients by Houghton et al.[62] The lack of renal or neurological side effects in these patients, despite low level expression of antigen in some normal tissues, might be due to quantitative or organizational differences in antigen expression, or to differential antibody access to tumor and normal tissue. Another novel glycolipid precursor structure has been identified on human B lymphocyte-derived Burkitt's lymphoma cells by the monoclonal 38-13 of Wiels et al.[63] By screening human cell lines and tissues sections, the antibody was shown to possess exclusive reactivity with Burkitt's lymphoma (15 of 26 lines), irrespective of Epstein-Barr virus (EBV) expression, and to red blood cells from certain individuals (designated ^{pk}), which express a common neutral glycolipid structure.[64] Recently, this antibody was coupled to ricin A and gelonin toxins and its cytotoxicity assayed in vitro. Cytotoxic activity was specific and effective despite a very low number of antigenic sites, indicating the potential utility of glycolipids as targets of antibody-directed tumor therapy.[65] Monoclonal antibodies have also identified a novel glycolipid precursor, a gangliotriaosylceramide (asialo GM-2), on Hodgkin's Disease cell lines,[66] a neuroectodermal tumor-associated GD2 glycolipid,[67] and a lymphocytic leukemia associated GD3 ganglioside.[68]

3. Neosynthesis

Monoclonal antibodies have identified additional novel human tumor associated glycolipids which have been termed neoglycolipids.[55] Alterations in membrane glycopeptides also probably occur via neosynthesis, as evidenced by the appearance of increased N-asparagine-linked carbohydrate chains of glycoproteins on transformed vs. nontransformed progenitor cells.[69] Neosynthesis of both glycolipid and glycopeptide structures is believed to be due to transformation-associated induction of specific glycosyl transferases. Induction of a specific fucosyl-transferase in the livers of rats treated with the chemical carcinogen N-2-acetylaminofluorene was shown by Hakomori's group.[70] This alteration could account for abnormal expression of fucose-containing fucolipids and fucogangliosides commonly detected in various human cancers, notably those deriving from endodermal epithelial origin.[55] Cancers expressing fucose-containing glycolipids (cancers of the gastrointestinal tract, pancreas, lung, and mammary glands) are also the most common and lethal human cancers. Several laboratories are currently engaged in purifying and characterizing these glycolipids, and one promising approach to the production of highly tumor-specific antibodies is the use of these purified components in immunization protocols.[71]

One cancer-associated fucosolipid of interest, termed gastrointestinal-associated cancer antigen (GICA), has been identified by Koprowski et al.,[72] using a monoclonal generated to human colorectal adenocarcinoma cells. Antibody N-19-9 activity has apparent specificity for colorectal adenocarcinoma, gastric, and pancreatic cancers; it also showed limited reactivity to loci of normal glandular epithelia of pancreas and gastric mucosae,[73] and to meconium.[74] Magnani et al.[74,75] have identified the antigenic component as a monoganglioside, further characterized as a sialylated form of the Lewis a (Le^a) blood group structure. Synthesis of this sialosyl Le^a structure, although not truly tumor specific, may be uniquely enhanced in transformed cells. Recent biochemical analyses of Liepkalns et al.[76] led to the proposal that synthesis of GICA, and possibly other fucosolipids, may be associated with dividing, undifferentiated tumor cell populations, and that fucosolipids may play a role in tumor cell division.

Monoclonal antibodies which identify blood group X-related fucosolipid determinants also show apparent human tumor association. The embryonic antigen SSEA-1 has been identified as an X structure.[77] A panel of monoclonals produced to a human small cell lung carcinoma and cross reactive with lung adenocarcinoma and squamatous carcinoma also recognize X structure.[78] A systematic analysis of human normal and tumor-associated structure X glycolipid has been done by Hakomori's group, elucidating a family of adenocarcinoma-associated fucosylated X structures.[79] A panel of monoclonals which recognize different epitopes of these structures was also generated. Some monoclonals have been produced by the unique approach of immunization with defined, purified membrane and glycolipid fractions adsorbed to the bacterium *Salmonella minnesota.*[71] The resultant antibodies are more specific for finely delineated carbohydrate structures, distinguishing sialylated and nonsialylated mono- and difucosylated Lewis X type 2 chain structures. One antibody, FH4, reacts exclusively with nonsialylated di- and trifucosylated type 2 chain, while monoclonals FH5 and FH18 show preferential reactivity to trifucosylated type 2 chain.[80] The defined epitopes are highly associated with human gastrointestinal tumors and fetal gastrointestinal epithelia. Expression in normal adult tissue is limited to gastric parietal cells, intestinal Paneth cells, pyloric epithelia and kidney proximal convoluted tubuli, and Henle's loop.

The monoclonal antibody CSLEXI, produced by immunization with membranes of human stomach adenocarcinoma tissue, reacts with sialosyl Lewis X structure, regardless of the carrier carbohydrate.[81] This antibody reacts with 41% of human stomach, lung, colon, and esophagus adenocarcinoma cell lines tested, and 68% of human tumor tissue sections. CSLEXI antigen is also found, however, in normal esophageal mucosa, colon crypts, pancreatic acinar cells, hepatic cells, kidney proximal tubules, Henle's loop, and granulocytes.

CSLEXI-reactive glycolipid fractions were used to immunize and generate additional monoclonals and one antibody, FH6, shows a more restricted reactivity.[82] FH6 binds sialyl X restricted to fucoganglioside carriers, a sialylated derivative of the FH4 antigen designated fucoganglioside 6B.[71] FH6 expression is highly tumor-associated, reacting with tissue sections of differentiated but not nondifferentiated tumors of stomach (66%), colon (33%), lung (50%), breast (86%), and kidney (55%).[82] Fetal epithelia showed weak staining suggesting an oncofetal property; reactivity of normal adult tissue was limited to granulocytes and kidney proximal tubuli. Production of this highly restricted, tumor-associated antibody is an impressive example of how a rational design approach can be utilized for development of specific, clinically relevant antibodies to biochemically identifiable target structures. If a high level of specificity can be attained by these approaches and followed up with experiments in vivo, select carbohydrate antigens may provide sufficiently restricted targets to be exploited as tumor-associated antigens.

C. Anomolous/Altered Major Histocompatibility (MHC) Antigens

The MHC locus (H-2 locus of mice, HLA locus of man) class I genes comprise a large multigene family which encodes, for transplantation antigens, a set of highly polymorphic allogeneic surface antigens constituitively expressed on most body cells. These antigens impart an individually identifiable antigen phenotype, matching of which is required for successful tissue transplantation.[83] Novel antigens on chemically,[84] virally,[6-7] irradiation,[8] and ultraviolet (UV) light-induced[9] tumors have been identified on the basis of transplantation rejection by syngeneic recipients, but the biochemical nature of many of these antigens is not known. There is evidence that some of these unique antigens may, in fact, be anomolously expressed or altered tissue transplantation antigens.[85] Indeed, an early described mouse T cell leukemic antigen, T1, is an anomolously expressed MHC class I gene product normally restricted to certain mouse strains and to an early thymic T cell developmental stage. In this common mouse leukemia, strains that are normally T1 negative express T1 antigens specifically on transformed cells.[14] In more recent years, human antigen equivalents of thymocyte-restricted T1 have been described on the basis of specifically reactive monoclonals,[86,87] and association of this antigen with human adult T cell lymphocytic leukemias (T-ALL) has also been reported.[88] One of these monoclonals, anti-OKT6, bound peripheral T cells from 20% of T-ALL patients.[88]

Tumor-associated alterations in class I antigen expression may be due to enhanced or activated expression of normally silent genes, as in the case of T1. Alterations in surface MHC antigen phenotype may also be due to quantitative shifts in normal class I gene expression, or even to expression of completely novel class I components.[85] Attenuation, loss of normal expression, and expression of new components have been reported for in vitro cultured tumor cell lines. Screening of lines with specific anti-MHC antibodies of T cell clones, for example, has turned up novel variants[89] at a frequency of 10^{-5} to 10^{-6}. These infrequent variant situations are not relevant to practical clinical applications. To be useful, abnormal structures common to all (or at least most) cells derived from a common transformed progenitor are required. If such situations do occur, however, why are MHC-aberrant tumors not recognized and eliminated by the host immune system, which operates by distinction of self from nonself or altered histocompatibility antigens?[90] Supporters of the controversial immune surveillance hypothesis would maintain that such a system does operate to eliminate nascent autochthonous tumors.[91] If such tumors do arise, then, their survival would only be expected in immune compromised hosts. It is of interest, therefore, that the arisal of one class of tumor which consistently expresses unique tumor antigens, based on transplantation rejection studies, is associated with the induction of an immune-suppressed state. Kripke[9] has described a murine tumor system in which UV light-induced skin fibrosarcomas express unique surface antigens. UV exposure also induces specific and transferrable immune suppression, affecting the T cell arm of the immune response. UV-treated mice, therefore, develop progressive fibrosarcomas, but when tumors are transplanted to nonUV-treated mice they regress, and these regressor mice become specifically immunized.

Two recent reports indicate that unique tumor antigens of a UV-induced C3H fibrosarcoma are class I MHC structures.[92,93] Four distinct tumor transplantation antigen epitopes of the C3H (H-2^k) fibrosarcoma 1591 have been identified by a panel of specificity reactive cloned cytolytic T cell lines (CTLL).[94] More recently, two monoclonal antibodies, generated to 1591, have identified unique MHC class I molecules on this tumor.[92,93] The 1591 tumor grows progressively in UV-treated, immune-compromised hosts, but it regresses when transplanted to normal syngeneic mice. The monoclonal antibodies CP28 and CP34 bind 1591, but not 37 other UV-induced fibrosarcomas, or 14 of 14, 1591 variants which have lost transplantation immunogenicity concurrent with loss of reactivity with the anti-tumor CTLL. The antibodies also fail to bind normal adult and embryonic C3H tissues screened, but did show cross reactivity with certain allogeneic class I molecules: CP28 bound cells expressing H-$2^{b,d,f,q,s,v}$ alleles, and CP3F4 bound cells from strains that bear H-$2^{d,q,s,v}$ alleles.[92] These antibodies immunoprecipitated a characteristic class I molecular complex of 48 kdalton and 12 kdalton (B-2 microglobulin, associated with class I antigens), which was confirmed by tryptic peptide analyses and two-dimensional electrophoresis. Genetic mapping studies with H-2 recombinant strains and tissue distribution analyses indicated reactivity with a public (i.e., broadly expressed) specificity of class I molecules. Normally expressed H-2^k molecules continued to be expressed by the tumor. Further biochemical analyses of 1591 surface antigens by McMillan et al. revealed a minimum of two novel class I antigens.[93] By tryptic peptide analysis and cross blocking RIA using CP28 and panels of monoclonals to characterized H-2 molecules they identified the two structures: one, recognized by CP28, is an apparently mosaic structure (part H-$2K^k$, part H-$2D^k$), and the other is a structure closely related to, but not identical to, the H-$2L^d$ molecule. The mechanism(s) for the generation of these structures remain uncertain — possibilities include mutation, derepression of normally silent genes (as in TL), or, as seems plausible for the CP28 defined mosaic structure, genetic recombination. It also remains to be ascertained whether such mechanisms are of a general significance, at least for this tumor type. Wider studies of other murine UV-induced fibrosarcomas using the antibody approach and molecular characterization at the gene level are required. It is of note, however, that evidence exists for increased susceptibility to UV-induced skin cancers in immune suppressed human tissue transplant recipients.[95] In a study of 290 cadaveric renal allograft patients who were followed up for 2 to 9 years, 28 cancers developed; 93% of these cancers were skin derived.[96] The biochemical nature of the MHC and other antigens of these human tumors is of obvious interest.

D. Viral Antigens

Viruses cause multiple cancers in animals, and many virally transformed cells bear characteristic surface antigens.[97] The fms oncogene product (see Section II.B) is encoded by feline sarcoma virus-transformed cells, and a variety of other viruses, including murine leukemia virus, SV-40 virus,[98] and polyoma virus,[99] characteristically express virus at the surface of the cells they transform. Viruses are also implicated in the genesis of certain human cancers, and human cellular homologs to identified animal retroviral oncogenes have been reported (see Section II.A.3). Many studies indicate a causal relationship between chronic hepatitis B virus infection and hepatocellular carcinoma,[100] and infection with EBV, a herpes virus, is associated with Burkitt's lymphoma and undifferentiated nasopharyngeal cancers.[101] There is evidence for an inductive role of the human T cell leukemia virus (HTLV-1) retrovirus in cutaneous T cell lymphoma and a form of T cell leukemia prevalent in Japan.[102] Herpes virus has been implicated in cervical cancer etiology, and there is evidence for human papilloma virus infection in the genesis of some UV-associated skin cancers.[103]

These viruses only infect human (or other primate) cells, however, rendering experimental analyses difficult or impossible. To investigate the possible existence of specific virus-associated antigens in these human cancers, monoclonal antibodies to viral particles or transformed cells have been made and screened in vitro on virus-producing human cell lines and human tumor specimens. Specific cytotoxic T cell reactivity patterns to EBV-infected cells have indicated that EBV transformation results in expression of membrane-associated transformation antigens, termed lymphocyte-derived membrane antigens (LYDMA).[101] It is of note that newly diagnosed patients with nasopharyngeal carcinoma showed impaired EBV-specific T cell mediated immunity when compared to long-term survivors and EBV-immune controls who do not have the disease.[104] The monoclonal approach has been implemented by laboratories attempting to identify these LYDMA antigens. One monoclonal produced to EBV B95-8 virions by Hoffman et al.[105] detected a 250 kdalton glycoprotein specifically expressed by human and marmoset virus-producing cells. Thorley-Lawson et al.[101] have produced monoclonal 17D6 against EBV-transformed cells and immunoprecipitated a 45 kdalton antigen. A monoclonal produced to another virus, HTLV-1, was specific for the viral internal protein p19 and specifically precipitated p19 from radiolabeled HTLV-1-producing cells.[106] This antibody bound three of twelve human cutaneous T cell lymphoma lines and one of two cultured Sezary syndrome cutaneous T cell leukemias, but it did not bind any of six fresh lymphoma specimens. The binding site was determined to be at the internal membrane face. More recently, a survey of adult T cell leukemia-lymphoma (ATL) patients in Okinowa showed that all patients with this clinicopathological diagnosis (ATL) showed serum antibody reactivity to HTLV-1 antigens.[107]

E. Autologous Antibody-Defined Tumor Antigens

The data mentioned to this point have been derived from tumor antigen studies utilizing rodents or investigations of human antigens as discerned by the immunization of rodents with human cells. An alternative approach to the elucidation of human tumor antigens is the analysis of autologous patient sera including the use of the patient's lymphocytes for hybridoma generation. Difficulties in establishment of human-rodent hybridomas, and in finding a suitable human myeloma fusion partner, have hampered this approach. However, technical modifications have resulted in some apparent success. The rationale for this approach is that novel antigen expression should be recognized by the host immune system which may be sufficiently primed to recognize TSA, but remain ineffective for complete tumor elimination. Autologous sera of cancer patients has been analyzed by Old's group for a decade, which has obtained some evidence for antigens of class I (restricted to the patient's autologous tumor), class II (present on some allogeneic tumors), and class III (present on a wide range of normal and malignant human tissues).[14] Class I and class II type antigens occur in approximately 10% of patients. More recently, the fusion of cancer-patient lymphocytes to murine myeloma cells has been attempted by Old's group[108,109] and others[110-113] in order to characterize these autologous antigens. Autologous antibodies which show preferential binding to malignant human lung,[113] breast,[111,112] melanoma,[109] and colon[110] have been reported, and one antimelanoma monoclonal derived from a fusion with autologous patient lymphocytes has been used to identify a unique class I 90 kdalton melanoma antigen.[114] Fusions using peripheral blood lymphocytes from autologously immunized human colorectal cancer patients resulted in several monoclonals to apparently tumor-specific colon epithelial cell surface antigens.[110] Two thirds of these monoclonal-producing cell lines were determined not to be mouse-human hybridomas, but transformed diploid human B cell lines stable for over 1 year in culture. It will be of interest to see whether further analysis in this area will be able to identify additional unique or tissue-specific tumor antigens, and to see how improvement of techniques will affect this approach.

F. Evidence for Other Tumor-Specific Antigens

Antigens encoded by activated cellular oncogenes, retroviral associated v-oncogenes, other viral sequences or cellular genes for MHC antigens, and glycosylation enzymes are focal areas in the ongoing investigation of TSA. In addition, a wide variety of partially characterized or uncharacterized human cancer antigens have been reported, as reviewed elsewhere.[115] These putative TSA, which continue to be reported, are identified by screening monoclonals produced from rodents immunized with human tumor cell lines or human cancer biopsy tissue. Antibodies that do not bind normal human tissue, but show selective binding to tumor cell lines and/or tissue sections, are tentatively classified as tumor specific; wider screening and follow-up biochemical analyses are required to determine whether these structures detected are true TSA. By this approach, human tumor antigens have been described for prostate,[116] breast,[117,118] melanoma,[119,120] glioma,[121] bladder,[122,123] pancreas,[124] ovary,[125,126] lung,[129,130] colon,[131] and leukocytes.[132,133]

III. NORMAL TISSUE DIFFERENTIATION ANTIGENS AS TUMOR-ASSOCIATED ANTIGENS

A. Definition of Differentiation Antigens

Differentiation antigens are normal antigens whose expression is restricted by tissue lineage and developmental stage, "antigens that appear only on certain cell types, whose expression appears to be conditional on a pathway of differentiation".[134] T1 antigens, whose expression is restricted to a particular developmental stage of the T cell lineage, is an example. There is usually no direct association of these tissue antigens with the malignant phenotype, but a tumor clonally derived from a particular tissue type may continue to express antigens characteristic of the normal progenitor tissue. Tissue differentiation antigens which are markers of tissues that are both nonessential to survival of the whole organism and frequent targets of malignancies present possible alternative targets for diagnostic and therapeutic applications of monoclonal antibodies. Examples of such tissues are breast and prostate. Antigens expressed on tumor cells derived from later developmental stages, but not on regenerative stem cell pools, such as growth-factor receptors characteristically expressed on mature, proliferative T cells, also may provide good targets.[135] In cases where continued maintenance of some antigenically characterized normal adult tissue is essential to host survival, or where antigen expression is not completely restricted to that tissue (i.e., cross reactivity with other related or unrelated tissue occurs), manipulation of schedules and methods of antibody administration may be possible. Preliminary clinical trials with monoclonals to tumor-associated differentiation structures have resulted in documented cancer remissions,[62,136,137] and one trial with melanoma patients has shown that antibody treatment may be effective in the absence of absolute tumor specificity.[62] A final consideration in this approach is that the absence of a direct role of these antigens in the maintenance of the transformed phenotype means that altered malignant clones deriving from the original tumor may lose antigen expression, and that antibody treatment may promote the arisal of such "escaping clones".[138] Treatment of cancer with monoclonals to normal tissue antigens in such situations will probably best be considered as an adjunctive approach, requiring great care in administration and patient follow-up.

B. Oncofetal Antigens

Oncofetal antigens (OFA) and embryonic antigens are those antigens characteristically expressed during embryonic and fetal stages of normal tissue development and expressed anomolously in certain tumors. In normal tissue their expression is reduced or absent after completion of organogenesis. They have been found in a wide variety of chemically and virally induced tumors,[139] and characteristic OFA also have been shown for certain human cancers. Carcinoembryonic antigen (CEA) was first described in 1965 as a 200 kdalton glycoprotein restricted to fetal and malignant gastrointestinal tissue.[140] More recent analyses have shown CEA to be structurally heterogeneous and monoclonals to distinct CEA epitopes, related perhaps to individuals or to disease stages, may aid in the definition of tumor-restricted forms. CEA, although a secreted glycoprotein, has been used as a target antigen in imaging studies with radiolabeled antibodies.[11] A study utilizing CEA as a target for antibody-mediated neutron-capture therapy in a hamster model has also been reported.[141] Other human tumor-associated antigens, many of them lipid or peptide-associated carbohydrate structures,[59] may also be OFA. These include SSEA-1[77] and FH4,5, and 6 antigens (see Section II.C).

Recently, Rettig et al.[142] described monoclonal K21, generated to a human teratocarcinoma cell line and a placental tissue membrane preparation, which bound teratocarcinoma cell lines, but not any normal adult tissues. Its fetal expression was restricted to intestine and bronchus, and the target antigen was identified as lacto-N-fucopentaose III (X-hapten). A monoclonal to a putative peptide OFA also has been reported by Payne and Coggin.[143] By immunization of mice with irradiated syngeneic fetal cells, an antibody which recognizes a developmental stage-specific embryonic antigen expressed on mouse, rat, and human fetal and tumor cells was produced. This monoclonal, which identified a 44 kd and a 200 kd peptide, was absorbed by a variety of human carcinomas, but not by normal adult human tissue.

C. Leukocyte Differentiation Antigens

The tissue which was first studied systematically for differentiation antigen expression, and which probably remains the most completely analyzed, is leukocytic tissue. Leukemic and nonleukemic T lymphocytes from mouse thymus provided a reliable and accessible source of large numbers of easily handled cells for initial transplantation antigen studies.[144] Leukocytic tissue antigens in mouse,[145,146] rat,[147] and man[135-137,148-150] have also provided some of the earliest tumor-associated targets for trials with monoclonal antibodies. A monoclonal antibody against a normal human myelomonocytic differentiation antigen, cross reactive with rat myelomonocytic cells, has been used to eliminate most antigen-positive leukemic cells in rats with acute nonlymphocytic leukemia without side effects.[147] In the mouse, Bernstein et al.[145] showed that a monoclonal antibody to the T cell Thy 1.1 differentiation alloantigen, when injected into (129 $\times$ AKR) F_1 mice bearing subcutaneously inoculated Thy 1.1 positive AKR SL2 leukemia cells, resulted in prolonged survival of mice and delayed the onset of systemic disease. When antibody treatment was accompanied by surgical excision of the subcutaneous primary, some mice were cured. A monoclonal antibody to the alternative allele, Thy 1.2, has also been shown to be effective in reduction of T-cell leukemia.[146]

Human T-cell differentiation antigens have provided the first targets for antitumor monoclonal antibodies in clinical trials. Treatment of an adult T-cell leukemia patient with a murine monoclonal antibody to a normal T cell antigen resulted in a marked, but transient, decline in circulating leukocytes.[151] Antibodies to Leu 1, another human T-cell differentiation antigen which is expressed on the majority of peripheral circulating T cells, have also been used for treatment of patients with cutaneous T-cell lymphoma and chronic lymphocytic leukemia.[150] These attempts resulted in transient declines of circulating antigen-positive cells with little toxicity. Another marker of peripheral T cells which may provide a sufficiently restricted target antigen in some leukemic patients is the T cell surface receptor for the lymphokine growth factor interleukin-2 (IL-2).[135] Waldmann et al. have conducted a clinical trial with a monoclonal to the human T-cell IL-2 receptor, designated anti-Tac.[152] IL-2 receptors occur only on mature, activated T cells, and cell lines from adult T-cell leukemic patients show a tenfold increase in surface receptor expression.[153] In the trial, one of three patients showed two remission periods following two courses of therapy. More recently, the antibody was linked to the alpha-particle emitting radionuclide bismuth-212, with the rationale of developing a radioimmunotherapeutic reagent effective in killing cells to whose surface it specifically bound.[154] Specific killing of surface antigen positive cells was observed in vitro in cytotoxicity assays.

Monoclonal antibody to the unique antigen-binding portion of B cell immunoglobulin, termed idiotype, has been used clinically with some objectively documented success.[136,137] Surface immunoglobulin is a normally expressed B lymphocyte differentiation antigen present on mature, immunocompetent B lymphocytes. The uniqueness of idiotypes for specific B-cell clones apparently makes it an ideal target for the treatment of mature B-cell malignancies via the monoclonal approach. Immunoglobulin is restricted to the B-cell lineage, but antibodies to idiotypic determinants, unique for each B-cell clone, will not cross react with other normal B-cell clones which are essential for normal survival. Consequently, all cells clonally derived from a common tumor cell, which express idiotype, can be targeted by the monoclonal approach, while the remainder of the functionally important B-cell repertoire is spared. Meeker et al.[136] and Miller et al.[137] have produced "tailor-made" monoclonals to idiotype present on biopsy material from 11 B cell lymphoma patients. Following treatment with the antibodies, 1 of 11 patients has been reported to be in complete remission for 42 months. Of the other 10 patients, 5 showed objectively documented partial remissions. Another group has also produced anti-idiotype monoclonals for treatment of two patients, both of whom showed specific antibody targeting, but limited clinical effect.[155] Expression of idiotype is not essential for the maintenance of the malignant phenotype and, thus, failures of clinical trials may be due to "escape" by arisal of nonidiotype positive variant clones.[138] As B cell idiotype is distinct in its clonality of expression, these clinical trials are prototypes for production of effective, tailor-made monoclonals for individual human cancers. Designed production of antibodies to clonally distinctive antigen receptors of T lymphocytes[156] is also plausible.

D. Nonleukocytic Human Tissue Differentiation Antigens

1. Introduction

Characterization of normal tissue differentiation antigens of nonleukocytic tissues is also progressing directly and indirectly through the generation of antitumor monoclonals which actually identify normal structures.[16] Several laboratories previously investigating tumor-specific antigens are now pursuing the identification and detailed analysis of tissue-specific developmental surface antigen expression; thoughtful application may provide another rational approach to the development of clinically useful anti-cancer monoclonals. The antibody approach is currently providing useful information about antigen structures of prostate, breast, colorectal, pancreatic, renal, and neuroectodermal cells.

2. Prostate

Carroll et al.[157,158] and others[159-161] have used the hybridoma technology to generate monoclonal antibodies which identify normal human prostate tissue differentiation antigens. One useful prostatic marker is a 34 kdalton cytoplasmic and secreted protein found in both normal and malignant prostate and called prostate antigen (PA).[162] Frankel et al.[160] have produced PA-specific monoclonals, but the lack of surface antigen expression may limit its usefulness for most monoclonal applications in vivo.

In a separate study, Frankel et al.[159] immunized BALB/c mice with membrane preparations of human benign prostate hyperplastic tissue and obtained three sets of antibodies that characterize stromal tissue antigens, prostate epithelial antigens, and polyepithelial antigens which are present on epithelia derived from a variety of tissue sources. Two antibodies detected stromal tissue antigens, one of which also reacted with prostatic and other organ

Table 2
REACTIVITY OF MURINE MONOCLONAL ANTIBODIES WITH HUMAN CELL LINES

	Hybridoma cell lines		
	F77-129 (1:50)	F77-21 (1:10)	F77-55 (1:50)
Prostate carcinoma			
PC-3	3+	3+	3+
Du-145	NT	NT	2+
Breast carcinoma			
MCF-7	2+	2+	2+
BT-20	3+	3+	3+
MB231	1+	2+	1+
HSO-584T	0	0	0
Colon carcinoma			
SW260	1+	1+	0
HI-135	0	0	0
Ovarian carcinoma			
McDonald	1+	1+	0
Renal carcinoma			
Pasteur	0	0	0
Melanoma			
H130M	0	0	0
S85A	0	0	0
G-361	NT	NT	0
Hematopoietic tumors			
CEM (T cell)0	0	0	
HL-60 (AML)	0	0	0
U937 (histiocytic)	0	0	0
SB (B cell)	0	0	0

Note: Unpurified F77-21, F77-55, and F77-129 supernatants were tested by FACS. The criteria used were: 0, no fluorescence above control; 1+, slight fluorescence above control; 2+, intermediate fluorescence above control; 3+, strong fluorescence; NT, line not tested.

endothelial cells, the other bound myoepithelial and muscle cells. Tissue section immunoperoxidase analysis showed restricted binding of two antibodies to both normal and malignant prostate epithelia with some cross reactivity to normal salivary gland. Antigens detected by four other monoclonals were termed polyepithelial; these defined three distinct protein antigens expressed differentially on a spectrum of normal epithelium. Ware et al.[161] have generated panels of anti-human prostate tissue monoclonals by immunization of mice with a human prostate adenocarcinoma cell line, PC-3. One antibody, anti-Pro 3, identified a 54 kd protein present on normal prostate, benign prostatic hyperplasia, and, to a lesser extent, on malignant prostate tissue; it is also present on the surface of cultured PC-3 cells. We have also produced antibodies to human prostate cell surface antigens by immunizing mice with PC-3 human prostate carcinoma cells.[157] When tested on a panel of human cell lines by indirect immunofluorescence staining and FACS analysis, supernatants of three distinct hybridomas from the same fusion (F77-21, 55, and 129) showed restricted binding to prostate and breast epithelial cell lines (Table 2). Analysis of human tissue section staining by an immunoperoxidase technique confirmed the epithelial cell staining in malignant human prostate and breast (Figure 1). Variable low-level staining of endothelia in other tissues also

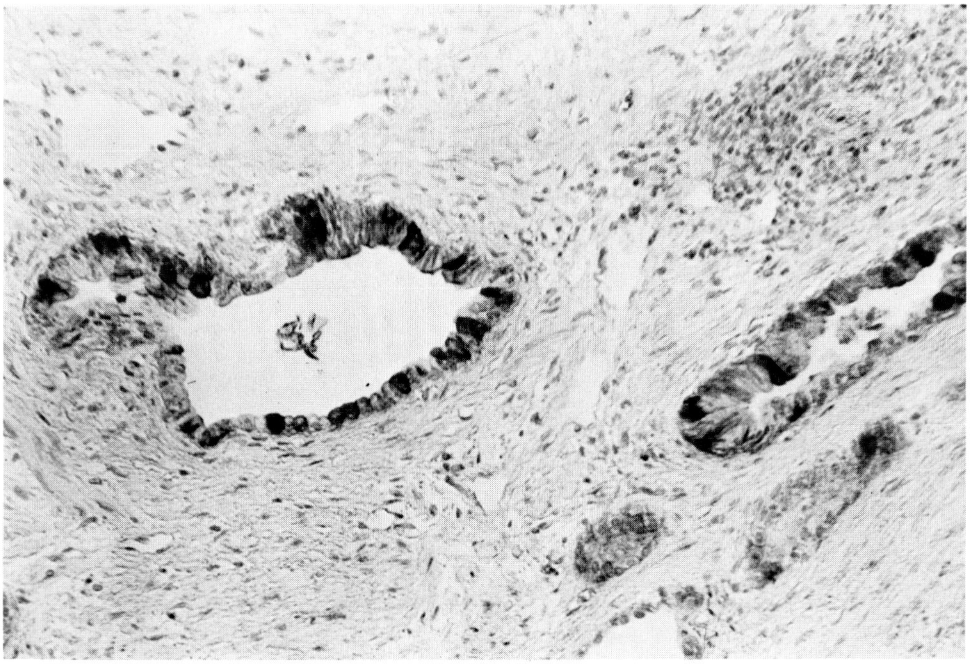

FIGURE 1. Immunoperoxidase staining of a paraffin section of normal human prostate tissue stained with F77-129 antibody. Magnification × 31.

occurred, the nature of which will require further investigation prior to any clinical application. On PC-3 cells, the antigen is present in high quantity, an estimated 10^5 antibody binding sites per cell, and is heat stable, indicative of a carbohydrate nature. The antigen, similar to p54 described by Ware et al.,[161] modulates from the cell surface upon incubation with antibody. Preliminary paired-label biodistribution studies were done in nude mice bearing xenografted PC-3 prostate tumor and antigenically irrelevant G-361 melanoma tumor using ^{125}I-labeled F77-129, an IgG3 antibody and an isotype-matched ^{131}I-labeled control antibody. Table 3 shows the specific localization of F77-129 in the PC-3 tumor of these mice at 24 and 72 hr post injection (no specific localization to G-361 tumor occurred — data not shown). These data indicate the ability of appropriate monoclonals to target relevant antigenic structures. In the development of these anti-prostate monoclonals, we considered antibodies which bound nonmalignant, as well as malignant, prostate because prostate is a high frequency organ of human cancer[164] and survival of this tissue is not essential to the prolonged survival of the organism. The primary question requiring further investigation is that of cross reactivity with other tissue, most notably breast epithelia and other tissue endothelium, as has been observed with our anti-prostate antibodies, those of Frankel et al. and other monoclonals developed to breast and various epithelial tissues (see below).

3. *Breast*

Several laboratories have been involved in the definition of human breast tissue antigens by the monoclonal technique. Papsidero et al.[165] generated antibodies to human breast carcinoma cell lines (MCF-7 and Sk-Br-3), two of which identified antigens whose expression appeared restricted to normal and malignant breast epithelium. The tissue specificity of one of these antibodies (F36/22) was further investigated. It bound a high percentage of breast carcinomas, normal differentiated mammary ductal epithelia, and milk fat globule mem-

Table 3
SPECIFIC LOCALIZATION OF F77-129 MONOCLONAL ANTIBODY

	Localization index[a]	
Tissue	**24 hr**	**72 hr**
Tumor[b]	8.8	9.1
Liver	0.9	0.9
Spleen	2.0	1.0
Lung	1.5	0.9
Heart	1.8	0.7
Kidney	1.7	1.0
Skin	2.3	1.5
Muscle	2.4	1.3
Bone	1.9	1.6

[a] Localization index (LI) expresses the localization of ^{125}I-labeled F77-129 relative to that of a ^{131}I-labeled antibody of identical isotype which does not bind to the PC-3 antigen, following intravenous injection into PC-3 tumor-bearing mice.

$$LI = \frac{\%/g \text{ of organ (specific/nonspecific)}}{\%/g \text{ of blood (specific/nonspecific)}}$$

[b] PC-3 tumor (2×10^6 to 5×10^6 cells) was injected subcutaneously in the dorsolateral region of nude mice 20 to 30 days prior to injection of radiolabeled antibody.

branes; it was also reactive with adenocarcinomas derived from certain tissue types (ovary, colon, stomach, and prostate), but not with their normal tissue counterparts.[166] Thompson et al.[167] generated an antibody to the MCF-7 carcinoma cell line which showed similar reactivity; it bound 10/10 malignant breast cell lines and was absent from 41/43 cell lines of different tissue origin; however, further histological analysis revealed that it bound normal breast epithelia and also epithelia of respiratory tract tissues, prostate, pancreas, and salivary glands. Menard et al.[168] generated two antibodies with superimposable activity of an apparently more restricted nature. Antibodies MBr1 and MBr2, also produced following immunization with the MCF-7 cell line, bound normal and malignant breast ductal epithelial cells and post-partum breast milk; the only non-breast tissue for which limited binding was noted was skin apocrine sweat glands. Recently, this antigen has been biochemically analyzed and determined to be a glycosphingolipid of the blood group H antigen series, abundant in teratocarcinoma cells and present in breast epithelia, but otherwise limited in normal human adults.[169] Another antibody generated to the MCF-7 cell line designated 15A8 was recently reported by White et al.[170] It bound a surface structure present on 28 of 31 human mammary carcinomas tested, and also reacted more weakly with normal breast epithelia, esophageal epithelia, kidney renal proximal tubule, and salivary glands. One other group has concentrated on the production of antibodies to human breast milk fat globule membranes and antigenic characterization of normal breast epithelial in cell subsets.[171] Three antibodies (LICR-LON-M8, M18 and M24) identified three antigens differentially distributed on normal breast lumenal epithelia; these markers were postulated to identify distinct developmental or functional (e.g., secretory vs. nonsecretory) states.

4. Neuroectodermal Antigens

Old's group has used a systematic approach to identify normal differentiation antigens of previously uncharacterized tissues by establishment of extensive panels of human tumor cell lines and mouse monoclonal antibodies generated to them.[127,172,175,177-179]

Houghton et al.[172] used a panel of 42 monoclonal antibodies against melanocytes to study melanocyte differentiation antigen expression. The antibodies were used as a typing sera on over 40 melanoma cell lines and on cultured nonmalignant melanocytes obtained from newborn foreskin or adult skin. Melanocytes from newborn and adult skin differ morphologically; newborn cells are bipolar, whereas adult cells are polydendritic. The pattern of serological reactivity with the anti-melanocyte/melanoma monoclonals also differed for these two normal cell subsets. Distinct cellular subsets were also detected when melanoma cell lines were typed with the antibodies. Based on these patterns of reactivity, typing antibodies were grouped in four categories defining differentiation antigen subsets.

1. Antigens not expressed on newborn or adult melanocytes, but expressed by subsets of melanoma (four markers), proposed to be very early markers of a melanocyte precursor class
2. Antigens detected on normal newborn, but not adult melanocytes, and classified as intermediate stage antigens (two markers)
3. Antigens detected on adult melanocytes and only weakly, or not at all, on most newborn melanocytes and designated late stage markers (two markers),
4. Antigens detected equally on newborn and adult melanocytes, and also on most melanoma cell lines.

When antibodies identifying these early, intermediate, and late stage antigens were used to type a panel of 25 human melanoma cell lines, 5 lines were found to express only the early markers, 10 to express intermediate markers, and 10 to express late stage antigens. These serological markers correlated with variations in morphology, pigmentation, and enzyme tyrosinase activity, and enabled Houghton et al. to propose a surface antigen lineage map. These melanocyte subset antigens are concordant with those designated by a different approach, analysis of two-dimensional electrophoretic patterns of [^{3}H] glucosamine-labeled glycoproteins.[173] Loms Ziegler-Heitbrock et al.[174] also used monoclonals to show that melanocyte differentiation antigen expression could be modulated by treatment of cell lines with the differentiating tumor promoter 12-O-tetradecanoylphorbol-13-acetate (TPA).

One of the monoclonals (R24) which identified class 4 melanoma antigens in Houghton's study has been used in clinical trials with melanoma patients.[62] R24 was generated by Dippold et al.[175] and identifies a restricted neuroectodermal marker present on melanocytes, astrocytes, melanomas, astrocytomas, and a subset of sarcomas. It also mediates biological activities including human complement fixation and antibody-dependent cell-mediated cytotoxicity. On the basis of these properties, R24 was chosen for clinical therapeutic trials. Twelve melanoma patients with objectively measurable disease, shown to express R24 antigen by biopsy and immunofluorescence, were treated with three dose levels of antibody (8, 80, or 240 mg/m^2) over a period of 2 weeks. Major regression was observed in three patients as evaluated by measurement of tumor size 6 weeks after initiation of therapy. Inflammatory reactions at the tumor site were observed in patients treated with doses 80 mg/m^2, and tumor biopsies during and after treatment showed infiltration of lymphocytes and mast cells, mast cell degranulation, and complement deposition. Despite reactivity of the antibody to normal melanocytes and astrocytomas, side effects were mild and readily controlled by antihistamines. Differential accessibility and reactivity of normal vs. tumor cells may be a relevant factor. These results support proposed clinical in vivo application of monoclonals which react with tumor-associated (rather than tumor-specific) tissue differentiation antigens.

A neuroectodermal tissue antigen is the apparent target of a monoclonal antibody, CG12, generated against the human glioma cell line, LN-18, by Schnegg et al.[121] This antibody bound 10 of 18 glioma lines, 5 of 5 melanoma lines and one of one neuroblastoma line tested, and its reactivity could be absorbed with both normal and fetal brain homogenates. Monoclonal anti-neuroblastoma antibodies of Kennett and Gilbert[176] showed similar cross reactivity with glioblastoma and fetal brain cells.

Cairncross et al.[177] have used monoclonal antibodies to human astrocytoma cell lines to characterize differentiation antigens on subsets of astrocytes. Serological analysis identified nine distinct antigenic systems. Two monoclonals, A010 and AJ8, subdivided 16 cultured astrocytomas (with two exceptions) into mutually exclusive astrocytoma subsets. Using a panel of cultured cells, binding of monoclonals to surface astrocytoma antigens and to glial fibrillary acidic protein (GFA), an internal protein of mature differentiated astrocytes, permitted antigenic classification of astrocyte precursors ($AJ8^+$, $A010^-$, GFA^-), immature astrocytes ($AJ8^-$, $A010^+$, GFA^-), and mature astrocytes ($AJ8^-$, $A010^+$, GFA^+).

5. Kidney

Ueda et al.[178] used a similar approach for the analysis of renal tissue differentiation antigens. A total of 17 mouse monoclonal antibodies were generated to human renal cancer cell lines, identifying 9 cell surface antigen systems. Although a few showed apparent restriction to malignant and nonmalignant adult and fetal kidney epithelial cells, further analysis on an expanded cultured cell panel revealed less-restricted specificity.[179] Staining of tissue sections by indirect immunofluorescence and immunoperoxidase analysis indicated binding of these antibodies to discrete regions of the kidney. Antibody S23 binds a 120 kdalton glycoprotein identified as adenosine deaminase binding protein,[180] which is present on kidney proximal tubule cells, and has also been detected in frozen sections of prostate, breast, and colon.[179] Antibody S4, which immunoprecipitates a 160 kdalton glycoprotein, binds both glomerular and proximal tubule cells; it also binds fetal kidney and some neuroblastoma and choriocarcinoma lines, but shows restricted binding to normal adult tissue. It was reported in the interstitial matrix of some tissues including placenta, myometrium, and fetal lung. More information about the nature of this reactivity and its occurrence in normal adult tissues will be needed for the determination of the practical utility of this antibody. These monoclonals and others have permitted antigenic classification of distinct subsets of renal cancer similar to that of the neuroectodermal markers.

6. Bladder

Eleven distinct systems were identified by production of mouse monoclonals to human bladder cancer or bladder papilloma lysates.[122] Binding studies using extensive panels of malignant and normal cultured cells and frozen tissue sections showed one antibody, designated JP165, with highly restricted specificity for normal adult and fetal bladder and renal tissues, and a subset of bladder and renal cancers. Other antibodies showed less restricted specificity.

7. Ovary

Old's group has employed the technique utilized to identify tumor associated normal tissue antigens for melanocyte, astrocyte, renal, and bladder cells for ovarian cells as well. Using human ovarian and endometrial carcinoma lines as immunogens, several reactive monoclonals were produced.[127] Most showed no cross reactivity with normal tissues, similar to previous findings of other groups.[125,126,128] One antibody, MH94, binds to carcinoma cell lines derived from ovary, uterus, colon, breast, lung, cervix, and pancreas, and also binds to epithelial cells of normal tissue sections, predominantly to secretory epithelial cells.

8. Colorectal

Mouse monoclonals generated against human colorectal carcinoma cells have identified normal tissue Lewis blood group alloantigens[72] and the oncofetal antigen CEA,[181] both of which may provide useful targets in selective situations. Another monoclonal antibody to a human stomach adenocarcinoma bound normal colonic epithelium, and it also bound normal superficial epithelium of several other tissues.[182]

9. Pancreas

Metzgar et al.[183] generated monoclonals to a human pancreatic tumor cell line, HPAF. Two antibodies reacted with four of five pancreatic tumor cell lines and also bound normal pancreatic tissues on frozen sections. Antibody Du-Pan-2 defined an antigen on adult pancreatic ductal epithelial cells, but not present on frozen sections of other normal tissues or tumors derived from nonpancreatic tissues. This antigen has since been identified as a carbohydrate rich, neuraminidase-sensitive mucin-like structure.[184] Antibody Du-Pan-3 was somewhat less restricted, reacting with both adult and fetal pancreatic cells and some nonpancreatic tumors (colon, lung, renal), but not with cells of normal adult or fetal nonpancreatic tissue. Two other monoclonals recently generated to the pancreatic cell lines COLO-357 and CAPAN-1 were also reported to react with normal (C54-0) or inflamed (C1-N3) pancreatic tissue.[124]

10. Other Tissue-Specific Antigens

The approach in the above studies has been similar: generation of monoclonals to malignant and normal human cellular material, with subsequent biochemical characterization of target antigens and analysis of the restriction of specificity. Most strategies have aimed at identification of cell surface components, as these are accessible to antibody in intact cells. Another approach to directing antibody to normal tissue-associated antigens has been used by Order et al.[185] These investigators have launched in vivo diagnostic and therapeutic trials with iodinated (^{131}I) antibody directed to a secreted tissue (and tumor) associated protein, ferritin. Ferritin production is characteristic of particular tissues, and is a tumor-associated protein in hepatoma, Hodgkins Disease, lung cancer, neuroblastoma, acute myelogenous leukemia, and breast and pancreatic carcinomas.[185,186] Clinical trials with ^{131}I-labeled rabbit anti-human ferritin showed tumor localization in a variety of ferritin-bearing tumor types and unmaintained (3 to 9 months) remissions in four of five hepatoma patients. Patients received 100 to 150 mCi doses of antibody, and tumor remissions were documented by clinical, biochemical, and radiographic evidence. Side effects were not reported to be serious. These studies thus provide an additional example of the utility of a tumor-associated, but nontumor-specific, antigen as an anti-tumor antibody target. Secreted, nonmembrane forms of tissue-specific products, such as ferritin and the oncofetal antigen CEA, may be acceptable targets for imaging and for therapeutic approaches not requiring direct cell contact and/or internalization.

IV. CONSIDERATIONS OF THE NATURE OF ANTIGEN EXPRESSION AND ACCESSIBILITY

This review has focused on the current evidence for the existence of TSA and other tumor-associated antigens which may provide useful targets for in vivo applications of monoclonals. The biology of expression at both the cellular and whole organism level also must be considered carefully before and throughout the clinical application of monoclonal antibodies. Factors which must be considered are

1. Cross-reactive antigen expression on non-tumor cells
2. Intraclonal generality (or variability) of antigen expression within a given tumor

3. Interclonal generality (or variability) of expression for tumors of a common tissue and/or developmental stage derivation
4. Shedding or secretion of antigen
5. Modulation of antigen from the cell surface consequent to antibody binding.

A. Cross-Reactive Antigens

We have already discussed the importance of tumor restricted specificity, and the in vitro screening procedures used to ensure this specificity. Most monoclonals which have been thoroughly screened on human biopsy tissue sections do show some cross reactivity, often to unrelated tissues, due to recognition of both related and unrelated antigen structures. It is the nature of monoclonals to recognize one limited, distinct epitope of an often complex antigen; consequently, there may be significant binding to a common epitopic determinant of an unrelated molecule and tissue.[187] Careful and thorough in vitro screening on human cell lines and tissue sections can indicate these cross reactivities and guide selection of antibodies for administration. Antibody to Burkitt's lymphoma antigen[63] (see Section II.B.2), for example, may be administered only to individuals with P^k negative erythrocytes. Following the in vitro screen, additional factors may come into play in the in vivo environment, resulting in more, or perhaps less, stringent application. Two studies attest to an in vivo utility better than might have been expected from in vitro analyses. In the first study, performed by Ballou et al.,[188] an iodinated monoclonal anti-SSEA-1 antibody was administered to MH-15 teratocarcinoma-bearing mice. Despite the higher concentration of SSEA-1 antigen on normal kidney relative to tumor, as determined by tissue immunoperoxidase analysis, antibody injected in vivo showed no significant localization in kidney. Anti-SSEA-1, but not an isotype (IgM) matched control antibody, did show significant tumor localization. Also, there was no notable accumulation in brain or salivary glands, which also express SSEA-1 antigen. The second system is a clinical trial of an anti-melanoma antibody by Houghton et al.[62] The anti-GD 3 ganglioside antibody used showed cross reactivity to normal tissue including astrocytes, retina, and skin melanocytes, yet remissions were obtained without notable damage to non-tumor tissue. These findings are probably due to differences in antigen accessibility at the cellular and whole organism level, and differential antibody processing by cells. Tumor vascular anatomy and tissue interstitial space may play a role[189,190] as may differential availability of antibody for binding at the cell surface.[49] Internal vs. external cell expression, antigen masking, antibody-induced modulation, and internalization vs. static binding (see below) and quantitative variations in antigen expression are all relevant factors. An understanding of these factors, together with the use of selective schedules and procedures of antibody administration (e.g., intralymphatic injection of antibody, see Chapter 8) may permit less stringent requirements for the application of antibodies to tumor-associated antigens.

B. Intraclonal Variability of Expression

We have discussed how cell surface oncogene-encoded TSA, essential to the maintenance of the transformed phenotype, are ideal targets for antibody therapy; they are expressed on every cell derived from the original progenitor clone, and loss of antigen by a genetic event would result in loss of malignancy. Most of the antigens discussed, however, are not integral parts of the malignant state, and creation of antigen-negative clonal variants may occur. Such variants are known to arise in tumor cell cultures in vitro. Varient MHC antigen expressing murine tumor clones, for example, were estimated to occur at a frequency of 10^{-5} to 10^{-6} in vitro.[89] Non-heritable quantitative variations in antigen expression unrelated to cell cycle stage have also been shown in vitro and have been correlated with differential susceptibility to immune lysis by relevant antibody.[191] Clinical evidence for tumor-cell antigen variant subpopulations also exists. Phenotypic heterogeneity has been observed in autologous primary and metastic lesions[192] and among different metastases in the same patient.[193] These findings indicate that differential antigen expression due to arisal of antigen-negative variants or to the existence of nonheritable quantitative heterogeneity of expression may result in malignant cell subpopulations with different antibody binding properties. This has obvious implications for planned diagnostic and therapeutic applications and indicates an adjunct role of antibody treatment in such situations. An additional consideration is that antibody administration may in itself select for antigen-negative variants. Meeker et al.[136] postulated that alterations in idiotypic expression occurred in two patients treated with anti-idiotype, and that this may have played a significant role in their failure to respond clinically. Follow-up studies of idiotypic variants from one patient indicated a role of antibody treatment in induction of somatic mutation of the idiotype-encoding gene.[138]

C. Interclonal Variability of Expression

Certain tumor types may characteristically express common antigens, facilitating development of broad spectrum reactive monoclonals. Such an approach would be possible when using tissue differentiation antigens as targets, for example. In other systems, however, heterogeneity of TSA expression may occur, such as with unique antigens characterizing UV elicited fibrosarcomas or unique idiotypic determinants of B cell lymphomas. In the latter case, an understanding of the biochemical nature of the antigen facilitates attempts to produce, screen, and select for appropriate antibody reactivity. The feasibility of this approach has been exemplified by the B cell lymphoma/anti-idiotype trials in which monoclonal antibodies were "tailor-made" for 11 patients using tissue from biopsies.[137] In a survey of 15 different anti-idiotypes on 100 different lymphomas, no cross reaction was observed. Monoclonals for chosen patients were successfully elicited, however, using cells from tumor biopsy or purified idiotype protein.

D. Antigen Shedding

Most of the antigens discussed in this review are cell surface components which are both localized and accessible, making them ideal targets for systemically circulating antibody. Some secreted proteins have also been used as tumor markers for immunoscintigraphy and even therapy with some success. Generally, however, existence of secreted or shed cell surface antigenic material is considered an obstacle to the in vivo administration of antibody. Shed antigen can result in diminished tumor to nontumor antibody localization ratios, clinically adverse circulating antigen-antibody complexes, and possibly false positive diagnoses due to accumulation of material shed (or secreted) from the tumor at nontumor sites.[11] Many tumor cell surface markers may also be shed (e.g., sialosyl Lewis a and X; see Section II.B.3), and it will be important to determine the effects of shed antigen on planned protocols for particular antigens. At the clinical level, a model analysis of this factor was performed by Meeker et al.[136] in an anti-idiotype trial of B cell lymphoma patients. Serum idiotype levels were monitored before and during antibody treatment of individual patients and plasmapheresis was utilized to lower these levels. Plasmapheresis was helpful in removing serum idiotype prior to antibody administration for two of three patients with high serum idiotype levels, and these investigators stressed the usefulness of this procedure. They considered persistent serum idiotype to be the primary cause of therapy failure in one patient. Similar monitoring of serum antigen levels for patients with different tumor-associated antigens during plasmapheresis and antibody administration will be needed when shed antigen is a factor.

E. Antigen Modulation

Some antigens, such as murine T cell leukemia T1 antigen, are modulated off the cell surface as a consequence of antibody binding. Many other cell surface antigens are not affected in this manner. Depending on the type of approach envisioned, this could be a positive or a negative factor. The behavior of cell surface antigen subsequent to antibody binding, therefore, must be understood for each antigen-monoclonal combination. For some imaging and therapeutic approaches, maintained presence of bound antibody on the cell surface is desired. Loss of antigen-antibody complexes from the cell surface to extracellular compartments would be undesirable, but complex internalization, resulting in internalization of antibody conjugated material as well, could be beneficial. Kozak et al.,[154] for example, utilized bismuth-212 labeled antibody to a T cell surface component which internalizes subsequent to antigen-antibody binding for specific intracellular targeting of an alpha particle-emitting isotope.

These factors and others need to be considered for each candidate antibody-antigen system for monoclonal-mediated tumor diagnosis and therapeutics. The complexities involved in these applications, as well as in understanding the basic nature of tumor-antigen expression, are apparent. The areas of current research as outlined will undoubtedly lead to a more comprehensive knowledge of transformation-associated changes in tumor cells and in tumor hosts, and of basic differentiation antigen components for particular tissues. Hopefully, careful monitoring of specificity and the factors modifying specificity at each step of in vitro and in vivo antibody investigations will lead to the elucidation of some useful targets for antibody-mediated diagnosis and therapy.

REFERENCES

1. **Ehrlich, P. A.,** A general review of the recent work in immunity, in *The Collected Works of Paul Ehrlich,* Himmelweit and Marquadt, Eds., Pergamon Press, New York, 1956, 442.
2. **Gorer, P. A.,** The genetic and antigenic basis of tumor transplantation, *J. Pathol.,* 44, 691, 1937.
3. **Gross, L.,** Intradermal immunization of C3H mice against a sarcoma that originated in an animal of the same line, *Cancer Res.,* 3, 326, 1943.
4. **Foley, E. J.,** Antigenic properties of methylcholanthrene-induced tumors in mice of the strain of origin, *Cancer Res.,* 13, 835, 1953.
5. **Prehn, R. T. and Main, J. M.,** Immunity to methylcholanthrene-induced sarcomas, *J. Natl. Cancer Inst.,* 18, 769, 1957.
6. **Klein, A.,** Tumor antigens, *Annu. Rev. Microbiol.,* 20, 223, 1966.
7. **Klein, G.,** Tumor immunology, in *Immunology 80,* Fougereau, M. and Duasset, J., Eds., Academic Press, New York, 680, 1980.
8. **Sjogren, H. O.,** Transplantation methods as a tool for detection of tumor-specific antigens, *Prog. Exp. Tumor Res.,* 6, 289, 1965.
9. **Kripke, M. L.,** Immunologic mechanisms in UV radiation carcinogenesis, *Adv. Cancer Res.,* 34, 69, 1981.
10. **Rosenberg, S. A. and Terry, W. D.,** Passive immunotherapy of cancer in animals and man, *Adv. Cancer Res.,* 25, 323, 1977.
11. **Sfakianakis, G. N. and DeLand, F. H.,** Radioimmunodiagnosis and radioimmunotherapy, *J. Nucl. Med.,* 23, 840, 1982.
12. **Hellstrom, K. E., Brown, J. P., and Hellstrom, I.,** Monoclonal antibodies to tumor antigens, *Contemp. Top. Immunobiol.,* 11, 117, 1980.
13. **Hewitt, H. B., Blake, E. R., and Walder, A. S.,** A critique of the evidence for active host defense against cancer, based on personal studies of 27 murine tumors of spontaneous origin, *Br. J. Cancer,* 33, 241, 1976.
14. **Old, L. J.,** Cancer immunology: the search for specificity. G. H. A. Clowes Memorial Lecture, *Cancer Res.,* 41, 361, 1981.
15. **Kohler, G. and Milstein, C.,** Continuous cultures of fused cells secreting antibody of predefined specificity, *Nature (London),* 256, 495, 1975.
16. **Beverly, P. C. L.,** Antibodies and cancer therapy, *Nature (London),* 297, 358, 1982.
17. **Greene, M. I.,** The genetic and cellular basis of regulation of the immune response to cancer antigens, *Contemp. Top. Immunobiol.,* 11, 81, 1980.
18. **Drebin, J. A., Perry, L. L., Carter, R., and Greene, M. I.,** Regulation of the immune response to antigens on the malignant cell surface, *Springer Semin. Immunopathol.,* 5, 175, 1982.

19. **Weinberg, R. A.,** Oncogenes of spontaneous and chemically induced tumors, *Adv. Cancer Res.*, 36, 149, 1982.
20. **Bishop, J. M.,** Cellular oncogenes and retroviruses, *Annu. Rev. Biochem.*, 52, 301, 1983.
21. **Duesberg, P. H.,** Activated proto-onc genes: sufficient or necessary for cancer?, *Science*, 228, 669, 1985.
22. **Doolittle, R. F., Hunkapillar, M. W., Hood, L. E., Davare, S. G., Robbins, K. L., Aaronson, S. A., and Antoniades, H. N.,** Simian sarcoma virus onc gene, v sis, is derived from the gene (or genes) encoding a platelet derived growth factor, *Science*, 221, 275, 1983.
23. **Waterfield, M. D., Sirace, G. T., Whittle, N., Sroobant, P., Johnson, A., Wasteson, A., Westermark, B., Hildin, C. H., Huang, J. S., and Deuel, T. F.,** Platelet derived growth factor is structurally related to the putative transforming protein p28 of simian sarcoma virus, *Nature (London)*, 304, 35, 1983.
24. **Heldin, C. H. and Westmark, B.,** Growth factors: mechanisms of action and relation to oncogenes, *Cell*, 37, 9, 1984.
25. **Downward, J., Yarden, Y., Mayes, E., Scare, G., Totty, N., Stockwell, P., Ullrich, A., Schlessinger, J., and Waterfield, M. D.,** Close similarity of epidermal growth factor receptor and v-erb-B oncogene sequences, *Nature (London)*, 307, 521, 1984.
26. **Padhy, L. C., Shih, C., Cowing, D., Finkelstein, R., and Weinberg, R. A.,** Identification of a phosphoprotein specifically induced by the transforming DNA of rat neuroblastomas, *Cell*, 28, 865, 1982.
27. **Drebin, J. A., Stern, D. F., Link, V. C., Weinberg, R. A., and Greene, M. I.,** Monoclonal antibodies identify a cell-surface antigen associated with an activated cellular oncogene, *Nature (London)*, 312, 545, 1984.
28. **Shih, C., Padhy, L. C., Murray, M., and Weinberg, R. A.,** Transforming genes of carcinomas and neuroblastomas introduced into mouse fibroblasts, *Nature (London)*, 290, 261, 1981.
29. **Drebin, J. A., Link, V. C., Stern, D. F., Weinberg, R. A., and Greene, M. I.,** Down-modulation of an oncogene protein product and reversion of the transformed phenotype by monoclonal antibodies, *Cell*, 41, 695, 1985.
30. **Drebin, J. A., Link, V. C., Weinberg, R. A., and Greene, M. I.,** Inhibition of tumor growth by a monoclonal antibody reactive with an oncogene-encoded tumor antigen, *Proc. Natl. Acad. Sci. U.S.A.*, 83, 9129, 1986.
31. **Schecter, A. L., Stern, D. F., Vaidyanathan, L., Decker, S. J., Drebin, J. A., Greene, M. I., and Weinberg, R. A.,** The neu oncogene: an erb B related gene encoding a 185,000-Mr tumour antigen, *Nature (London)*, 312, 513, 1984.
32. **Bargmann, C. I., Hung, M. C., and Weinberg, R. A.,** The neu oncogene encodes an epidermal growth factor receptor-related protein, *Nature (London)*, 319, 226, 1986.
33. **Yamamoto, T., Ikawa, S., Akiyama, T., Semba, K., Nomura, N., Miyajima, N., Saito, T., and Toyoshima, K.,** Similarity of protein encoded by the human c-erb-B-gene to epidermal growth factor receptor, *Nature (London)*, 319, 230, 1986.
34. **Porzig, K. J., Barbacid, M., and Aaronson, S. A.,** Biological properties and translational products of three independent isolates of feline sarcoma virus, *Virology*, 92, 91, 1979.
35. **Frankel, A. E., Gilbert, J. H., Porzig, K. J., Scolnick, E. M., and Aaronson, S. A.,** Nature and distribution of feline sarcoma virus nucleotide sequences, *J. Virol.*, 30, 821, 1979.
36. **Anderson, S. J., Furth, M., Wolff, L., Rusietti, S. K., and Sherr, C. J.,** Monoclonal antibodies to the transformation specific glycoprotein encoded by the feline retroviral oncogene v-fms, *J. Virol.*, 44, 696, 1982.
37. **Anderson, S. J., Gonda, M. A., Rettenmeir, C. W., and Sherr, C. J.,** Subcellular localization of glycoproteins encoded by the viral oncogene v-fms, *J. Virol.*, 51, 730, 1984.
38. **Manger, R., Najita, L., Nichols, E. J., Hakomori, S., and Rohrschneider, L.,** Cell surface expression of the McDonough Strain of feline sarcoma virus fms gene product (gp 140 fms), *Cell*, 39, 327, 1984.
39. **Braun, M. S., Andersen, R. G. W., and Goldstein, J. L.,** Recycling receptors: the roundtrip itinerary of migrant membrane proteins, *Cell*, 32, 663, 1983.
40. **Hampe, A., Gobet, M., Sherr, C. J., and Gailbert, F.,** Nucleotide sequence of the feline retroviral oncogene v-fms shows unexpected homology with oncogenes encoding tyrosine-specific protein kinases, *Proc. Natl. Acad. Sci. U.S.A.*, 81, 85, 1984.
41. **Roussel, M. F., Rettenmier, C. W., Look, A. T., and Sherr, C. J.,** Cell surface expression of v-fms coded glycoproteins is required for transformation, *Mol. Cell Biol.*, 4, 1999, 1984.
42. **Rettenmier, C. W., Roussel, M. F., Quinn, C. O., Kitchingman, G. R., Look, A. T., and Sherr, C. J.,** Transmembrane orientation of glycoproteins encoded by the v-fms oncogene, *Cell*, 40, 971, 1985.
43. **Rettenmier, C. W., Chen, J. H., Rousell, M. F., and Sherr, C. J.,** The product of the c-fms proto-oncogene a glycoprotein with associated tyrosine kinase activity, *Science*, 228, 320, 1985.
44. **Stanley, E. R., Guilbert, L. J., Tushinki, R. J., and Bartelmey, S. H.,** CSF-1-a mononuclear phagocyte lineage-specific hemopoietic growth factor, *J. Cell Biochem.*, 21, 151, 1983.

45. **Sherr, C. J., Rettenmeier, C. W., Sacca, R., Roussel, M. F., Look, A. T., and Stanley, E. R.,** The c-fms proto-oncogene product is related to the receptor for the mononuclear phagocyte growth factor, CSF-1, *Cell,* 41, 665, 1985.
46. **Prakash, K., McBride, O., Swan, D. L., Devare, S. G., Tronick, S. R., and Aaronson, S. A.,** Molecular cloning and chromosomal mapping of a human virus related to the Maloney murine sarcoma virus transforming gene, *Proc. Natl. Acad. Sci. U.S.A.,* 79, 5210, 1982.
47. **Swan, D. C., McBride, O. W., Robbins, K. C., Keithley, D. A., Reddy, E. P., and Aaronson, S. A.,** Chromosomal mapping of the simian sarcoma virus oncogene analogue in human cells, *Proc. Natl. Acad. Sci. U.S.A.,* 79, 4691, 1982.
48. **Magnani, J. L.,** Carbohydrate differentiation and cancer-associated antigens detected by monoclonal antibodies, *Biochem. Soc. Trans.,* 12, 543, 1984.
49. **Hakamori, S.,** Tumor-associated carbohydrate antigens, *Annu. Rev. Immunol.,* 2, 103, 1984.
50. **Kannazi, R., Stroup, R., Cochran, N. A., Urdal, D. L., Young, W. W., and Hakamori, S.,** Factors affecting expression of glycolipid tumor antigens: influence of ceramide composition and coexisting glycolipid on the antigenicity of gangliotriasyluramide in murine lymphoma cells, *Cancer Res.,* 43, 4997, 1983.
51. **Hakamori, S. and Murakami, W. T.,** Glycolipids of hamster fibroblasts and derived malignant-transformed cell lines, *Proc. Natl. Acad. Sci. U.S.A.,* 59, 254, 1968.
52. **Kijimoto, S. and Hakomori, S.,** Enhanced glycolipid: galactosyltransferase activity in contact-inhibited hamster cells, and loss of this response in polyoma transformants, *Biochem. Biophys. Res. Commun.,* 44, 557, 1971.
53. **Den, H., Sela, B. A., Roseman, S., and Sachs, L.,** Blocks in ganglioside synthesis in transformed hamster cells and their revertants, *J. Biol. Chem.,* 249, 659, 1974.
54. **Robbins, P. W. and McPherson, I.,** Control of glycolipid synthesis in a cultured hamster cell line, *Nature (London),* 229, 569, 1971.
55. **Hakamori, S. and Kannagi, R.,** Glycosphingolipids as tumor-associated and differentiation markers, *J. Natl. Cancer Inst.,* 71, 231, 1983.
56. **Hakamori, S.,** Blood group ABH and Ii antigens of human erythrocytes: chemistry, polymorphism, and their developmental change, *Semin. Hematol.,* 18, 39, 1981.
57. **Teizi, T.,** The blood group Ii system: a carbohydrate antigen system defined by naturally monoclonal or oligoclonal autoantibodies of man, *Immunol. Commun.,* 10, 127, 1981.
58. **Kapadia, A., Feizi, T., Jewell, D., Kelling, J., and Slavin, G.,** Immunocytochemical studies of blood group A, H, I and i antigens in gastric mucosal of infants with normal gastric histology and of patients with gastric carcinoma and chronic benign peptic ulceration, *J. Clin. Pathol.,* 34, 320, 1981.
59. **Feizi, T.,** Demonstration by monoclonal antibodies that carbohydrate structures of glycoproteins and glycolipids are onco-developmental antigens, *Nature (London),* 314, 53, 1985.
60. **Nudelman, E., Hakomori, S., and Kannagi, R.,** Characterization of a human melanoma associated ganglioside antigen defined by a monoclonal antibody 4.2, *J. Biol. Chem.,* 257, 12752, 1984.
61. **Pukel, C. S., Lloyd, K. O., Travassos, L. R., Dippold, W. G., Oettgen, H. F., and Old, L. J.,** GD_3 a prominent ganglioside of human melanoma: detection and characterization by mouse monoclonal antibody, *J. Exp. Med.,* 155, 1133, 1982.
62. **Houghton, A. N., Mintzer, D., Cordon-Cardo, C., Welt, S., Fliegel, B., Vadhan, S., Carswell, E., Melamed, M. R., Oettgen, H. F., and Old, L. J.,** Mouse monoclonal IgG3 antibody detecting GD_3 ganglioside: a phase I trial in patients with malignant melanoma, *Proc. Natl. Acad. Sci. U.S.A.,* 82, 1242, 1985.
63. **Wiels, J., Lenoir, G. M., Fellows, M., Lipinski, M., Solomon, J. C., Jedard, C., and Tursz, T.,** A monoclonal antibody with anti-Burkitt lymphoma specificity, *Int. J. Cancer,* 29, 653, 1982.
64. **Lipinski, M., Nudelman, E. D., Wills, J., and Parson, M.,** Monoclonal antibody defining a Burkitt's lymphoma associated antigen detects carbohydrate in neutral glycolipid, *J. Immunol.,* 129, 2301, 1982.
65. **Wiels, J., Juqua, S., Dujardin, P., LePecq, J., and Tursz, T.,** Properties of immunotoxins against a glycolipid antigen associated with Burkitt's lymphoma, *Cancer Res.,* 44, 129, 1984.
66. **Kriep, B., Monner, D. A., Burrichler, H., Diehl, V., and Mulradt, P. F.,** Gangliotriaosylceramide (asialo GM2), a glycosphingolipid marker for all lines from patients with Hodgekin's disease, *J. Immunol.,* 131, 1591, 1983.
67. **Cahan, L. D., True, E. I., Singh, R., and Cassidenti, A.,** Identification of human neuroectodermal tumor antigen (OFA-1-1) as ganglioside GD2, *Proc. Natl. Acad. Sci. U.S.A.,* 79, 7629, 1982.
68. **Siddiqui, B., Buehler, J., DeGregorio, M. W., and Macher, B. A.,** Differential expression of ganglioside GD3 by human leukocytes and leukemia cells, *Cancer Res.,* 44, 5262, 1984.
69. **Warren, L., Buck, C. A., and Tuszynski, G. P.,** Glycopeptide changes and malignant transformation: a possible role for carbohydrate in malignant behavior, *Biochim. Biophys. Acta,* 516, 97, 1978.
70. **Holmes, E. H. and Halomori, S.,** Enzymatic basis for changes in fucoganglioside during chemical carcinogenesis, *J. Biol. Chem.,* 258, 3706, 1983.

71. **Fukushi, Y., Nudelman, E., Levery, S. B., Rauvala, H., and Hakomori, S.,** Novel fucolipids accumulating in human adenocarcinoma III. A hybridoma antibody (FH6) defining a human cancer-associated difucoganglioside, *J. Biol. Chem.,* 259, 10511, 1984.
72. **Koprowski, H., Steplewski, Z., Mitchell, K., Herlyn, M., Herlyn, D., and Fuhrer, P.,** Colorectal carcinoma antigens detected by hybridoma antibodies, *Somatic Cell Genet.,* 5, 957, 1979.
73. **Atkinson, B. E., Ernst, C. S., Herlyn, M., Steplewski, Z., Sears, H. F., and Koprowski, H.,** Gastrointestinal cancer-associated antigen in immunoperoxidase assay, *Cancer Res.,* 42, 4820, 1982.
74. **Magnani, J. L., Brockhaus, M., Smith, D. F., Ginsburg, V., Blaszczyk, M., Mitchell, K. F., Steplewski, Z., and Koprowski, H.,** A monoganglioside is a monoclonal antibody-defined antigen of colon carcinoma, *Science,* 212, 55, 1981.
75. **Magnani, J. L., Nilsson, B., Brockhaus, M., Zoof, D., Steplewski, Z., Kaprowski, H., and Ginsburg, V.,** A monoclonal antibody defined antigen associated with gastrointestinal cancer is a ganglioside containing sialylated lacto-N-fucopentaose II, *J. Biol. Chem.,* 257, 14365, 1982.
76. **Liepkalns, V. A., Herrero-Zabaleta, E., Fondaneche, M. C., and Burtin, P.,** Alterations in expression and synthesis of glycolipid antigens in human colonic tumor cell lines, *Cancer Res.,* 45, 2255, 1985.
77. **Gooi, H. C., Feizi, T., Kapadia, A., Knowles, B. B., Salter, D., and Evans, J. M.,** Stage-specific enzyme antigens involves $\alpha 1 \rightarrow 3$ fucosylated type 2 blood group chains, *Nature (London),* 292, 156, 1981.
78. **Huang, L. C., Brockhaus, M., Magnani, J. L., Cuttitta, F., Rosen, S., Minna, G. D., and Ginsburg, V.,** Many monoclonal antibodies with an apparent specificity for certain lung cancers are directed against a sugar sequence found in lacto-N-fucopentoase III, *Arch. Biochem. Biophys.,* 220, 318, 1983.
79. **Hakomori, S., Nudelman, E., Kannozi, R., and Levery, S. B.,** The common structure in fucosyllactosamino lipids accumulating in human adenocarcinomas, and its possible absence in normal tissue, *Biochem. Biophys. Res. Commun.,* 109, 36, 1982.
80. **Fukushi, Y., Hakomori, S., Nudelman, E., and Cochran, N.,** Novel fucolipids accumulating in human adenocarcinoma, II. Selective isolation of hybridoma antibodies that differentially recognize mono-, di- and trifucosylated type 2 chain, *J. Biol. Chem.,* 259, 4681, 1984.
81. **Fukushima, M., Hirota, M., Terasaki, P. I., Wakisaka, A., Togashi, H., Chia, D., Sagama, N., Fukushi, Y., Nudelman, C., and Hakomori, S.,** Characterization of sialosylated Lewis X as a new tumor-associated antigen, *Cancer Res.,* 44, 5279, 1984.
82. **Fukuski, Y., Kannagi, R., Hakamori, S., Shepard, T., Kalander, B. G., and Singer, J. W.,** Location and distribution of difucoganglioside in normal and tumor tissues defined by its monoclonal antibody FH6, *Cancer Res.,* 45, 3711, 1985.
83. **Benacerraf, B.,** The genetic control of specific immune responses, *Harvey Lect.,* 67, 109, 1976.
84. **Lennox, E.,** The antigens of chemically induced tumors, *Immunology 80,* Fougereau, M. and Dausset, J., Eds., Academic Press, New York, 1980, 659.
85. **Goodenow, R. S., Vogel, J. M., and Linski, R.,** Histocompatibility antigens on murine tumors, *Science,* 230, 777, 1985.
86. **Knowles, R. W. and Bodmer, W. F.,** A monoclonal antibody recognizing a human thymus leukemia-like antigen associated with B-2 microglobulin, *Eur. J. Immunol.,* 12, 676, 1982.
87. **Terhorst, C., Van Agthoven, A., leClair, K., Snow, P., Reinherz, E., and Schlossman, S.,** Biochemical studies of the human thymocyte cell surface antigens T6, T9 and T10, *Cell,* 23, 771, 1981.
88. **Reinherz, E. L. and Schlossman, S. F.,** Derivation of human T cell leukemias, *Cancer Res.,* 41, 4767, 1981.
89. **Doherty, P. C., Knowles, B. B., and Wettstein, P. J.,** Immunological surveillance of tumors in the context of major histocompatibility complex restriction of T cell function, *Adv. Cancer Res.,* 42, 1, 1984.
90. **Schwartz, R.,** The role of gene products of the major histocompatibility complex in T cell activation and cellular interactions, in *Fundamental Immunology,* Paul, W., Ed., Raven Press, New York, 1984, 379.
91. **Stutman, O.,** in *Origins of Human Cancer,* Hiatt, H. H., Watson, H. D., and Winsten, J. A., Eds., Cold Spring Harbor Laboratories, New York, 1977, 729.
92. **Phillips, C., McMillan, M., Flood, P. M., Murphy, D. B., Forman, J., Lancki, D., Womack, J. E., Goodenow, R. S., and Schreiber, H.,** Identification of a unique tumor-specific antigen as a novel class I major histocompatibility molecule, *Proc. Natl. Acad. Sci. U.S.A.,* 82, 5485, 1985.
93. **McMillan, M., Lewis, K. D., and Rooner, D. M.,** Molecular characterization of novel H-2 class I molecules expressed by a C3H UV-induced fibrosarcoma, *Proc. Natl. Acad. Sci. U.S.A.,* 82, 5485, 1985.
94. **Wortzel, R. D., Phillips, C., and Schreiber, H.,** Multiple tumor-specific antigens expressed on a single tumor cell, *Nature (London),* 304, 165, 1983.
95. **Shiel, A. G. R.,** in *Tissue Transplantation,* Vol. 3, Morris, P. J., Ed., Edinburgh, 1982, 242.
96. **Hardie, I. R., Strong, R. W., Hartley, L. J. C., Woodruff, P. W. H., and Clunie, G. J.,** Skin cancer in Caucasian renal allograft recipients in a subtropical climate, *Surgery,* 87, 177, 1980.
97. **Klein, G.,** Ed. *Viral Oncology,* Raven Press, New York, 1980.

98. **Mora, P. T.**, The immunopathology of SV-40 induced transformation, *Springer Semin. Immunopathol.*, 5, 7, 1982.
99. **Benjamin, T. L., Carmichael, G. G., and Schauffhausen, B. S.**, The hr-t gene of polyoma virus, *Cold Spring Harbor Symp. Quant. Biol.*, 44, 263, 1979.
100. **Robinson, W. S., Miller, R. H., Klote, L., Marion, P. L., and Lee, S. C.**, Hepatitis B virus and hepatocellular carcinoma, in *Viral Hepatitis and Liver Disease*, Vyas, G. N., Dienstag, J. L., and Hoofnagle, J. F., Eds., Grune and Stratton, Orlando, Fla., 1984, 245.
101. **Thorley-Lawson, D. A., Edson, C. M., and Geilinger, K.**, Epstein-Barr virus antigens: a challenge to modern biochemistry, *Adv. Cancer Res.*, 36, 295, 1982.
102. **Poiesz, B. J., Ruscetti, F. W., Gazdar, A. F., Bunn, P. A., Minna, J. D., and Gallo, R. C.**, Detection and isolation of type C retrovirus particles from fresh and cultured lymphocytes of a patient with cutaneous T cell lymphoma, *Proc. Natl. Acad. Sci. U.S.A.*, 77, 7415, 1980.
103. **Kirchner, H.**, Immunologic surveillance and human papillomoviruses, *Immunol. Today*, 5, 272, 1984.
104. **Moss, D. G., Chan, S. H., Burrows, S. R., Chew, T. S., Kane, R. A., Staples, J. A., and Kunarathiem, N.**, Epstein-Barr virus specific T-cell response in nasopharyngeal carcinoma patients, *Int. J. Cancer*, 32, 301, 1983.
105. **Hoffman, G. J., Lazarowitz, S. G., and Hayward, S. D.**, Monoclonal antibody against a 250,000-dalton glycoprotein of Epstein-Barr virus identifies a membrane antigen and a neutralizing antigen, *Proc. Natl. Acad. Sci. U.S.A.*, 77, 2979, 1980.
106. **Robert-Guroff, M., Ruscetti, F. W., Posner, L. E., Poiesz, B. J., and Gallo, R. C.**, Detection of the human T cell lymphoma virus p19 in cells of some patients with cutaneous T-cell lymphoma and leukemia using a monoclonal antibody, *J. Exp. Med.*, 154, 1957, 1981.
107. **Clark, J. W., Robert-Guroff, M., Ikehara, O., Henzan, E., and Blattner, W. A.**, Human T cell leukemia-lymphoma virus type 1 and adult T cell leukemia-lymphoma in Okinawa, *Cancer Res.*, 45, 2849, 1985.
108. **Cote, R. J., Morrissey, D. M., Oettgen, H. F., and Old, L. J.**, Analysis of human monoclonal antibodies derived from lymphocytes of patients with cancer, *Fed. Proc. Fed. Am. Soc. Exp. Biol.*, 43, 2465, 1984.
109. **Houghton, A. N., Brooks, H., Cote, R., Taormina, M. C., Oettgen, H. F., and Old, L. J.**, Detection of cell surface and intracellular antigens by human monoclonal antibodies, *J. Exp. Med.*, 158, 53, 1983.
110. **Haspel, M. V., McCabe, R. P., Pomato, N., Janesch, N. J., Knowlton, J. V., Peters, L. C., Hoover, H. C., and Hanna, M. G.**, Generation of tumor cell reactive human monoclonal antibodies using peripheral blood lymphocytes from actively immunized colorectal carcinoma patients, *Cancer Res.*, 45, 3951, 1985.
111. **Iman, A., Drushella, M. M., Taylor, C. R., and Tokes, Z.**, Generation and immunohistological characterization of human monoclonal antibodies to mammary carcinoma cells, *Cancer Res.*, 45, 263, 1985.
112. **Schlom, J., Wunderlich, D., and Teramoto, U.**, Generation of human monoclonal antibodies reactive with human mammary carcinoma cells, *Proc. Natl. Acad. Sci. U.S.A.*, 77, 6841, 1980.
113. **Sikora, K., Alderson, T., Ellis, J., Phillips, J., and Watson, J.**, Human hybridomas from patients with malignant disease, *Br. J. Cancer*, 47, 135, 1983.
114. **Real, F. X., Mattes, M. J., Houghton, A. N., Oettgen, H. F., Lloyd, K. O., and Old, L. J.**, Class 1 (unique) tumor antigens of human melanoma. Identification of a 90,000 dalton cell surface glycoprotein by autologous antibody, *J. Exp. Med.*, 159, 1217, 1984.
115. **Lloyd, K. O.**, Human tumor antigens: detection and characterization with monoclonal antibodies, in *Basic and Clinical Tumor Immunology*, Herberman, R. B., Ed., Martinus Nijhoff Publishers, Boston, 1983, 159.
116. **Starling, J. J. and Wright, G. L.**, Disulfide bonding of a human prostate tumor-associated membrane antigen recognized by monoclonal antibody D83.31, *Cancer Res.*, 45, 804, 1985.
117. **Colcher, D., Horan Hand, P., Nuti, M., and Schlom, J.**, A spectrum of monoclonal antibodies reactive with human mammary tumor cells, *Proc. Natl. Acad. Sci. U.S.A.*, 78, 3199, 1981.
118. **Nuti, M., Teramoto, Y. A., Mariani-Constantini, R., Horan Hand, P., Colcher, D., and Schlom, J.**, A monoclonal antibody (B72.3) defines patterns of distribution of a novel tumor-associated antigen of human mammary carcinoma cell properties, *Int. J. Cancer*, 29, 539, 1982.
119. **Reisfeld, R. A.**, Monoclonal antibodies to human malignant melanoma, *Nature (London)*, 298, 325, 1982.
120. **Woodbury, R. G., Brown, J. P., Yey, M., Hellstrom, I., and Hellstrom, K. E.**, Identification of a cell surface protein, p97, in human melanomas and certain other neoplasms, *Proc. Natl. Acad. Sci. U.S.A.*, 77, 2183, 1980.
121. **Schnegg, J. F., Diserens, A. C., Carrel, S., Accolla, R. S., and de Tribolet, N.**, Human glioma-associated antigens detected by monoclonal antibodies, *Cancer Res.*, 41, 1209, 1981.
122. **Fradet, Y., Cordan-Cardo, C., Thompson, T., Daly, M. E., Whitmore, W. F., Lloyd, K. O., Melamad, M. R., and Old, L. J.**, Cell surface antigens of human bladder cancer defined by mouse monoclonal antibodies, *Proc. Natl. Acad. Sci. U.S.A.*, 81, 224, 1984.
123. **Starling, J. J., Sieg, S. M., Beckett, M. L., Schellhammer, P. F., Ladaga, L. E., and Wright, G. L.**, Monoclonal antibodies to human prostate and bladder tumor-associated antigens, *Cancer Res.*, 42, 3084, 1982.

124. **Schmiegel, W. H., Kalthoff, H., Arndt, R., Gieseking, J., Greten, H., Kloppel, G., Krieker, C., Ladak, A., Lampe, V., and Ulrich, S.**, Monoclonal antibody defined human pancreatic cancer-associated antigens, *Cancer Res.*, 45, 1402, 1986.
125. **Bast, R. C., Feeney, M., Lazarus, H., Nadler, L. M., Calvin, R. B., and Knapp, R. C.**, Reactivity of a monoclonal antibody with human ovarian carcinoma, *J. Clin. Invest.*, 68, 1331, 1981.
126. **Bhattachariga, M., Chatterjee, S. K., Barloco, J. J., and Fugi, H.**, Monoclonal antibodies recognizing tumor-associated antigen of human ovarian mucinous cystadenocarcinomas, *Cancer Res.*, 42, 1650, 1982.
127. **Mattes, M. J., Cordon-Cardo, C., Lewis, J. L., Old, L. J., and Lloyd, K. O.**, Cell surface antigens of human ovarian and endometrial carcinoma defined by mouse monoclonal antibodies, *Proc. Natl. Acad. Sci. U.S.A.*, 81, 568, 1984.
128. **Tagliabue, E., Menard, S., Della Torre, G., Barbanti, P., Mariani-Constantini, R., Porro, G., and Colnaghi, M. I.**, Generation of monoclonal antibodies reacting with human epithelial ovarian cancer, *Cancer Res.*, 45, 379, 1985.
129. **Bernal, S. D., Mabry, M., Stahel, R. A., Griffin, J. D., and Speak, J. A.**, Selective cytotoxicity of the SM1 monoclonal antibody towards small cell carcinoma of the lung, *Cancer Res.*, 45, 1026, 1985.
130. **Cuttita, F., Rosen, S., Gazdar, A. F., and Minna, J. D.**, Monoclonal antibodies that demonstrate specificity for several types of human lung cancer, *Proc. Natl. Acad. Sci. U.S.A.*, 78, 4591, 1981.
131. **Sears, H. F., Herlyn, D., Steplewski, Z., and Koprowski, H.**, Effects of monoclonal antibody immunotherapy with gastrointestinal adenocarcinoma, *J. Biol. Resp. Mod.*, 3, 138, 1984.
132. **Aoto, F., Chang, D., Hill, N. O., and Khan, A.**, Monoclonal antibody against myeloid leukemia cell line (KG-1), *Cancer Res.*, 43, 1093, 1983.
133. **Ritz, J., Pesando, J. M., Notis-McConarty, J., Lazarus, H., and Schlossman, S. F.**, A monoclonal antibody to human acute lymphoblastic leukemia antigen, *Nature (London)*, 283, 583, 1980.
134. **Boyse, E. A., Old, L. J., and Scheid, M.**, Selective gene action in the specification of cell surface structure, *Am. J. Pathol.*, 65, 439, 1971.
135. **Waldmann, T. A., Longo, D. L., Leonard, W. J., Depper, J. M., Thompson, C. B., Kronke, M., Goldman, C. K., Sharrow, S., Bongiovanni, K., and Greene, W. C.**, Interleukin-2 receptor (TAC antigen) expression in HTLV-1-associated adult T cell leukemia, *Cancer Res.*, 45, 4559, 1985.
136. **Meeker, T. C., Lowder, J., Maloney, D. G., Miller, R. A., Thielemans, K., Warnke, R., and Levy, R.**, A clinical trial of anti-idiotype therapy for B cell malignancy, *Blood*, 65, 1349, 1985.
137. **Miller, R. A., Maloney, D. G., Warnke, R., and Levy, R.**, Treatment of B-cell lymphoma with monoclonal anti-idiotype antibody, *N. Engl. J. Med.*, 306, 517, 1982.
138. **McCleary, M. L., Meeker, T. C., Levy, S., Lee, E., Trela, M., Sklar, J., and Levy, R.**, Clustering of extensive somatic mutations in the variable region of an immunoglobulin heavy chain gene from a human B cell lymphoma, *Cell*, 44, 97, 1986.
139. **Hellstrom, K. E. and Brown, J. P.**, Tumor antigens, in *The Antigens*, Vol. 5, Sela, M., Ed., Academic Press, New York, 1979, 1.
140. **Gold, P. and Freedman, S. O.**, Specific carcinoembryonic antigens of the human digestive system, *J. Exp. Med.*, 122, 267, 1965.
141. **Goldenberg, D. M., Sharkey, R. M., Primus, F. J., Mizusawa, E., and Hawthorne, F. M.**, Neutron-capture therapy of human cancer: *in vivo* results on tumor localization of boron-10-labeled antibodies to carcinoembryonic antigen in the GW-39 tumor model system, *Proc. Natl. Acad. Sci. U.S.A.*, 81, 560, 1984.
142. **Rettig, W. J., Cordon-Cardo, C., Ng, J. S. C., Oettgen, H. F., Old, L. J., and Lloyd, K. O.**, High molecular weight glycoproteins of human teratocarcinoma defined by monoclonal antibodies to carbohydrate determinants, *Cancer Res.*, 45, 815, 1985.
143. **Payne, W. J. and Coggin, J. H.**, Mouse monoclonal antibody to embryonic antigen: development, cross-reactivity with rodent and human tumors and preliminary polypeptide characterization, *J. Natl. Cancer Inst.*, 75, 527, 1985.
144. **Boyse, E. A. and Old, L. J.**, The immunogenetics of differentiation in the mouse, *Harvey Lect.*, 71, 23, 1975.
145. **Bernstein, I. D., Tam, M. R., and Nowinski, R. C.**, Mouse leukemia: therapy with monoclonal antibodies against a thymus differentiation antigen, *Science*, 207, 68, 1980.
146. **Kirsch, M. E. and Hammerling, U.**, Immunotherapy of murine leukemias by monoclonal antibody. I. Effect of passively administered antibody on growth of transplanted tumor cells, *J. Immunol.*, 127, 805, 1981.
147. **Johnson, R. J. and Shih, H. S.**, Monoclonal antibody against a differentiation antigen on human leukemia cells: cross-reactivity with rat leukemia and suppression of rat leukemia in vivo *J. Immunol.*, 131, 2930, 1983.
148. **Dillman, R. O., Shawler, D. L., Sobel, R. E., Collings, H. A., Beauregard, J. C., Wormsley, S. B., and Royston, I.**, Murine monoclonal antibody therapy in two patients with chronic lymphocytic leukemia, *Blood*, 59, 1036, 1982.

149. **Levy, R. and Miller, R. A.,** Tumor therapy with monoclonal antibodies, *Fed. Proc. Fed. Am. Soc. Exp. Biol.,* 42, 2650, 1983.
150. **Miller, R. A. and Levy, R.,** Response of cutaneous T cell lymphoma to therapy with hybridoma monoclonal antibody, *Lancet,* 2, 226, 1981.
151. **Miller, R. A., Maloney, D. G., McKellop, J., and Levy, R.,** *In vivo* effects of murine hybridoma monoclonal antibody in a patient with T cell leukemia, *Blood,* 58, 78, 1981.
152. **Leonard, W. J., Depper, J. M., Uchiyama, T., Smith, K. A., Waldmann, T. A., and Greene, W. C.,** A monoclonal antibody that appears to recognize the receptor for human TCGF: partial characterization of the receptor, *Nature (London),* 300, 267, 1982.
153. **Depper, J. M., Leonard, W. J., Kronke, M., Waldmann, T. A., and Greene, W. C.,** Augmented T cell growth factor receptor expression in HTLV-infected human leukemic T cells, *J. Immunol.,* 133, 1691, 1984.
154. **Kozak, R. W., Atcher, R. W., Gansow, O. A., Friedman, A. M., Hines, J. J., and Waldmann, T. A.,** Bismuth-212-labeled anti-Tac monoclonal antibody: α-particle emitting radionuclides as modalities for radioimmunotherapy, *Proc. Natl. Acad. Sci. U.S.A.,* 83, 474, 1986.
155. **Rankin, E. M., Hekman, A., Somers, R., and Bokkel Huinink, W.,** Treatment of two patients with B cell lymphoma with monoclonal anti-idiotype antibodies, *Blood,* 65, 1373, 1985.
156. **Reinherz, E. L., Acuto, O., Fabbi, M., Bensussan, A., Milanese, C. L., Rayer, H. D., Meuer, S. C., and Schlossman, S. F.,** Clonotypic surface structure on human T lymphocytes: functional and biochemical analysis of the antigen receptor complex, *Immunol. Rev.,* 81, 95, 1984.
157. **Carroll, A. M., Zalutsky, M., Shatten, S., Bhan, A., Perry, L., Sobotka, C., Benacerraf, B., and Greene, M. I.,** Monoclonal antibodies to tissue-specific cell surface antigens. I. Characterization of an antibody to a prostate tissue antigen, *Clin. Immunol. Immunopathol.,* 33, 268, 1984.
158. **Carroll, A. M., Zalutsky, M. R., Benacerraf, B., and Greene, M. I.,** Monoclonal antibodies to tissue-associated antigens as anti-tumor reagents, *Surv. Synth. Pathol. Res.,* 3, 189, 1984.
159. **Frankel, A. E., Rouse, R. V., and Herzenberg, L. A.,** Human prostate specific and shared differentiation antigens defined by monoclonal antibodies, *Proc. Natl. Acad. Sci. U.S.A.,* 79, 903, 1982.
160. **Frankel, A. E., Rouse, R. V., Wang, M. C., Chu, T. M., and Herzenberg, L. A.,** Monoclonal antibodies to a human prostate antigen, *Cancer Res.,* 43, 3714, 1982.
161. **Ware, J. L., Paulson, D. F., Parks, S. F., and Webb, K. S.,** Production of monoclonal antibody anti-Pro3 recognizing a human prostatic carcinoma antigen, *Cancer Res.,* 42, 1215, 1982.
162. **Wang, M. C., Valenzuela, L. A., Murphy, G. P., and Chu, T. M.,** Purification of a human prostate specific antigen, *Invest. Urol.,* 17, 159, 1979.
163. **Webb, K. S., Ware, J. L., Parks, S. F., Briner, W. A., and Paulson, D. F.,** Monoclonal antibodies to different epitopes on a prostate tumor associated antigen, *Cancer Immunol. Immunother.,* 14, 155, 1983.
164. **Silverberg, E.,** Cancer statistics, *Cancer,* 31, 13, 1981.
165. **Papsidero, L. D., Croghan, G. A., O'Connell, M. J., Valenzuela, L. A., Nemoto, T., and Chu, T. M.,** Monoclonal antibodies (F36/22 and M7/105) to human breast carcinoma, *Cancer Res.,* 43, 1741, 1983.
166. **Croghan, G. A., Papsidero, L. D., Valenzuela, L. A., Nemoto, T., Penetrante, R., and Ming Chu, T.,** Tissue distribution of an epithelial and tumor-associated antigen recognized by monoclonal antibody F36/22, *Cancer Res.,* 43, 4980, 1983.
167. **Thompson, C. H., Jones, S., Whitehead, R. H., and McKenzie, I. F. C.,** A human breast tissue-associated antigen detected by a monoclonal antibody, *J. Natl. Cancer Inst.,* 70, 409, 1983.
168. **Menard, S., Tagliabue, S., Fossati, G., and Colnaghi, M. I.,** Generation of monoclonal antibodies reacting with normal and cancer cells of human breast, *Cancer Res.,* 43, 1295, 1983.
169. **Bremer, E. G., Levery, S. B., Sonnino, S., Ghidoni, R., Canevari, S., Kannagi, R., and Hakomori, S.,** Characterization of glycosphingolipid antigen defined by monoclonal antibody MBr1 expressed in normal and neoplastic epithelial cells of human mammary gland, *J. Biol. Chem.,* 259, 14773, 1985.
170. **White, C. A., Dulbecco, R., Allen, R., Bowman, M., and Armstrong, B.,** Two monoclonal antibodies selective for human mammary carcinoma, *Cancer Res.,* 45, 1337, 1985.
171. **Edwards, P. A. W. and Foster, C. S.,** Monoclonal antibodies that bind to normal and neoplastic breast epithelial cells distinguish subsets of normal breast epithelial cells, in *Monoclonal Antibodies and Cancer,* Boss, B. D., Langman, R., Trowbridge, I., and Dulbecco, R., Eds., Academic Press, Orlando, 1983, 285.
172. **Houghton, A. N., Eisenger, M., Albino, A. P., Cairncross, J. G., and Old, L. J.,** Surface antigens of melanocytes and melanomas: markers for melanocyte differentiation and melanoma subsets, *J. Exp. Med.,* 156, 1755, 1982.
173. **Tai, T., Eisinger, M., Ogata, S., and Lloyd, K. O.,** Glycoproteins as differentiation markers in human malignant melanoma and melanocytes, *Cancer Res.,* 43, 2773, 1983.
174. **Loms Ziegler-Heitbrock, H. W., Munker, R., Johnson, J., Petersmann, I., Schmoeckel, C., and Reithmuller, G.,** In vitro differentiation of human melanoma cells analyzed with monoclonal antibodies, *Cancer Res.,* 45, 1344, 1985.

175. **Dippold, W. G., Lloyd, K. O., Li, L. T. C., Ikeda, H., Oettgen, H. F., and Old, L. J.,** Cell surface antigens of human malignant melanoma. Definition of six antigenic systems with mouse monoclonal antibodies, *Proc. Natl. Acad. Sci. U.S.A.*, 77, 6114, 1980.
176. **Kennett, R. H. and Gilbert, F. M.,** Hybrid myelomas producing antibodies against a human neuroblastoma antigen present on fetal brain, *Science*, 203, 1120, 1978.
177. **Cairncross, J. G., Mattes, M. J., Beresford, H. R., Albino, A. P., Houghton, A. N., Lloyd, K. O., and Old, L. J.,** Cell surface antigens of human astrocytoma defined by mouse monoclonal antibodies: identification of astrocytoma subsets, *Proc. Natl. Acad. Sci. U.S.A.*, 79, 5641, 1982.
178. **Ueda, R., Ogata, S., Morrissey, D. M., Finstad, C. L., Szkudlavek, J., Whitmore, W. F., Oettgen, H. F., Lloyd, K. O., and Old, L. J.,** Cell surface antigens of renal cancer defined by mouse monoclonal antibodies: identification of tissue-specific glycoproteins, *Proc. Natl. Acad. Sci. U.S.A.*, 78, 5122, 1981.
179. **Finstad, C. L., Cordon-Cardo, C., Bander, N. H., Whitmore, W. F., Melamed, M. R., and Old, L. J.,** Specificity analysis of mouse monoclonal antibodies defining cell surface antigens of human renal cancer, *Proc. Natl. Acad. Sci. U.S.A.*, 82, 2955, 1985.
180. **Andy, R. J., Finstad, C. L., Old, L. J., Lloyd, K. O., and Kornfeld, R.,** The antigen identified by a mouse monoclonal antibody raised against human renal cancer cells is the adenosine deaminase binding protein, *J. Biol. Chem.*, 259, 12844, 1985.
181. **Herlyn, M., Basczyk, M., Sears, H. F., Verrill, H., Lindgren, J., Colcher, D., Steplewski, D., Schlom, J., and Koprowski, H.,** Detection of carcinoembryonic antigens and related antigens in sera of patients with gastrointestinal tumors using monoclonal antibodies in double-determinant radioimmunoassays, *Hybridoma*, 2, 329, 1983.
182. **Togashi, H., Teraski, P. I., Chia, D., Kukes, G., Kasai, K., Suyama, N., Fukushima, K., and Hirota, M.,** A monoclonal antibody (STO-1), against a stomach adenocarcinoma-associated antigen, *Cancer Res.*, 44, 3952, 1984.
183. **Metzgar, C. S., Gaillard, M. T., Levine, S. J., Tuck, F. L., Bossen, E. H., and Borowitz, M. J.,** Antigens of human pancreatic adenocarcinoma cells defined by murine monoclonal antibodies, *Cancer Res.*, 42, 601, 1982.
184. **Lan, M. S., Finn, O. J., Fernsten, D. D., and Metzgar, R. S.,** Isolation and properties of a human pancreatic adenocarcinoma-associated antigen Du-PAN-2, *Cancer Res.*, 45, 305, 1985.
185. **Order, S. E., Klein, J. L., and Leichner, P. K.,** Anti-ferritin IgG antibody for isotopic cancer therapy, *Oncology*, 38, 154, 1981.
186. **Eshhar, Z., Order, S. E., and Katz, D.,** Ferritin is a Hodgkin's Disease associated antigen, *Proc. Natl. Acad. Sci. U.S.A.*, 71, 3956, 1974.
187. **Haspel, M. V., Orodera, T., Prabhakar, B. S., McClintock, P. R., Essani, K., Ray, U. R., Yagihashi, S., and Nottins, A. L.,** Multiple organ reactive monoclonal autoantibodies, *Nature (London)*, 304, 73, 1983.
188. **Ballou, B., Jaffe, R., Taylor, R. J., Solter, D., and Hakala, T. R.,** Tumor radio-immunolocation: differential antibody retention by antigenic normal tissue and tumor, *J. Immunol.*, 132, 2111, 1984.
189. **Izzo, M. J. and Bale, W. F.,** Preferential localization and rate of loss of labeled allo-antibody from rat tumors and skin transplants carrying the corresponding alloantigen, *Cancer Res.*, 36, 2868, 1976.
190. **Key, M. E., Bernhard, M. I., Hoyer, L. C., Foon, K. A., Oldham, R. K., and Hanna, M. G.,** Guinea pig line 10 hepatocarcinoma model for monoclonal antibody serotherapy: *in vivo* localization of a monoclonal antibody in normal and malignant tissues, *J. Immunol.*, 130, 1451, 1983.
191. **Taupier, M. A., Klarney, J. F., Liebson, P. J., Loken, M. R., and Schreiber, H.,** Nonrandom escape of tumor cells from immune lysis due to intraclonal fluctuations in antigen expression, *Cancer Res.*, 43, 4050, 1983.
192. **Natali, P. G., Cavaliere, R., Bigotti, A., Nicotra, M. R., Russo, C., Ng, A. K., Giacomini, P., and Ferrone, S.,** Antigenic heterogeniety of surgically removed primary and autologous metastases of the same patient, *J. Immunol.*, 130, 1462, 1983.
193. **Albino, A. P., Lloyd, K. O., Houghton, A. N., Oettgen, H. F., and Old, L. J.,** Heterogeniety in surface antigen and glycoprotein expression of cell lines derived from different melanoma metastases of the same patient, *J. Exp. Med.*, 154, 1764, 1981.

Chapter 3

DEVELOPMENT OF MONOCLONAL ANTIBODIES FOR THE DIAGNOSIS AND TREATMENT OF TUMORS

Su Metcalfe

TABLE OF CONTENTS

I. INTRODUCTION

The tumor cell is a paradox, causing life-threatening disease by its own commitment to growth and immortality. The essential change between a tumor cell and its normal cell counterpart occurs when the initial tumor cell divides and each daughter cell inherits a perpetual commitment to divide again. The resultant logarithmic expansion of cell numbers forms the tumor growth. Most normal cells retain the ability to divide, and some function by division. Skin cells are constantly being lost and replenished by epithelial stem cells which divide continuously, but with only one daughter cell inheriting the commitment to divide, thus providing a linear increase in cell numbers to meet the linear rate of loss. Spermatozoa result from germ cells, each of which undergoes two meiotic and then three mitotic cell divisions: here the inherited ability to divide is rigorously controlled. It is when the inherited control of division is lost that the tumor cell emerges. The skin cell begins to replicate at a logarithmic rate resulting in cancer of the skin; the sperm cell persists in dividing and grows on as a seminoma in the testis.

The altered behavior of the tumor cell, with its perpetual commitment to cell division, follows altered genetic expression (as discussed in the previous chapter). In turn, cellular structures also become altered where these are governed by the abnormal gene expression. A structural change unique to a tumor cell is a tumor antigen; few are known. Where the tumor is caused by a virus, then viral antigens expressed on the transformed cells are true tumor antigens. Another example of a tumor antigen is that of myeloma cells (transformed B lymphocytes) which continue to express surface immunoglobulin idiotype. There are other antigens occurring on tumor cells (A, B, or O blood group antigens and carcinoembryonic antigen [CEA]) which are not present on the normal cell counterpart. However, since these are not unique to the tumor cell (e.g., normal cells express CEA during infection), they are not true tumor antigens. Irregular expression of antigen by tumor cells is due to abnormal enzyme activity, while in normal cells, it may result from normal (reversible) physiological responses. Surface changes on tumor cells result from over-elaborate, or incomplete, synthesis of structural components. In addition, reexpression or overexpression of genes may cause abnormal levels of protein products. For example, liver tumor cells often reexpress the gene for alpha feto protein (αFP). This gene should only be active during fetal life, being "closed" in the normal adult liver cell.

A distinctive structural change on the surface of a tumor cell creates the possibility of "seeing" that cell against a background of normal cells. The fine specificity of antibody in recognition of an antigenic epitope brings this possibility to a reality. Such specificity is provided by monoclonal antibodies; they are homogeneous in terms of molecular structure and antigenic specificity. A single clone of B lymphocytes secretes monoclonal antibody in vitro, but dies out after about fifty cell divisions, at which time the amount of antibody is too small for clinical use. Immortalization of the B lymphocyte results in the production of unlimited quantities of monoclonal antibody.

II. MONOCLONAL ANTIBODY PRODUCTION

There are two basically different means of immortalizing a B cell. Fusion with a tumor cell creates an immortal hybridoma.[1] Alternatively, tumor viruses can be used to transform the B cell with the same result.[2] In either case, the fundamental problem is first to obtain the B cell which is specific for the chosen antigen. This cell is rare in the normal lymphocyte population, approximately 1 in 500,000 cells, and it is usual to amplify the numbers by immunization. Good immunization should increase the frequency of the desired B cell type by an order of a thousandfold.

A. Hybridoma Method

1. Choice of Antigen

The choice of antigen is obviously important, but not necessarily simple. In the context of the applications discussed in this book, the isolated tumor antigen is ideal, but is often impractical, especially for proteins. Isolation of a membrane protein antigen often alters its conformation with corresponding alteration of the antigenic epitopes; however, carbohydrate structures are less sensitive to modification.

It is usual to use whole tumor cells or fragments of the tumor cell membrane for immunization. These materials present complicated arrays of antigens, the majority having value for targeting and imaging. However, in certain cases it is possible to simplify the number of antigens presented. For example, most adenocarcinoma cells, such as breast and colorectal carcinomata, express an antigenic epitope known as the Thomsen-Freidenriech (T) antigen.[3] The T antigen is also present on erythrocytes, but is not accessible because it is covered by sialic acid residues comprising the M and N blood group antigens.[4] After enzymatic treatment to remove sialic acid the T antigen is exposed, and desialylated erythrocytes are a rich source of immunizing material with a limited antigenic profile. By this method we have obtained monoclonal antibodies against T antigen and its immediate precursor, Tn.[5] A further advantage in using a simple antigenic profile is in reducing responses to species-specific immunodominant antigens. This is illustrated by the finding of Magnani[6] that one third of some 150 mouse monoclonal antibodies to human tumor cells are specific for lacto-N-fucopentose, clearly an antigenically dominant epitope in the profile of antigens on human cells as seen by the mouse immune system.

An alternative strategy in the therapeutic use of monoclonal antibodies is to influence the tumor cell indirectly, by interfering with the conditions necessary for their growth. Monoclonal antibodies are currently being developed which neutralize specific factors essential for stimulating tumor growth. Isolated growth factor provides a simple antigen for immunization. Alternatively, it is possible to envisage the use of antibodies which bind and block receptors for these factors. Antibodies against receptor are detected by their ability to block the effect of factor on factor-dependent cells, a method used to identify antibody against receptors for interleukin 2.[7]

2. Problems with Species and Immunization

The choice of species for immunization is largely limited by the availability of a suitable fusion partner. Fusion partners should normally be of the same species, although when mouse myeloma cells are fused with rat spleen cells, most of the rat chromosomes are lost, but that bearing the immunoglobulin gene is preferentially retained. Mouse-rabbit or mouse-human hybrids do not show this bias and so the chances of retaining a relevant chromosome bearing the immunoglobulin gene is very small. To date, most monoclonal antibodies are either mouse or rat in origin, reflecting the limited number of fusion partners. NSI (which secretes its own kappa chain)[8] and NSO (a non-secreting variant of NSI)[9] are mouse myelomas and Y3 (a light chain secretor)[10] and its non-secreting variant[11] YO, are rat myelomas. Each has been generated in the laboratory of Cesar Milstein who, with Georges Kohler, first produced monoclonal antibodies by the hybridoma method. These myelomas are now used worldwide. It is interesting that myeloma cells seem preferentially to immortalize those spleen cells involved in antibody secretion,[1] although it is important to note that not all myelomas are good secretors when hybridized. The possibility that nonmyeloma cell types might immortalize the B cell and express an acquired immunoglobulin gene has been explored; results indicate that synthesis of immunoglobulin ceases rapidly after fusion.

3. Immunization Procedure

After selecting a compatible strain of mouse or rat that is genetically matched to the myeloma fusion partner, several animals are immunized to increase the chance of one giving

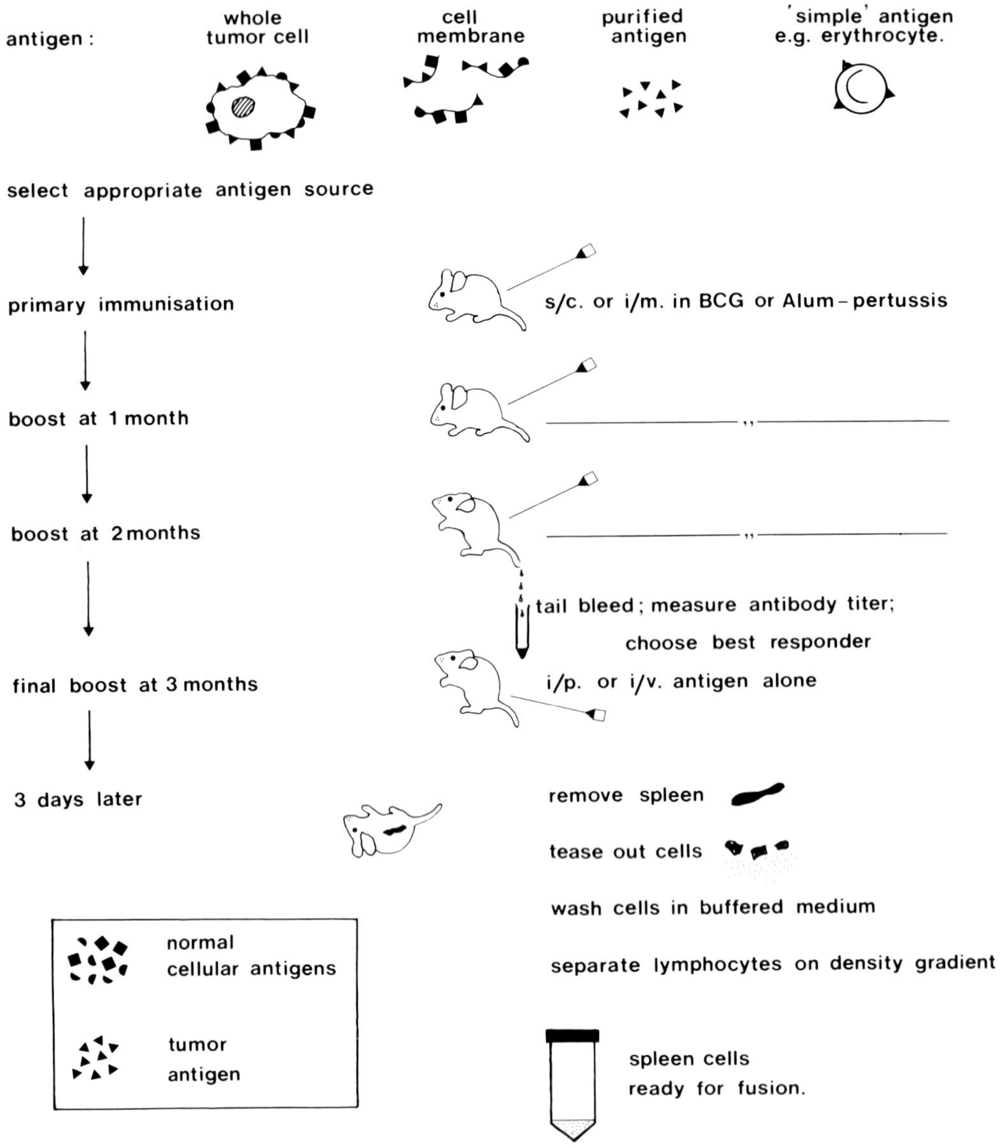

FIGURE 1. Immunization protocol.

a good response to the antigen. Genetic matching is necessary to enable a resultant hybrid to be grown as ascites in an immune-compatible host.

Methods of immunization vary in detail, but usually follow the protocol of three or four injections of antigen at monthly intervals (see Figure 1). Antibody titres of the serum are monitored after each immunization. Intramuscular or subcutaneous injection is preferred. BCG or B. pertussis may be mixed with the antigen as an adjuvant of lymphocytes to the injected site. Alum may also be added to provide a slow release of antigen over a prolonged period. Adjuvant should never be used in intraperitoneal immunization as peritonitis will result. Three days after a final boost of antigen alone, the animal is sacrificed and the spleen cells collected for fusion.

A recently described alternative method of immunization is to inject antigen into the animal's footpad.[12] This immunization route leads to localization of antigen-reactive lymphocytes in the popliteal lymph nodes. Thus, lymphocytes harvested from these nodes are rich in cells of the chosen antigenic specificity.

B. Cell Fusion

Once the lymphocytes have been collected, they are then fused with myeloma cells taken from a healthy, growing culture. Fusion is a somewhat random event when chemicals, or inactivated Sendaii virus are used, and the mechanics of these fusion processes have been explored in detail.[13] A new alternative is to induce cell-to-cell fusion by an electrical field,[14] an approach which is outlined later in this chapter.

1. Chemical Fusion

Polyethylene glycol (PEG) is the most commonly used fusogenic reagent, acting to destabilize cell membranes in a mixed pellet of myeloma cells and lymphocytes. The pellet is gently resuspended in 1 mℓ of PEG for 1 min, then the PEG is slowly diluted by addition of medium. Clearly, any reagent which destabilizes the cell membrane is potentially cytolytic: exposure to PEG must be brief and handling gentle to avoid irreversible damage. Only a small proportion of the cells fuse and, although the unfused spleen cells will eventually die, the many unfused myeloma cells must be eliminated to prevent them overgrowing the few hybrids. For this, the trick of using abnormal, mutant myeloma cells is employed. These cells are defective enzymatically (usually in thymidine kinase) and are unable to synthesize DNA in selective medium lacking thymidine. Those myeloma cells which have fused with spleen cells receive the wild-type complement of genes, including that for thymidine kinase, and continue to grow and divide in the selective conditions. Hence, after about six days, most of the cells in the culture are dead, but the occasional live hybrid cell can be seen. Over the next few weeks this hybrid divides and gradually overgrows the culture. An outline of this methodology is given in Figure 2.

From a fusion of 3×10^7 rat spleen cells, with 5×10^7 Y3 myeloma cells, we obtain a recovery of about 100 hybrids; an efficiency of one hybrid per 3×10^5 cells. If immunization has amplified the required cell type to about 1 in 500 spleen cells there is reasonable chance of obtaining a hybrid with the desired specificity.

When a single hybrid occurs in the culture, the resultant population of cells is monoclonal. Often, two or three hybrids occur in the same culture, and these have to be recloned to obtain each as a monoclonal culture. Different groups approach this problem in different ways; some seed the initial fusion into large numbers of small volume cultures (approximately 600 cultures of 100 μℓ volume) to favor the chances of monoclonal growth. We opt to culture in larger volume wells (1 mℓ) using a smaller number of cultures, simply to reduce the work load and related risk of infection during daily microscopic scoring of each well and feeding the individual cultures. When a clone is sufficiently large to cause a pH change in the medium (due to accumulation of lactic acid associated with respiration), a sample of supernatant is tested for antibody of desired specificity. A variety of assays are used and these are outlined in Figure 3; the type of assay — cell surface binding, radioimmune, ELISA, plaque, or hemagglutination — is selected according to the type of antigen and the nature of the antibody. If the assay reveals a specific antibody, then the hybrid is usually recloned either by limiting dilution or in agar.

In successful fusions the maintenance of a 100 or so discrete cultures and the testing of supernatants from each is a considerable workload, and a "time spacer" may be introduced. For this purpose, each clone is preserved by storage in liquid nitrogen. Supernatants from each clone are also stored frozen. Once the clones are preserved the supernatants can be tested at leisure. After testing, clones proven to be of the required specificity are recovered from liquid nitrogen and cultured for antibody production in quantity.

The objective is to secure large numbers of early cultures from a single clone which is

Source of Lymphocyte		Compatible myeloma partner
Mouse:	Balb/c	NS1 or NS 0
Rat:	DA	Y3
	LOU	YO
	AO	YO
Man:		LICR LON/HMy2

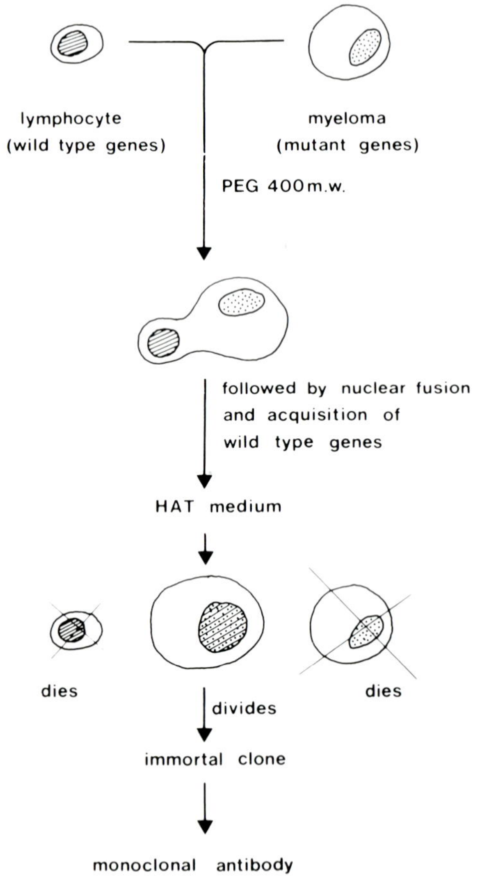

FIGURE 2. Hybridoma: cell fusion method.

stable in the production of the desired antibody. Large amounts of monoclonal antibody are usually required for clinical use. Antibody may be obtained direct from the culture supernatant (1 to 5 μg/mℓ) which contains few other proteins. Alternatively, a more concentrated source of antibody is obtained by intraperitoneal inoculation of hybridoma cells into rats or mice of compatible strain. The ascitic fluid can then be tapped off and this is relatively rich in monoclonal antibody (approximately 10 mg/mℓ). The major drawback with this approach is that the monoclonal antibodies become contaminated with other proteins including host antibodies. The means of antibody production, therefore, depends ultimately on its intended use and the technology available for purification.

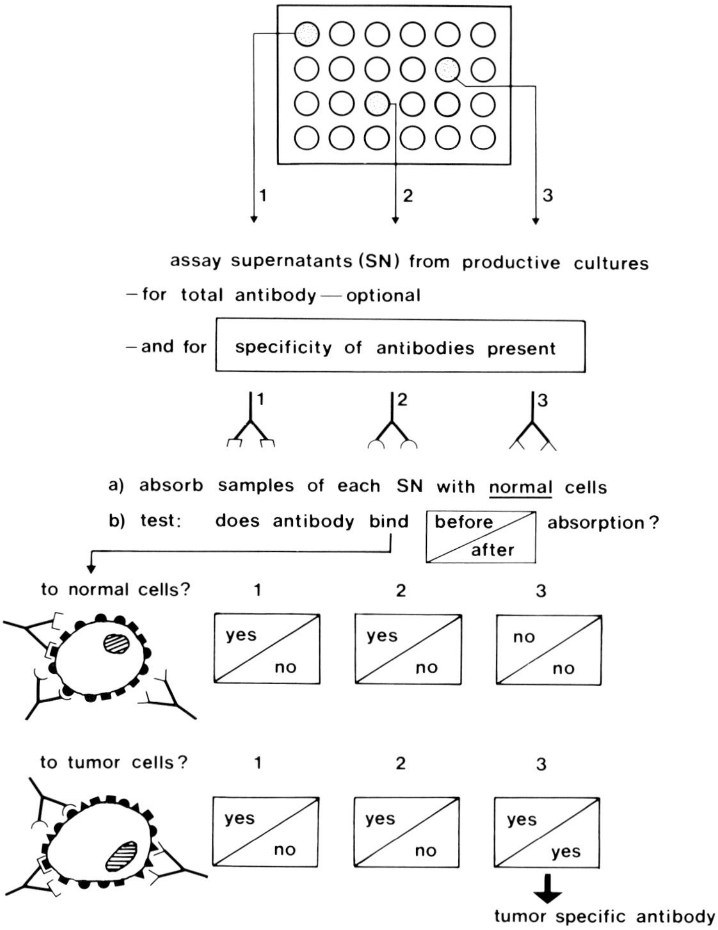

METHODS FOR DETECTING BOUND ANTIBODIES:

method		detection
Hemagglutination, direct or indirect:		Light microscopy.
Complement dependent cytolysis:		Isotope release (e.g. ^{51}Cr); vital stains.
Anti-immunoglobulin reagents labeled with:	fluorochromes:	Fluorescence microscopy.
	radioisotopes:	beta & gamma spectrometry.
	enzymes:	Add substrate ⟶ colored product – e.g. immunoperoxidase.
Staphylococcus aureus (Cowan I) protein A labeled as above:		as above

FIGURE 3. Some assays for antibodies in hybridoma culture supernatants.

2. Electrical Fusion

A different technique for inducing cell to cell fusion has been developed by Zimmerman and Pilwak.[15] Cells are subjected to an alternating electrical field, and during this process (dielectrophoresis) they form tight membrane contacts. A high-intensity field pulse then causes reversible electrical breakdown in the membrane contact zone resulting in fusion. The process and the precision required to achieve high yields of hybrids has been described in detail.[16] Some points to note are

1. Fusion is done on a glass slide containing wire electrodes, enabling the process to be observed and monitored microscopically
2. A relatively nonconducting solution (e.g., glucose or mannitol) is required to avoid heating effects
3. The myeloma cells need enzymatic treatment with pronase or dispase to overcome the problem of the different cell volumes of the small lymphocyte and the larger myeloma cell
4. A high yield of hybridomas may be achieved (50 to 80%), although the total numbers of cells used is reduced by several orders of magnitude compared to the chemical fusion methods.

The electrical fusion technique is particularly useful when only small numbers of cells are available, as after in vitro immunization.

C. Human Monoclonal Antibodies

Human myeloma cells suitable for human B cell fusions are now available,[17] although the efficiency of hybridization is relatively low (around 1 hybrid per 10^6 cells) and the incidence of relevant B cells is often low (1 per 6×10^6 cells for peripheral blood).

The importance of human monoclonal antibodies for treatment of patients is readily appreciated when the consequences of repeated injections of a foreign protein, such as mouse antibody, are recalled. Severe allergy, including anaphylactic shock, may result. In addition, the immuno-competent individual will develop antibodies against the foreign protein to neutralize and clear it from the circulation. Moreover, it should be remembered that immune clearance of human monoclonal antibodies may also occur because of allotype and idiotype polymorphism.

For humans deliberate immunization is rarely ethical and peripheral blood is the usual source of lymphocytes, though lymphocytes, spleen, and diseased tissue may be available when operative procedures are necessary for the patient. An alternative approach to immunization is in vitro culture of lymphocytes in the presence of the antigen.

Direct immortalization of human B cells can be achieved by viral transformation using Epstein-Barr virus (EBV). This method can result in some 50% efficiency of transformation, but the transformed cells are rapidly lost due to attack by cytotoxic T cells present in the culture, since these remain functionally active against viral-infected cells. Thus, it is necessary to clone early to dilute out the T lymphocytes. Alternatively, addition of Cyclosporin A to the culture will suppress the cytotoxic T cells.[18] Even when Cyclosporin A is used, an early cloning is required to isolate the immunoglobulin-secreting clones from overgrowth by nonsecreting B cells. Clearly any infective viral components must be destroyed before administration to humans; filtration, purification, DNAse and RNAse digestion, and UV irradiation are among the methods available to ensure safety.

III. PURIFICATION OF MONOCLONAL ANTIBODY

Ammonium sulfate precipitation is the standard method routinely used to isolate antibody from either culture medium or from ascitic fluid. Different proteins precipitate out in different concentrations of ammonium sulfate; these concentrations are expressed as the percentage of ammonium sulfate present compared to that of a saturated solution. Fibrinogen is precipitated at 30% saturation and is discarded. Each monoclonal antibody protein has its own precipitation point which is first established by precipitation with a dilution series of ammonium sulfate, followed by measuring antibody concentration in each fraction. Usually, precipitate from 30 to 50% ammonium sulfate is collected, and then reprecipitated at the appropriate ammonium sulfate concentration for the desired antibody. The second precipitate is then redissolved in saline and exhaustively dialyzed against phosphate-buffered saline. Any aggregates are removed by centrifugation at 100,000 *g* and the solution is sterilized by passage through a 0.45 μm filter. The antibody may be stored deep frozen at −70°C (to overcome the eutectic effect of concentrated protein on the freezing of water). Aliquots should be tested for sterility, absence of pyrogens, and specific activity.

Different subclasses of immunoglobulin have individual physicochemical properties which may be exploited for purification. For example, monoclonal rat IgG2c behaves as a euglobulin and may be precipitated at pH 6 in very dilute phosphate buffer, leaving most other serum components, including albumin, in solution. Alternatively, the pH profile of IgG2c binding to Staphylococcus protein A allows complete purification by elution at pH 4 after absorption at neutral pH. Another example is mouse IgG1, routinely purified by its pH-dependent binding to protein A from which it may be eluted pure at pH 5.0.

IV. PRACTICAL CONSIDERATIONS OF MONOCLONAL ANTIBODIES FOR CLINICAL USE

When monoclonal antibody is being considered for use clinically, its individual properties must be respected. For instance, the choice of an appropriate subclass enables production of a reagent efficient in complement-mediated cell lysis. An antibody of a different subclass will be suitable for imaging because it remains at the cell surface and does not fix complement. These aspects can be illustrated by a more detailed consideration of complement fixation. (Table 1 lists the types of antibody which are discussed.)

A. Fixation of Complement by Monoclonal Antibody

The biological method of targeting cells involves binding of antibody, followed by complement fixation and resultant cell lysis. This natural system can be used therapeutically, particularly if the underlying mechanism is well understood. Certain antibody subclasses are efficient at fixing complement, although it is extremely important to recognize that this is dependent on the species of complement. Complement fixation also depends on antigen density; this needs to be great enough to allow at least two molecules of bound IgG to be close enough to bind Clq, the first component of the classical complement cascade. Thus, if targetting of this type is planned (i.e., complement fixation) it must be ascertained that the antibody subclass, and the density of antigen on the target cell, are suitable to achieve cytolysis by complement. Even though the above conditions are fulfilled, there may be failure to lyse cells. This happens because antigens, after binding of antibody, can be physically relocated in the membrane by patching and capping and thereby avoid efficient complement fixation. This relocation of antigen is dependent upon multivalent antibody binding to multivalent antigen, resulting in the formation of a multimolecular lattice. Binding of *mono*valent antibodies cannot lead to lattice formation, and the subsequent escape by relocation is not possible. Certain monoclonal antibodies with high binding affinity are, therefore, more cytolytic in the monovalent form, and these can be produced by enzymic methods.[19] Monovalent antibody may also occur naturally in the hybridoma cell culture,[20] and cloning procedures can select for these. This can be understood when it is realized that the hybrid is, strictly speaking, biclonal, having immunoglobulin genes donated by both the myeloma cell and the spleen cell. Coexpression of these genes can permit production of hybrid immunoglobulin as the heavy and light chains assemble — part B cell and part myeloma. Thus, hybrid antibody, monovalent for B cell specificity, can be secreted. An example of a monovalent rat monoclonal antibody is CamPath 1[21] which binds to human lymphocytes and fixes complement efficiently. This has recently been used successfully in the clinic to intercept rejection of transplanted organs; its effectiveness in vivo depends on the fact that its antigenic target does not relocate by modulation.

Table 1
IMMUNOGLOBULIN CLASSES AND SUBCLASSES: BINDING TO PROTEIN A[a] AND COMPLEMENT FIXATION[b]

			Protein A	Complement
Human	Ig	M	−	+
		A1	−	−
		A2	?	−
		E	−	−
		G1	+	+
		G2	+	+
		G3	+, −[c]	+
		G4	+	−
Mouse	Ig	M	+, −[c]	+
		A	−	−
		E	−	−
		G1	weak	−, +[d]
		G2a	+	+
		G2b	+	+
		G3	+	?
Rat	Ig	M	+, −[c]	+
		A	+[e]	−
		E	−	−
		G1	weak	+, −[c]
		G2a	−	+
		G2b	weak	+
		G2c	+	−

Note: Binding to Protein A is extremely pH dependent. Data given refer to binding to Protein A linked to Sepharose® 4B at pH 7 to 8. Most of the data given refer to monoclonal antibodies and/or purified myeloma proteins. Polyclonal preparations may differ in characteristics from monoclonal materials.

[a] Classical binding to the Fc portion of the antibody.
[b] Classical pathway; heterologous complement.
[c] Different monoclonal antibodies of the same class/subclass can show either characteristic.
[d] Monoclonal antibodies are negative; purified IgG1 from immune serum can be positive.
[e] Binding to $F(ab')_2$ sites not excluded.

The idea of using hybrid antibody molecules leads to a further exploitation of the hybridoma method. For example, fusion of two different hybridomas, one with specificity for a tumor-cell antigen, and the second with specificity for a therapeutic targetting or imaging reagent can lead to a mixed assembly of immunoglobulin components possessing dual specificity. The antibodies would be capable of focusing together the therapeutic reagent and the target cell. These examples suffice to show that the natural versatility of antibody structure and its associated properties, together with the hybridoma methodology, open up possibilities for novel biological creations.

B. Crossreactive and Nonspecific Effects

Each antibody type can crossreact with sites other than the immunizing antigen. The size of the epitope in an antigenic polypeptide molecule is small — approximating a five or six amino-acid cluster. Given that proteins commonly range between 100 to 1000 amino acids, it is possible that a given antibody might crossreact with a similar epitope shape which happens to fortuitously occur on a different molecule. The possibility even arises that an antibody raised against a given immunogen might have greater affinity for epitopes on completely different molecules with a different tissue distribution. The practical implication is, of course, that each monoclonal antibody intended for therapeutic use must be rigorously screened to determine any crossreactivity of this type.

Antibodies can bind to cells other than the target cell in a nonspecific way, viz. through Fc receptors that occur on many cell types. This nonspecific binding can be appreciable. It can be avoided by use of IgM, which lacks available Fc, or by enzymatically modified IgG where the constant region (Fc) of the immunoglobulin is cleaved off to leave $F'(ab)_2$ (bivalent) or F′ab (monovalent) fragments. Of particular relevance are the receptors of human IgE on mast cells. Certain mouse immunoglobulin subclasses bind to this receptor and may induce allergic responses.

V. CONCLUSION

Monoclonal antibodies provide a new probe invaluable in biological systems, which, by being itself biological, is capable of exquisite sensitivity. Clinical exploitation of monoclonal antibodies has been taken up on two main fronts: by the oncologist to image and target tumor metastases and by the transplant surgeon to intercept rejection of transplanted tissues and organs.

Many different disciplines are united in the need for a fundamental understanding of antibody behavior in vivo, and of how the antibody molecule may be ''designed'' over and above that produced by the original B cell. Thus, the molecule may be tailored to possess properties desired by the clinician, in addition to maintaining specificity for the target antigen.

ACKNOWLEDGMENTS

I am indebted to Dr. Hugh ff. Davies for his constructive criticism of the manuscript and for the mouse artwork.

REFERENCES

1. **Milstein, C.,** Monoclonal antibodies from hybrid myelomas: theoretical aspects and some general comments, in *Monoclonal Antibodies in Clinical Medicine,* McMichael, A. J. and Fabre, J. W., Eds., 1982, chap. 1.
2. **Steinitz, M., Izak, G., Cohen, S., Ehrenfeld, M., and Flechner, I.,** Continuous production of monoclonal rheumatoid factor by E. B. V. transformed lymphocytes, *Nature (London),* 287, 443, 1980.
3. **Springer, G. F. and Desai, P. R.,** Cross-reacting carcinoma-associated antigens with blood group and precursor specificities, *Transplant. Proc.,* 9, 1105, 1977.
4. **Springer, G. F. and Desai, P. R.,** Common precursors of human blood group MN specificities, *Biochem. Biophys. Res. Commun.,* 61, 740, 1974.
5. **Metcalfe, S., Springer, G. F., Svvennsen, R. J., and Tegtmeyer, H.,** Monoclonal antibodies specific for human Thomson-Friedenreich (T) and T_n blood group precursor antigens, in *Protides of the Biological Fluids,* Peeters, H., Ed., Permagon Press, New York, 1984, 765.
6. **Magnani, J. L.,** Carbohydrate differentiation and cancer-associated antigens detected by monoclonal antibodies, *Biochem. Soc. Trans.,* 12, 543, 1984.

7. **Leonard, W. J., Depper, J. M., Uchiyama, T., Smith, K. A., Waldmann, T. A., and Greene, W. C.,** A monoclonal antibody that appears to recognize the receptor for human T-cell growth factor; partial characterization of the receptor, *Nature (London),* 300, 267, 1982.
8. **Kohler, G., Howe, S. C., and Milstein, C.,** Fusion between immunoglobulin-secreting and non-secreting myeloma cell lines, *J. Immunol.,* 6, 292, 1976.
9. **Galfre, G. and Milstein, C.,** Preparation of monoclonal antibodies: strategies and procedures, in *Methods in Enzymology,* Colowick, S. P., Kaplan, N. O., and Langone, J. J., Eds., Academic Press, New York, 73, 3, 1981.
10. **Galfre, G., Milstein, C., and Wright, B.,** Rat x rat hybrid myelomas and a monoclonal anti-Fd portion of mouse IgG, *Nature (London),* 277, 131, 1979.
11. **Kilmartin, J. V., Wright, B., and Milstein, C.,** Rat monoclonal antitubulin antibodies derived by using a new non-secreting rat cell line, *J. Cell. Biol.,* 93, 576, 1982.
12. **Holmdahl, R., Moran, T., and Andersson, M.,** A rapid and efficient immunisation protocol for production of monoclonal antibodies reactive with autoantigens, *J. Immunol. Methods,* 83, 379, 1985.
13. **Post, G. and Nicholson, G. L., Eds.,** *Membrane Fusion,* Elsevier, Amsterdam, 1978.
14. **Halfmann, H. J., Emeis, C. C., and Zimmermann, U.,** Electro-fusion of haploid Saccharomyces yeast cells of identical mating type, *Arch. Microbiol.,* 134, 1, 1983.
15. **Zimmermann, U. and Pilwak, G.,** Electrical breakdown of cell membranes, Abstract IV-19-(H), 140, *6th Int. Biophys. Congress,* Kyoto, Japan, 1978.
16. **Zimmerman, U. and Vienken, J.,** Electric field-induced cell-to-cell fusion, *J. Membr. Biol.,* 67, 165, 1982.
17. **Edwards, P. A. W., Smith, C. M., Neville, A. M., and O'Hare, M. J.,** A human-human hybridoma system based on a fast-growing mutant of the ARH-77 plasma cell leukaemia derived line, *Euro. J. Immunol.,* 12(8), 641, 1982.
18. **Sikora, K. and Neville, M.,** Human monoclonal antibodies. News and views, *Nature (London),* 300, 316, 1982.
19. **Glennie, M. J. and Stevenson, G. T.,** Univalent antibodies kill tumour cells in vitro and in vivo, *Nature (London),* 295, 712, 1982.
20. **Cobbold, S. P. and Waldmann, H.,** Therapeutic potential of monovalent monoclonal antibodies, *Nature (London),* 301, 460, 1984.
21. **Waldmann, H., Or, R., Hale, G., Weiss, L., Cividall, G., Samuel, S., Manor, D., Brautbar, C., Pollack, A., Rachmilewitz, E. A., and Slavin, S.,** Elimination of graft versus host disease by in vitro depletion of alloreactive lymphocytes using a rat antihuman lymphocyte antibody (CAMPATH-1), *Lancet,* 2, 483, 1984.

Chapter 4

RADIOIMMUNOSCINTIGRAPHY OF HUMAN CARCINOMA: CHARACTERIZATION OF MONOCLONAL ANTIBODIES*

Daniel F. Hayes, Eliot L. Friedman, and Donald W. Kufe

TABLE OF CONTENTS

* Supported by PHS Grant CA-38869 (DWK) and CA-01041 (DFH), awarded by the National Institutes of Health, DHHS, and by an American Cancer Society Faculty Research Award (DWK).

I. INTRODUCTION

The development of hybridoma technology has led to the application of monoclonal antibodies (MAbs) to the diagnosis and treatment of neoplastic diseases. One such application has been the use of radiolabeled MAbs for immunoscintigraphy of a variety of human cancers. Several recent studies have demonstrated that a number of factors related to the characteristics of both the radiolabeled MAb and the antigen with which it reacts affect the ultimate success of radioimaging tumors.

This review focuses on the preclinical evaluation of MAbs which are being considered for radioimmunoimaging trials. Several factors in evaluating a MAb for immunoscintigraphy are reviewed, including the importance of the sensitivity and specificity of the MAb, the cellular location of the antigen, the stability of the antigen-antibody complex, and the kinetics of the MAb-antigen interaction. Finally, the interrelationships between these factors are reviewed in terms of problems encountered with heterogeneous antigen expression. Comprehensive preclinical evaluation of each MAb should provide more efficient and successful clinical immunoscintigraphy trials.

II. SENSITIVITY AND SPECIFICITY OF MAb REACTIVITY

A. Preclinical Considerations

Tumor cells in both animals and humans express distinct cell surface antigens that distinguish them from normal tissues.[1-3] These tumor-associated antigens (TAA) are of biologic and clinical interest, since they may represent the target by which the host may identify and reject the neoplasm. However, the biological definition of a TAA is difficult, since the demonstration that an antigen is absent from normal tissues at all stages of embryonic development, and subsequent cellular differentiation, is nearly impossible. Nonetheless, within experimental limitations, many TAA have been described.[4-11] Although some of these antigens are of viral[4-6] or fetal[7-9] origin, more still remain undefined.

TAA may differ quantitatively and qualitatively from those antigens on normal cells.[1-3] Successful radioimmunoimaging depends on the ability of the antibody to reliably recognize these differences. Prior to the availability of MAbs, studies of TAA with conventional, hyperimmune polyclonal sera were hampered by the heterogeneity of the antibody populations employed and the amount of specific immunoglobulin that could be generated. Nonetheless, the use of radiolabeled antibodies directed against normal and malignant tissues was first attempted in the 1950s and 1960s.[12-15] The majority of the antibodies used in early clinical trials were constituents of goat or rabbit antisera to antigens such as carcinoembryonic antigen (CEA),[16-19] alpha fetoprotein,[20-22] ferritin, and human chorionic gonadatropin.[23-25] In fact, studies using anti-CEA successfully demonstrated the localization of malignant breast tumors.[16,18] In some of these studies,[16,18,19,24,25] the immunoglobulins were partially purified using affinity chromatography which resulted in limited increases in immunoreactivity.[26] Although localization of human tumors was achieved, the low level of labeled antibody bound to tumor and high background radioactivity[19] necessitated computer subtractions of blood-pool activity to define tumor sites.

In contrast to heterologous antisera, MAbs raised against tumor cell surface antigens have the potential to react with a high percentage of the tumor cells of interest, while not binding with cells of other tumors and normal tissues. Thus, use of MAbs for immunoscintigraphy could decrease nonspecific binding, obviate the need for background subtraction, and produce images of greater diagnostic utility. Therefore, preclinical evaluation with techniques such as radioimmunoassay (RIA), enzyme-linked immunoassay, and immunoperoxidase staining should be directed towards defining the sensitivity and specificity of a given MAb.

One group of MAbs, designated the DF series, was generated in our laboratory against a membrane-enriched fraction from a human metastatic mammary carcinoma. Initially, the hybridoma supernatants were screened by indirect RIA for reactivity with membrane-enriched extracts of normal livers and of metastatic breast carcinomas. Additionally, reactivity was monitored against cultured human breast cancer cells (MCF-7), cultured human hepatocellular carcinoma cells (HepG2), normal granulocytes, and purified carcinoembryonic antigen (CEA) and normal cross-reactive antigen (NCA). One MAb, an IgG_1 designated DF3, reacts with extracts of metastatic breast cancers and breast cancer cell lines, but does not react with normal liver, CEA, NCA, or granulocytes (Table 1). Subsequent biochemical analysis has demonstrated that MAb DF3 reacts with a 300 to 450 kdalton glycoprotein which is present in the human milk fat globule (HMFG) and in breast cancer cells.[27] Thus, MAb DF3 was chosen for more extensive evaluation with immunoperoxidase studies.

The immunoperoxidase technique permits an evaluation of the sensitivity and specificity of MAb reactivity with fresh or frozen tissue.[28] The method of tissue fixation can effect antigenicity. For example, the ovarian carcinoma-associated antigen CA125 is destroyed by paraffin fixation. Thus, characterization of this monoclonal antibody has required immunoperoxidase evaluation of frozen tissue.[29] In contrast, the DF3 antigen survives fixation. Therefore, several histologic types of human malignant mammary carcinomas were examined for reactivity with MAb DF3 using the ABC immunoperoxidase method and 5 μm sections of formalin fixed tissues.[30]

MAb DF3 is reactive with 78% of 32 infiltrating ductal carcinomas (IDC)[30] (Table 2). As shown in Figure 1, the proportion of tumor cells which stain within each of the 25 IDC ranges from a few to over 90%. Furthermore, the reactivity with MAb DF3 for these carcinomas is found within the cytoplasm and/or throughout the cellular membrane (Figure 2A and 2B). A similar staining pattern is observed for mammary carcinomas containing both infiltrating ductal and intraductal elements. Figure 3 compares MAb DF3 reactivity with infiltrating elements (Figure 3A) and intraductal elements (Figure 3B) of nine such tumors. The percent of reactive cells varies for individual tumors, but the infiltrating elements of each tumor display a higher degree of cytoplasmic and total membrane reactivity than the intraductal component. Similar staining patterns have been observed with *in situ,* medullary, and infiltrating lobular carcinomas (Figure 3C). While infiltrating lobular carcinomas and medullary carcinomas demonstrate only cytoplasmic staining, *in situ* carcinomas display varying degrees of cytoplasmic and apical border reactivity. Thus, these data indicate that MAb DF3 binds with most breast cancers and may be a useful agent for immunoscintigraphy.

Reactivity of a MAb with normal tissues might result in false-positive images and possible toxicity. When investigated rigorously, no TAA has been observed to be absolutely restricted to a malignant clone of cells. In addition to reactivity with a number of benign breast tumors (Table 2), MAb DF3 binds with certain normal tissues as well (Table 3). However, in contrast to the cytoplasmic and total membrane reactivity observed with the malignant breast tissues, MAb DF3 reacts primarily with the apical borders of all benign breast lesions and normal tissues. Figures 2C and 2D demonstrate the apical reactivity of MAb DF3 in fibroadenomas and fibrocystic disease, respectively. A similar pattern of reactivity has been observed with lactating breast tissue. Approximately 10 to 20% of normal ducts from breast tumor patients also display apical reactivity. However, none of five fibroadenomas (Figure 4A), only one of eight fibrocystic disease specimens (Figure 4B), and no normal duct cells demonstrate any evidence of cytoplasmic MAb DF3 reactive antigen. In similar fashion, MAb DF3 reactivity with normal tissue is also apical.

Table 4 summarizes the reactivity of MAb DF3 on the basis of cytoplasmic and total membrane staining. While 78% of malignant lesions display this pattern, only one of 13 benign lesions has more than apical reactivity. Thus, although some benign and normal tissues do express the DF3 antigen, reactivity of these with circulating MAb DF3 may be minimized due to the apical position of the antigen.

Table 1
INITIAL CHARACTERIZATION OF MONOCLONAL ANTIBODY DF3

		Reactivity[a]											
		Cell extracts							Live cells			Purified antigen	
Antibody	Isotype	Met 1[b]	Met 2[b]	Met 3[b]	Met 4[b]	Norm 2[c]	Norm 3[c]	Norm 6[c]	MCF-7[d]	HepG2[e]	Granulocytes[f]	CEA[g]	NCA[h]
3	IgG_1	− −	+ +	+ +	±	− −	− −	− −	+	− −	− −	− −	− −

Note: − −, <3 × background cmp; ±, < 6 × background cpm; +, <9 × background cpm; + +, > 9 × background cpm.

[a] By indirect radioimmunoassay.
[b] Partially purified membrane extracts of human breast cancer metastases to liver.
[c] Partially purified membrane extracts of normal human liver.
[d] Cultured human breast cancer cell line.
[e] Cultured human hepatocellular carcinoma cell line.
[f] Normal human granulocytes isolated by density centrifugation.
[g] Carcinoembryonic antigen.
[h] Normal cross-reacting antigen.

Table 2
REACTIVITY OF MAb DF3 WITH MALIGNANT AND BENIGN MAMMARY TUMORS[a]

Tissue	Total number tested	Number reactive with MAb DF3 (%)
Malignant		
Infiltrating ductal (IDC)	32	25 (78)
IDC + intraductal	12	12 (100)
Intraductal only	4	4 (100)
Infiltrating lobular	3	3 (100)
Medullary	1	1 (100)
Total	**52**	**45 (87)**
Benign		
Fibrocystic	8	8 (100)
Fibroadenoma	5	5 (100)
Total	**13**	**13 (100)**

[a] By immunoperoxidase staining.

Modified from Kufe, D., Inghirami, G., Abe, M., Hayes, D., Justi-Wheeler, H., and Schlom, J., *Hybridoma,* 3, 223, 1984. With permission.

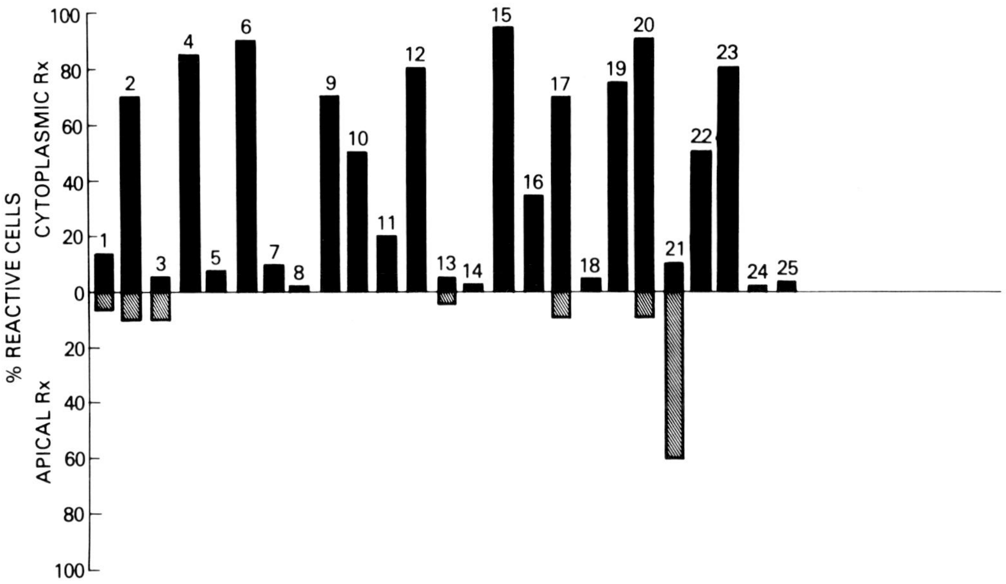

FIGURE 1. Reactivity of MAb DF3 with infiltrating duct carcinomas. Each numbered bar represents a different patient. The dark areas represent the percent of tumor cells with a cytoplasmic reaction. The striped areas represent the percent of tumor cells displaying MAb DF3 reactivity on apical borders. (From Kufe, D., Inghirami, G., Abe, M., Hayes, D., Justi-Wheeler, H., and Schlom, J., *Hybridoma,* 3, 223, 1984. With permission.)

B. Clinical Studies

Preclinical evaluation of specificity may not predict in vivo cross reactivity. For example, recent human trials of three separate MAbs have been complicated by unsuspected binding with normal granulocytes.[31,32] One of these, MAb B6.2, is an IgG_1 generated against a

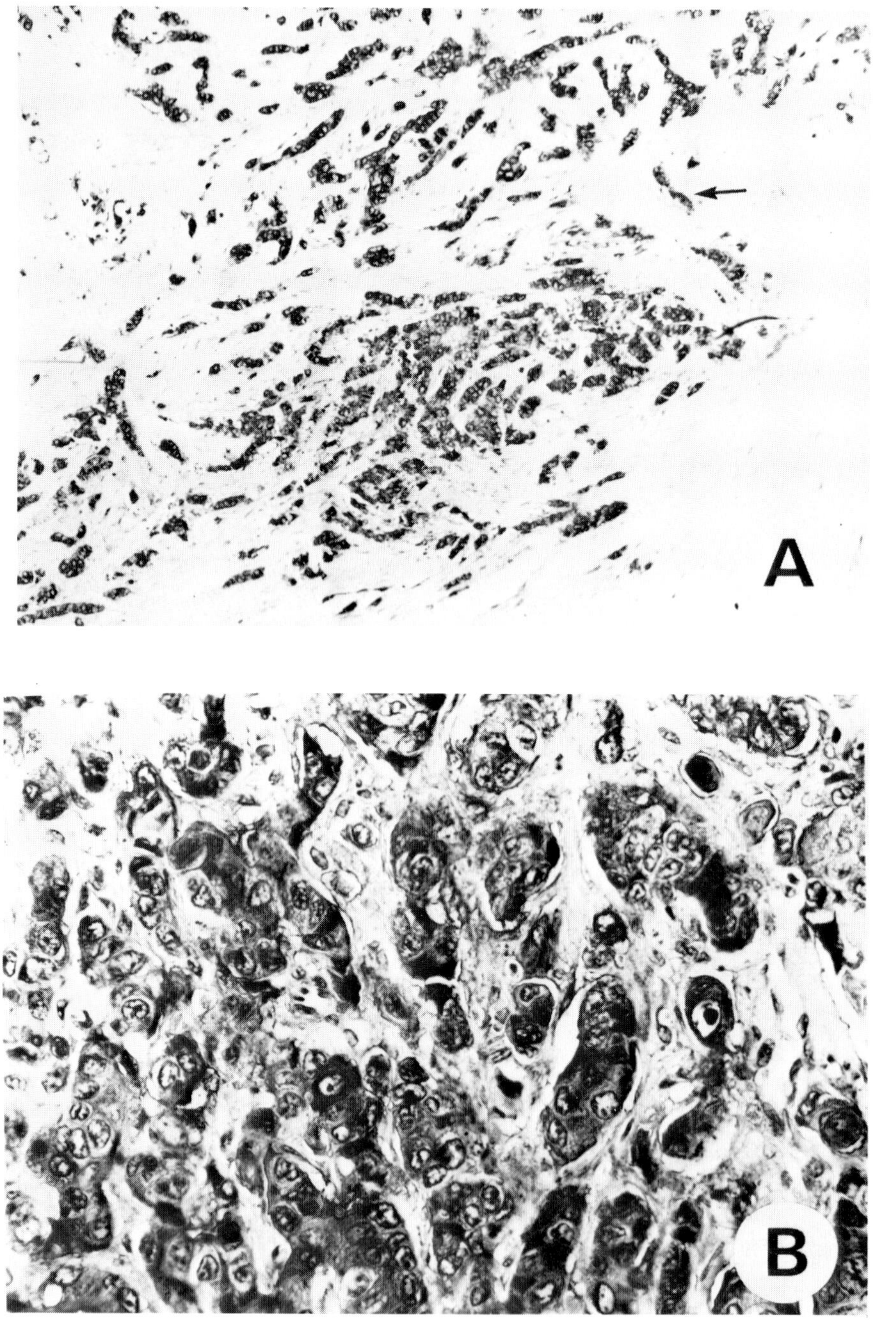

FIGURE 2. Reactivity of MAb DF3 with fixed tissue sections of mammary tumors using the ABC immunoperoxidase method: (A) infiltrating ductal carcinoma with strong cytoplasmic reactivity. (Magnification × 54); (B) higher magnification of (A), (Magnification × 330); (C) fibroadenoma showing MAb DF3 reactivity on apical borders of cells (arrow) — "S" is stroma; (D) fibrocystic disease showing apical staining of the cell lining of the cyst (large arrow) and normal gland (small arrow) (Magnification × 130). (From Kufe, D., Inghirami, G., Abe, M., Hayes, D., Justi-Wheeler, H., and Schlom, J., *Hybridoma,* 3, 223, 1984. With permission.)

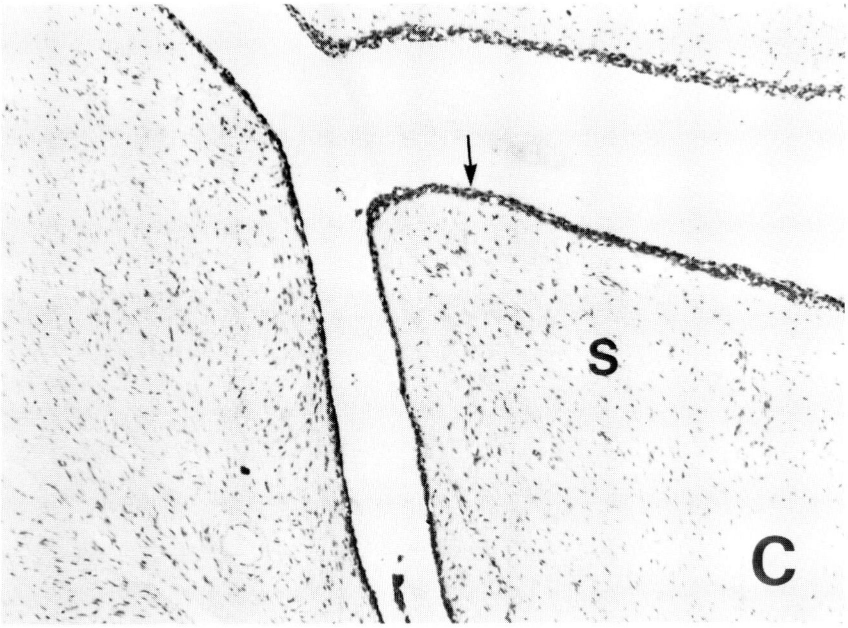

FIGURE 2C

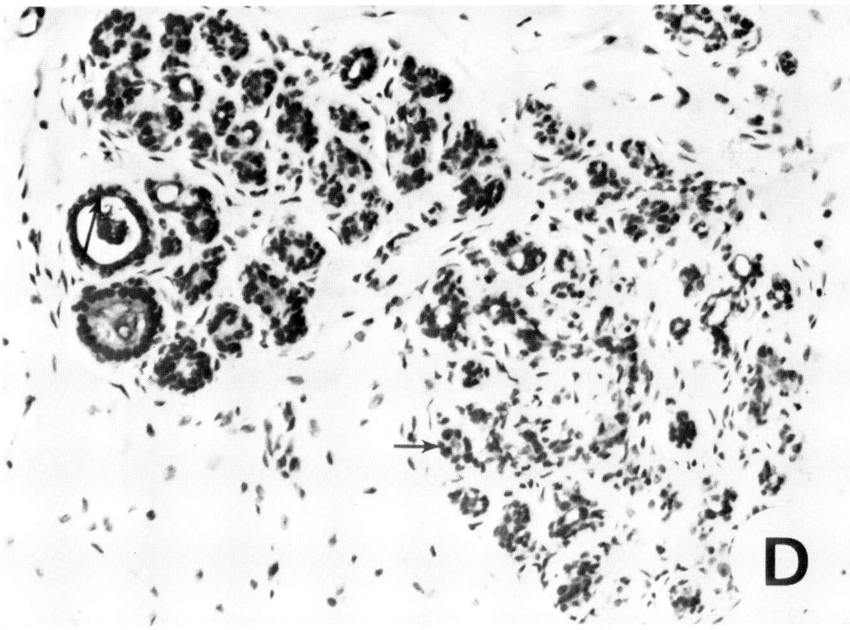

FIGURE 2D

membrane-enriched fraction of human metastatic mammary carcinoma cells.[33] Extensive preclinical investigations demonstrate that this MAb reacts with 74% of paraffin-fixed primary breast carcinomas and 50% of distal metastases.[33] Furthermore, none of 24 normal tissues, encompassing a broad range of epithelial organs, express the MAb B6.2-reactive

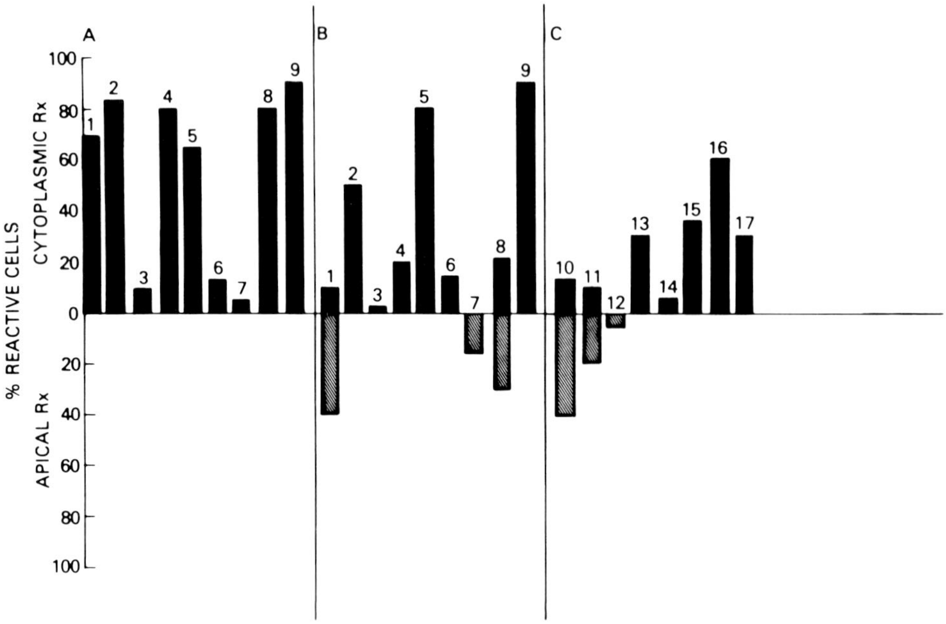

FIGURE 3. Reactivity of MAb DF3 with malignant mammary tumors. Each number represents a tumor from different patients. Panels A and B represent nine tumors with both infiltrating ductal elements (Panel A) and intraductal elements (Panel B). In Panel C, tumors 10 to 13 are *in situ* carcinomas, tumors 14 to 16 are infiltrating lobular, and tumor 17 is medullary. The dark areas represent the percent of tumor cells with cytoplasmic reaction; the striped areas represent the percent tumor cells displaying MAb DF3 reactivity on apical borders. (From Kufe, D., Inghirami, G., Abe, M., Hayes, D., Justi-Wheeler, H., and Schlom, J., *Hybridoma,* 3, 223, 1984. With permission.)

antigen. However, when ^{131}I-MAb B6.2 was evaluated as a scintigraphic agent in patients with metastatic breast cancer, skeletal images were observed in each of 13 patients investigated.[31]

Further evaluation demonstrated that MAb B6.2 reacts with granulocytes from normal subjects (Figure 5), and that radiolabeled B6.2 binds to granulocytes[31] from breast cancer patients (Table 5). MAb B6.2 was found to react with NCA, which is expressed on normal granulocytes. Thus, the skeletal uptake of radiolabeled MAb B6.2 prevented imaging of metastatic breast cancer in all but one patient.[31]

Similarly, Dillman et al.[32] have reported clinical studies of Indium-111 labeled MAbs 065 and 326, which react with CEA. Preclinical evaluation demonstrated excellent uptake of the radiolabeled MAb in colorectal carcinoma xenografts. However, these MAbs also crossreact with granulocytes.[32] Even with injections of relatively high doses of antibody (3 to 6 mg), specific images of metastatic carcinoma were not obtained in this study.

C. Potential Toxicity Due to Antibody Reactivity

Binding of an MAb to normal tissues could potentially result in toxicity. Adverse effects might occur through one of several mechanisms, including

1. Exposure of normal tissues to radioactivity
2. Removal of cross-reactive circulating cells,
3. Direct cytotoxicity of normal tissues by the MAb.

1. Exposure of Normal Tissues to Radioactivity

Binding of isotope-labeled MAb with antigen present on normal tissues would specifically

Table 3
REACTIVITY OF MAb DF3 WITH NORMAL HUMAN TISSUES[a]

Tissue	Total number tested	Number reactive with MAb DF3 (% reactive cells)	Type of cell reactive with MAb DF3
Stomach	2	1 (5)	Gastric glands
Duodenum	1	0	
Colon	3	0	
Liver	4	2 (10—25)	Epithelial cells along bile ducts
Fetal liver	1	0	
Gallbladder	3	2 (5—80)	Epithelial cells
Spleen	2	0	
Lung	7	3 (5—25)	Alveolar and bronchiolar cells
Heart	1	0	
Kidney	7	5 (15—100)	Convoluted distal and collecting tubules
Bladder	1	1 (10—30)	Transitional epithelial cells
Testis	1	1 (5)	Epithelial cells along seminiferous ducts
Uterus	1	1 (100)	Epithelial cells, cells of glands
Endocervix	2	2 (100)	Mucus-secreting glandular epithelial cells
Exocervix	3	0	
Skin	1	0	
Sebaceous gland	3	3 (50—70)	Alveolar cells
Sweat gland	3	3 (10—80)	Secretory tubule cells
Adrenal cortex	1	0	
Thyroid	1	1 (10)	Follicular cells
Bone marrow	2	0	

[a] By immunoperoxidase staining.

expose these tissues to radioactivity. However, radiation-induced cellular damage depends not only on the interaction of the antigen with the radiolabeled MAb, but on the dose and type of isotope used as well. In most immunoscintigraphic studies, the injected dose has been limited to 1 to 2 mCi. Furthermore, isotopes with relatively short half-lives (2 to 6 days) have generally been selected.[34] Thus, dosimetry calculations suggest that normal tissues will be exposed to insignificant levels of damaging radiation.[35] Choice of nuclides is discussed in more detail elsewhere in this book.

2. Removal of Circulating Cells Which Express a Crossreacting Antigen

Systemic symptoms associated with intravenous infusion of MAb, such as fever, chills, vascular instability, and dyspnea have been reported.[36] These symptoms may occur as a consequence of clearing of MAb aggregates, removal of immune complexes between MAb and circulating free antigen, and/or sequestration of normal circulating cells which bind the MAb.[36]

Therapeutic trials of intravenously injected antibody have demonstrated that if infused slowly, very large doses (200 to 1000 mg) of MAb can be injected safely.[37,38] However, systemic symptoms related to MAb binding of normal circulating cells may be related to dose. For example, no toxicity was observed in the MAb B6.2 immunoscintigraphy trial in which MAb bolus doses of 50 to 1050 μg were injected.[31] However, Dillman et al.[32] reported fever, chills, malaise, nausea, and vomiting after injection of 3 to 6 mg of MAbs 065 and 326. These symptoms were associated with decreases in circulating granulocytes, and the authors concluded that the observed toxicities were directly related to neutrophil sequestration.

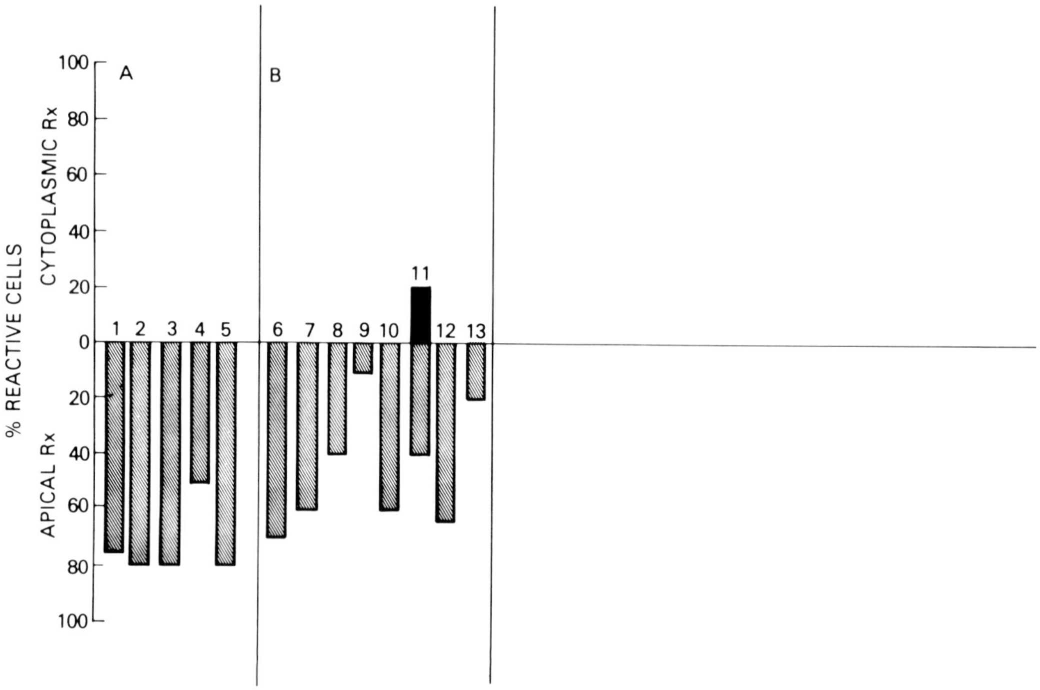

FIGURE 4. Reactivity of MAb DF3 with benign mammary tumors. Panel A represents five fibroadenomas, and Panel B represents eight fibrocystic disease specimens. The dark areas represent the percent of tumor cells with a cytoplasmic reaction; the striped areas represent the percent tumor cells displaying MAb DF3 reactivity on apical borders. (From Kufe, D., Inghirami, G., Abe, M., Hayes, D., Justi-Wheeler, H., and Schlom, J., *Hybridoma,* 3, 223, 1984. With permission.)

Table 4
CYTOPLASMIC AND/OR TOTAL MEMBRANE REACTIVITY OF MAb DF3 WITH HUMAN MAMMARY TUMORS[a]

Tissue	Total number tested	Number reactive with MAb DF3 (%)
Malignant		
Infiltrating ductal	32	25 (78)
Infiltrating and intraductal	12	9 (75)
Other	7	6 (86)
Total	**51**	**40 (78)**
Benign		
Fibroadenomas	5	0
Fibrocystic disease	8	1 (13)
Total	**13**	**1 (8)**

[a] By immunoperoxidase staining.

Modified from Kufe, D., Inghiromi, G., Abe, M., Hayes, D., Justi-Wheeler, H., and Schlom, J., *Hybridoma,* 3, 223, 1984. With permission.

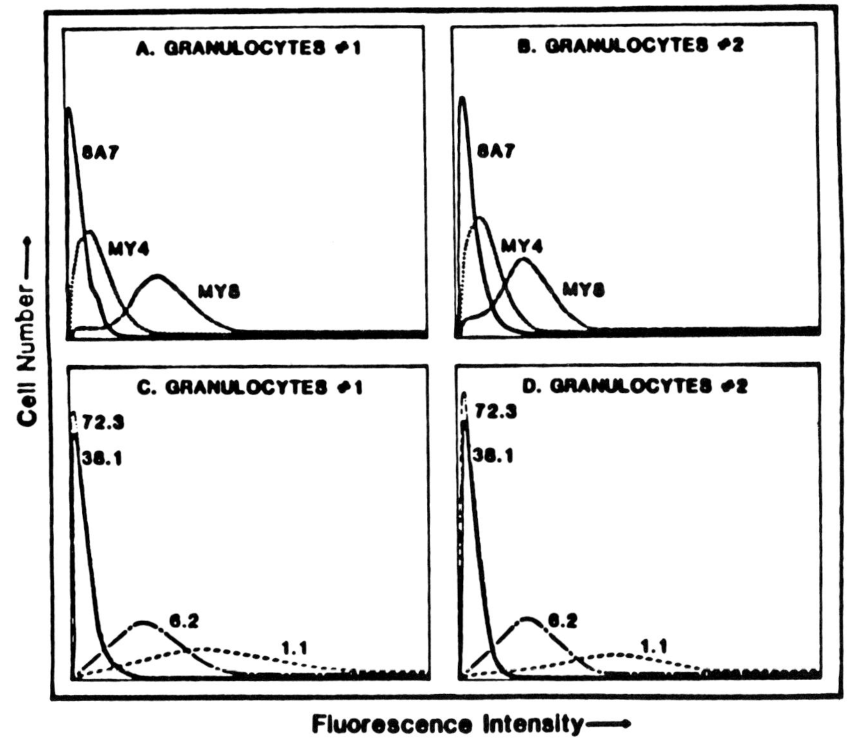

FIGURE 5. Reactivity of MAb B6.2 with human granulocytes. Human granulocytes were harvested from two normal donors by Ficoll-Hypaque differential sedimentation (A and C, Subject 1; B and D, Subject 2). In A and B, the cells were incubated with MAb 8A7 (negative control), MAb My4 or My8 (positive controls) and then fluoresceinated goat anti-mouse antibody). The cells were analyzed by fluorescein-activated cell sorting. Sections C and D are the same as A and B except MAb 72.3, 38.1, 6.2, or 1.1 was used instead of 8A7, My4, My8. (From Hayes, D. F., Zalutsky, M. R., Kaplan, W., Noska, M., Thor, A., Colcher, D., and Kufe, D. W., *Cancer Res.*, 46, 3157, 1986. With permission.)

Table 5
MAb B6.2 REACTIVITY WITH HEMATOPOIETIC CELLS FROM PATIENTS WITH BREAST CANCER[a]

Patient number	Circulating granulocytes[b]	Antibody molecules bound per cell: Granulocytes	Mononuclear leukocytes	Erythrocytes
1	5313	8700	1400	35
2	1120	1800	30	2
3	3540	2300	630	11

[a] In vitro live cell radioimmunoassay.
[b] Per mm^3.

From Hayes, D. F., Zalutsky, M. R., Kaplan, W., Noska, M., Thor, A., Colcher, D., and Kufe, D. W., *Cancer Res.*, 46, 3157, 1986. With permission.

3. Direct Cytotoxicity of Normal Tissues by the MAb

While ultimately MAbs may be used therapeutically, the exposure of normal, cross-reactive tissues to cytotoxic MAbs could result in necrosis of these "innocent bystanders".

Thus, evaluation of the MAb by an antibody-dependent cytotoxicity assay may be informative. Evaluation with a ^{51}Cr release assay[39] of MAb DF3 directed toward cultured target cells in the presence of human complement has demonstrated that this MAb is not cytotoxic (Table 6). In contrast, MAb B6.2 lyses MCF-7 mammary carcinoma cells in an antibody-dependent cell mediated cytotoxicity assay.[40] Nonetheless, although MAb B6.2 binds to normal human granulocytes, no neutropenia was observed in 13 patients following intravenous injection with this radioiodinated MAb.[31]

D. Regional Injection of Radiolabeled MAb

One means of preventing cross reactivity may be the use of regional injections followed by imaging. This approach could enhance tumor imaging by avoiding interference from binding of the radiolabeled MAb with normal tissues. In this regard, encouraging results have recently been obtained after radiolabeled MAbs were injected subcutaneously or intralymphatically for lymphoscintigraphy.[41,42] Likewise, intracavitary (pleural, pericardial, peritoneal) injection may be appropriate for selected tumor types.[43]

E. MAb Reactivity with Other Tumors

Several tumor-associated antigens are expressed in different histologic types of carcinomas.[44] However, recent studies have demonstrated that certain epitopes defined by MAbs may be relatively tumor-specific. For example, MAb 115D8, generated against a component of HMFG, reacts with the breast cancer-associated antigen which is also identified by MAb DF3.[44,45] However, immunoperoxidase evaluations with non-breast malignancies demonstrate that MAb 115D8 has a much broader pattern of reactivity than does MAb DF3. For example, MAb 115D8, but not MAb DF3, reacts with most colon carcinomas,[46] as demonstrated by immunoperoxidase studies[46,59] and live cell assays[30,46] (Table 7). These data indicate that MAbs against the same antigens may not necessarily demonstrate similar sensitivity and specificity, and that each MAb requires separate evaluation. Furthermore, the selection of a MAb which can be utilized to make specific tumor diagnoses, both histopathologically and radiologically, may ultimately be possible. The presence of distinct epitopes on the same antigen suggests that a MAb reactive with a "tumor-specific" epitope may be generated in the future.

III. LOCATION, CELL GROWTH DEPENDENCE, AND STABILITY OF REACTIVE ANTIGEN

A. Location

One important element for successful immunoscintigraphy is the availability of antigen for interaction with the radiolabeled MAb. In general, this requires cell surface expression by the tumor cell. Indirect immunofluorescence has been used to monitor expression of the DF3 antigen on the surface of MCF-7 breast carcinoma cells. The fluorescence histogram pattern of reactivity, compared with a nonreactive MAb of the same IgG_1 isotype,[30] is illustrated in Figure 6. MAb DF3 reacts with the surface of MCF-7 cells, and furthermore, fluorescent microscopy demonstrates diffuse distribution of the DF3 antigen on the cell surface. Live cell radioimmunoassay further confirms that MAb DF3 binds with an antigen on the surface of MCF-7 cells as well as BT-20 mammary carcinoma cells[30] (Table 7). Thus, the DF3 antigen is available on the cell surface for interaction with circulating MAb.

Interestingly, a recent investigation by Welt et al.[47] has demonstrated successful imaging of a melanoma xenograft in nude mice with radiolabeled MAb TA99. This MAb reacts with a 70 kdalton perinuclear antigen which is not present on the cell surface. Imaging of the xenograft was possible for up to 10 weeks, and 8% of the injected ^{125}I-MAb TA99 localized in the tumors. Thus, cell surface expression of the reactive antigen may not be essential for successful radioimmunoimaging.

Table 6
LACK OF IgG_1 MAb DF3 CYTOTOXICITY AGAINST THE MCF-7 BREAST CANCER CELL LINE

MCF-7 +	MAb DF3								
Human complement	**1.00 mg**	**0.32 mg**	**0.10 mg**	**0.03 mg**	**0.01 mg**	**0.003 mg**	**0.001 mg**	**0.0003 mg**	**0.0001 mg**
% Cell kill[a]	−10.2	−18.9	−13.3	−11.6	−4.2	−11.3	5.0	0.0	−3.9

Note: Negative values indicate no cytotoxicity.

[a] Value calculated as follows:

$$\frac{\text{chromium in cells treated with control MAb} - \text{chromium in cells treated with MAb DF3}}{\text{chromium in cells treated with control MAb} - \text{chromium in cells treated with 10\% Triton}} \times 100$$

Table 7
BINDING OF MAb DF3 TO THE SURFACE OF LIVE MAMMARY CARCINOMA CELLS[a]

Carcinoma	Cell line designation	CPM bound
Mammary	BT 20	3350
Mammary	MCF-7	
Passage 126		5750
Passage 142		9350
Passage 196		2050
Colon	LS174	150
Colon	WIDR	150

[a] By radioimmunoassay.

From Kufe, D., Inghirami, G., Abe, M., Hayes, D., Justi-Wheeler, H., and Schlom, J., *Hybridoma,* 3, 223, 1984. With permission.

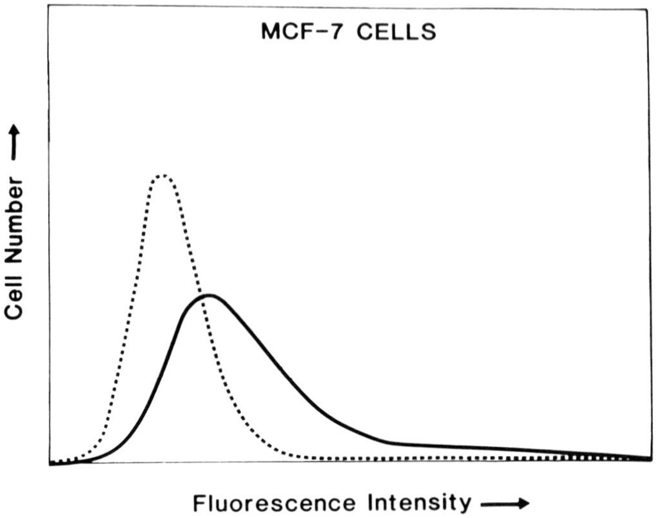

FIGURE 6. Immunofluorescence profiles of MCF-7 cells with MAb DF3 (thin line) and an isotype-identical control MAb 287 (broken line). (From Kufe, D., Inghirami, G., Abe, M., Hayes, D., Justi-Wheeler, H., and Schlom, J., *Hybridoma,* 3, 223, 1984. With permission.)

B. Cell Growth Dependence

Expression of surface antigens by tumor cells varies with both the age of the tumor cell line and the phase of the cell cycle. For example, surface expression of the DF3 reactive antigen varies with different passage levels of MCF-7 cells[30] (Table 7). In similar fashion, the cell surface binding of MAbs B6.2 and B38.1 has been monitored on MCF-7 mammary carcinoma cells[40] during logarithmic growth phase and at density-dependent arrest ($<5\%$ control DNA synthesis) (Figures 7 and 8). Antibody binding was monitored each day for seven consecutive days after passage. On the day after passage, both antibodies were strongly reactive with the MCF-7 cells (Figure 8). Over the following 7 days, the reactivities of MAbs B6.2 and B38.1 decreased progressively and were nearly undetectable on Day 7.

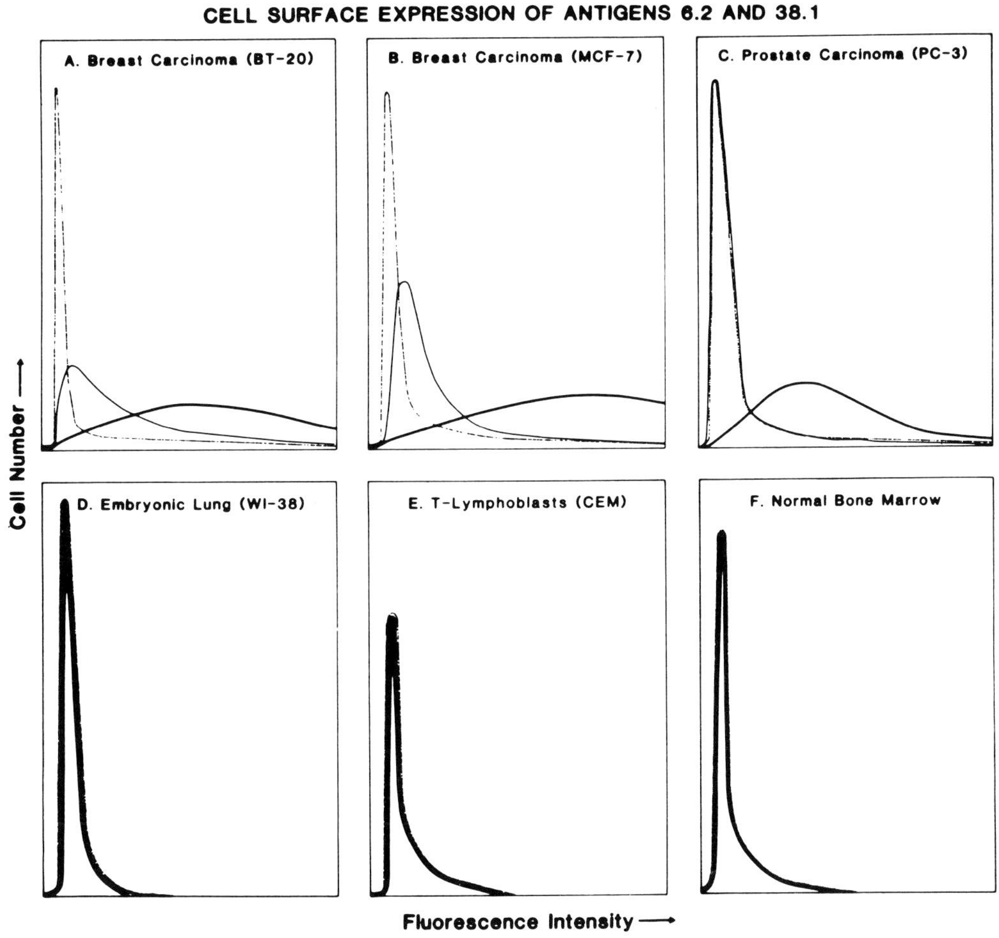

FIGURE 7. Immunofluorescence profiles of human cell lines with monoclonal antibodies B6.2 (thin line), B38.1 (thick line), and an isotype-identical control (broken line). (From Kufe, D. W., Nadler, L., Sargent, L., Shapiro, H., Hand, P., Austin, F., Colcher, D., and Schlom, J., *Cancer Res.*, 43, 851, 1983. With permission.)

Passage of these cells on Day 7 resulted in the reappearance of both antigens within 24 hr. One explanation for these results would be a cell cycle-related expression of the antigens detected by each of these MAbs.[40]

To further investigate the relationship of antigen expression to cell cycle phase, Day 7 cells at density-dependent arrest were passed and monitored 24 hr later for both DNA content and cell surface antigen expression. The relationship of DNA content to cell surface antigen expression is illustrated in Figure 9. While G_0-G_1 cells express background fluorescence, MAb B38.1 is reactive with cells in S phase. Differential binding with cells in S phase[40] is also observed for MAb B6.2. These data suggest that antigen expression, and thus successful tumor imaging, may be dependent on cell cycle kinetics. Since larger tumors may have a greater fraction of cells in the resting phase than smaller tumors,[40] more advanced neoplasms paradoxically might be less well imaged. The clinical impact of these in vitro observations has not been determined.

C. Stability

For immunoscintigraphy, the significance of cell surface antigen stability has not been established. Although some antigens may remain unaltered in the presence of a reactive

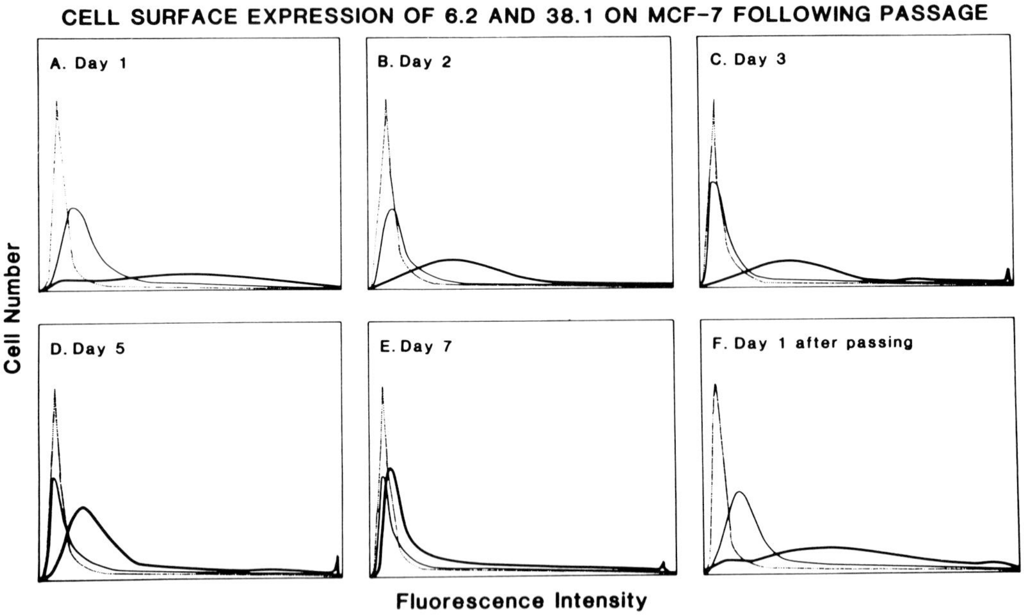

FIGURE 8. Immunofluorescence profiles of MCF-7 cells with monoclonal antibodies B6.2 (thin line), B38.1 (thick line), and an isotype-identical monoclonal antibody (broken line) at various times following passage. (From Kufe, D. W., Nadler, L., Sargent, L., Shapiro, H., Hand, P., Austin, F., Colcher, D., and Schlom, J., *Cancer Res.*, 43, 851, 1983. With permission.)

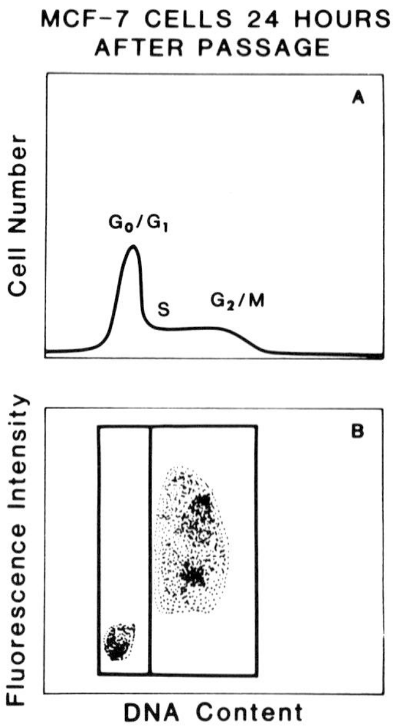

FIGURE 9. MCF-7 cells were grown to confluency and 24 hr after passage were stained with Hoechst dye (5 μg/mℓ for 1 hr at 37°C), and antibody B38.1. The cells were then stained with G/M FITC prior to analysis by (A) flow cytometry and (B) indirect immunofluorescence. (From Kufe, D. W., Nadler, L., Sargent, L., Shapiro, H., Hand, P., Austin, F., Colcher, D., and Schlom, J., *Cancer Res.*, 43, 851, 1983. With permission.)

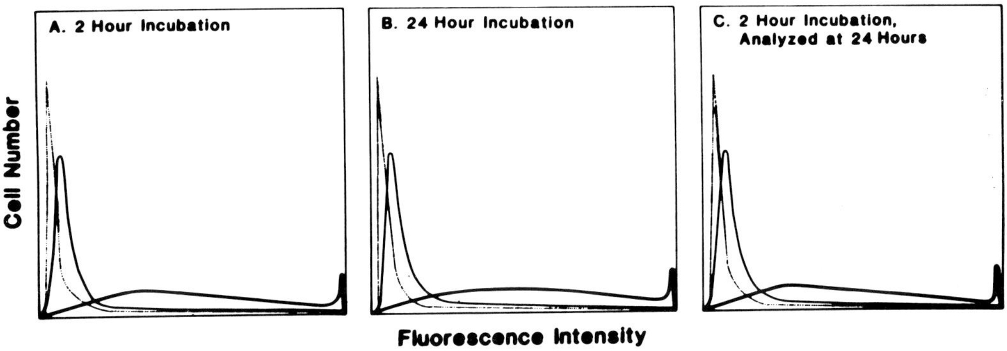

FIGURE 10. Immunofluorescence profiles of MCF-7 cells with monoclonal antibodies B6.2 (thin line), B38.1 (thick line), and an isotype-identical monoclonal antibody (broken line) following (A) a 2 hr incubation, and (B) a 24 hr incubation, and (C) a 2 hr incubation with an additional 22 hr in the absence of antibody. (From Kufe, D. W., Nadler, L., Sargent, L., Shapiro, H., Hand, P., Austin, F., Colcher, D., and Schlom, J., *Cancer Res.*, 43, 851, 1983. With permission.)

antibody,[48] others may be modulated internally or lost from the cell surface after binding with specific MAb. Furthermore, several TAA are shed into the circulation spontaneously.

1. Modulation

Internalization after exposure to specifically reactive MAb has been demonstrated for certain cell surface antigens.[49] Perhaps the most extensively characterized system is that of the common acute lymphocytic leukemia antigen (CALLA)[49,50] Loss of CALLA from the cell surface due to modulation has been suggested as one mechanism of resistance to treatment with anti-CALLA MAbs in patients with acute lymphocytic leukemia.[49,50] However, no data exist on the ability to image tumors which have undergone antigen internalization from exposure to radiolabeled MAbs. Conversely, theoretical considerations suggest that extrusion of the antigen from the cell surface after binding MAb might diminish or prevent imaging.

Thus, in vitro studies were undertaken to determine the effect of prolonged exposure of MCF-7 cells to MAbs B6.2 and B38.1 on the cell surface expression of the reactive antigens.[40] MCF-7 cells were incubated in the presence of MAb B6.2 or B38.1 for 2 or 24 hr and evaluated by indirect fluorescence analysis. The fluorescence patterns are similar for either duration of exposure as illustrated in Figure 10A and B. MCF-7 cells were also incubated with MAb for 2 hr, washed extensively, and then fed again with complete media. The cells were then incubated without MAb for an additional 22 hr, followed by indirect fluorescence analysis. The fluorescence profile (Figure 10C) is similar to that achieved during a 2- or 24-hr antibody incubation. Further, these profiles are identical to that obtained with a 30-min MAb incubation, suggesting that the membrane expression of the reactive antigens is stable despite continued exposure to antibody. Further, antigen-antibody complexes at the cell membrane remain stable in the absence of continued antibody exposure. This membrane stability of the antigen-antibody complex persists for >72 hr.[40]

The distribution of binding of MAb B6.2 on MCF-7 cells[40] is shown in Figure 11. This pattern remains unchanged despite continued antibody exposure over a 24-hr period. Furthermore, exposure of these cells to MAb B6.2 for 2 hr, and analysis by live-cell assay at 24 hr, results in a similar pattern of immunofluorescence. Identical results are obtained with antibody B38.1. These data indicate that no redistribution of antigens reactive with either antibody occurs. Thus, the evaluation of MCF-7 cells after saturation with either MAb B6.2 or MAb B38.1 has demonstrated that these cell surface antigens remain as integral components of the cell membrane without internalization or release of the antigen-antibody complex.[40]

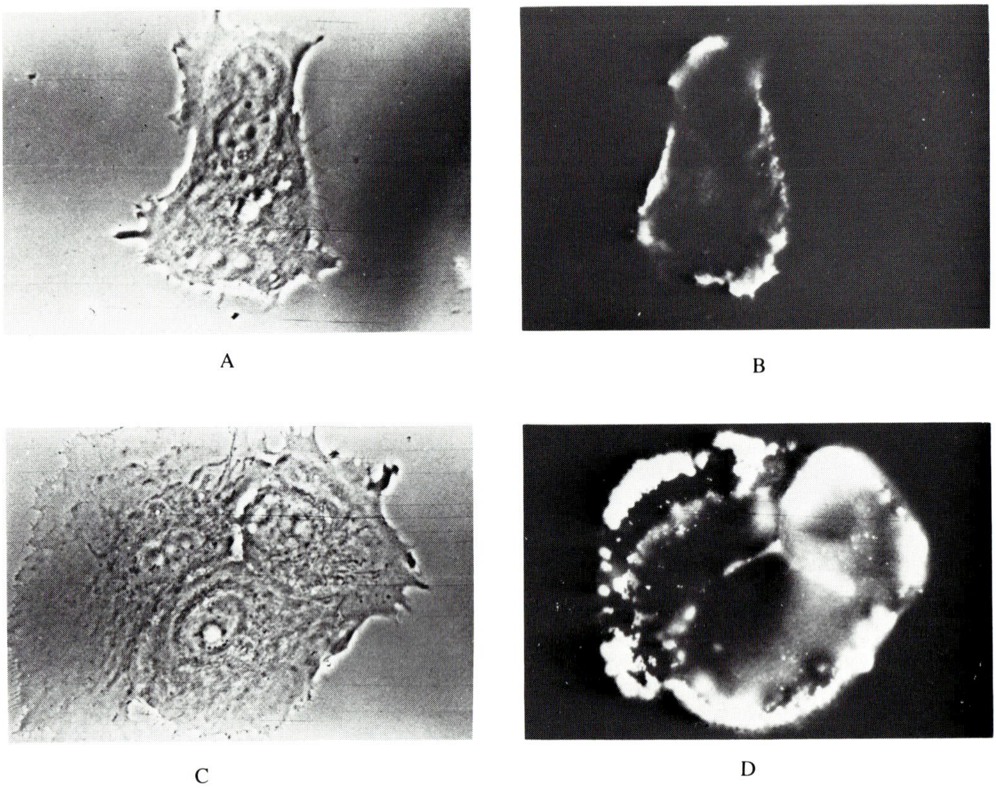

FIGURE 11. Phase contrast (A and C) and immunofluorescence staining (B and D) of MCF-7 cells following exposure to monoclonal antibody B6.2 for (A and B) 2 hr and (C and D) 24 hr. (From Kufe, D. W., Nadler, L., Sargent, L., Shapiro, H., Hand, P., Austin, F., Colcher, D., and Schlom, J., *Cancer Res.*, 43, 851, 1983. With permission.)

Although cell surface antigen stability may be of importance in immunoscintigraphy, the investigation of MAb TA99 by Welt et al.[47] suggests that it is not essential. In fact, the intracellular MAb TA99 reactive antigen may be available for interaction with the radiolabeled MAb because the antigen is shed from the cytoplasm, resulting in satisfactory images. These data require further investigation.

2. *Spontaneous Release of Cell Surface Antigen*

Interaction with circulating antigen shed from tumor cells may interfere with MAb localization. For example, Nadler et al.[51] required large doses of MAb 89 to overcome circulating "blocking factors" in order to achieve localization of a cytotoxic antilymphoma antibody. In contrast, immunoscintigraphy of colorectal cancer using an anti-CEA MAb has been successful in patients with serum CEA levels of 3000 ng/mℓ and more.[52] Thus, the presence of circulating antigen is not a sufficient indication to disregard a MAb for radioimmunoimaging.

IV. MAb-ANTIGEN BINDING KINETICS

The ability to image tumor using a radiolabeled MAb in vivo depends upon the presence of antigen in an appropriate location for interaction with the MAb. However, the characteristics of the MAb-antigen interaction are an important factor in dictating the fraction of MAb, and thus the radiolabel, which remains in the tumor following exposure of the antigen to the antibody. With directly labeled antibody, one can determine the affinity constant (K_a)

of the MAb for the reactive antigen expressed by a given cell line. Kennel et al.[53] have systematically analyzed several MAbs and suggested that those with affinity constants less than 10^8 per mole will not localize sufficiently in specific tumors to allow imaging with satisfactory resolution.

Haskell et al.[54] have confirmed these findings in an investigation of two MAbs (MAb 23 and MAb 202) which react with the same epitope on CEA. At physiologic molarity, MAb 202 has an affinity for CEA nearly twice that of MAb 23 (1.1×10^9 per mole vs. 5.7×10^8 per mole). Imaging results with radiolabeled MAb 202 are dramatically better than those with MAb 23.

However, these investigators have cautioned that the determination of K_a can be affected by experimental conditions, including the relative purity of the MAb preparation[53] and alterations in ionic strength of the buffer system.[54] For example, the affinity of MAb 23 is diminished by two logs when tested in physiologic molarity rather than low molarity buffers, while other MAbs are less affected (MAb 202) or unaffected (MAbs 35 and 192) by buffer changes.[54]

The apparent affinity of the unlabeled antibody may be modified following radiolabeling. For example, the affinity of unlabeled MAb DF3 for the reactive antigen in MCF-7 cells[60] is 1.2×10^9 per mole. However, certain methods of iodination diminish binding of MAb DF3 with the reactive antigen in MCF-7 cells, possibly due to exposure to high concentrations of oxidant.[60] Thus, the specific binding characteristics of the individual MAb, either in its native state or following modifications, may influence the success of immunoscintigraphy.

V. HETEROGENEITY

Expression of a TAA is highly influenced by tumor heterogeneity. Immunoperoxidase studies[30] have demonstrated that MAb DF3 reactivity with breast tumors is distinct from that for other antibreast MAbs such as B1.1, B6.2, and B72.3. Additionally, breast cancers from separate patients, and even metastatic lesions in multiple sites within the same patient, display heterogenous DF3 phenotypes[30] (Table 8). Furthermore, different areas within a single lesion variably express DF3 antigen (Figure 12). Thus, a single antibody may not be sufficient to achieve adequate imaging of all tumor sites in different individuals, or even within a single patient. Therefore, a ''cocktail'' of MAbs, each of which recognizes a distinct antigen or epitope, may enhance the sensitivity of radiodetection without compromising specificity. For example, the ovarian carcinoma-associated antigen identified by MAb DF3 (DF3-0) is distinct from CA125, an ovarian carcinoma-associated antigen[55] reactive with MAb OC125. Furthermore, immunoperoxidase staining demonstrates that MAb DF3 reacts with 95% of benign, borderline, and malignant tumors (serous, mucinous, endometrioid) of the ovary.[56] Malignant tumors contain cytoplasmic and total membrane DF3 antigen, while benign tumors express the antigen only on apical surfaces. This antigen is detectable by immunofluorescence on the cell surface of five of six cultured human ovarian carcinoma cell lines. The extent of ovarian carcinoma cell surface reactivity[56] with MAb DF3 is equivalent to, or greater than, that obtained with MAb OC125 (Figure 13). Furthermore, uptake of ^{125}I-labeled MAb DF3 by human ovarian carcinoma xenografts in athymic mice is 5.4- and 6.2-fold higher than the respective uptake noted in liver and control tumor. These findings suggest that DF3-0 antigen is similar, if not identical, to the antigen detected in human breast carcinomas by MAb DF3, and that the use of MAb DF3 may be complementary with OC125 in immunodetection of human epithelial ovarian carcinomas.[56]

The potential utility of such a ''cocktail'' of MAbs is supported by other investigations. Krizan et al.[57] observed that binding of five separate MAbs with cell surface antigens on human melanoma cells is complementary. The percentage of cells which were detected in an in vitro indirect immunofluorescence assay was enhanced when all five MAbs, combined

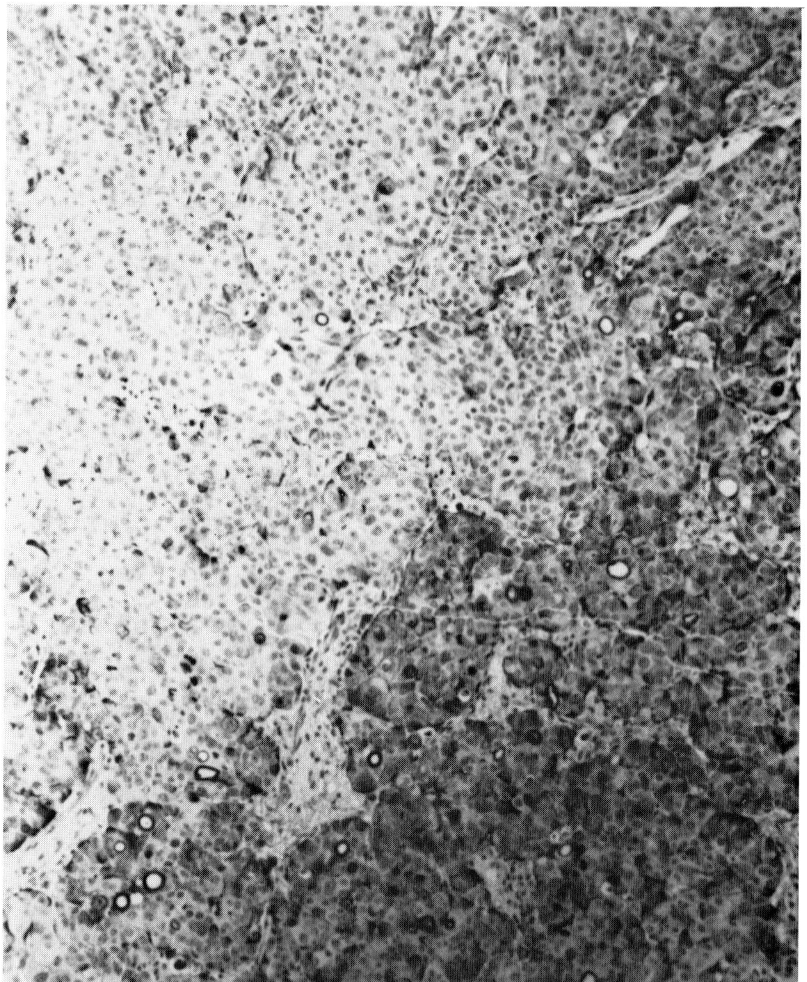

A

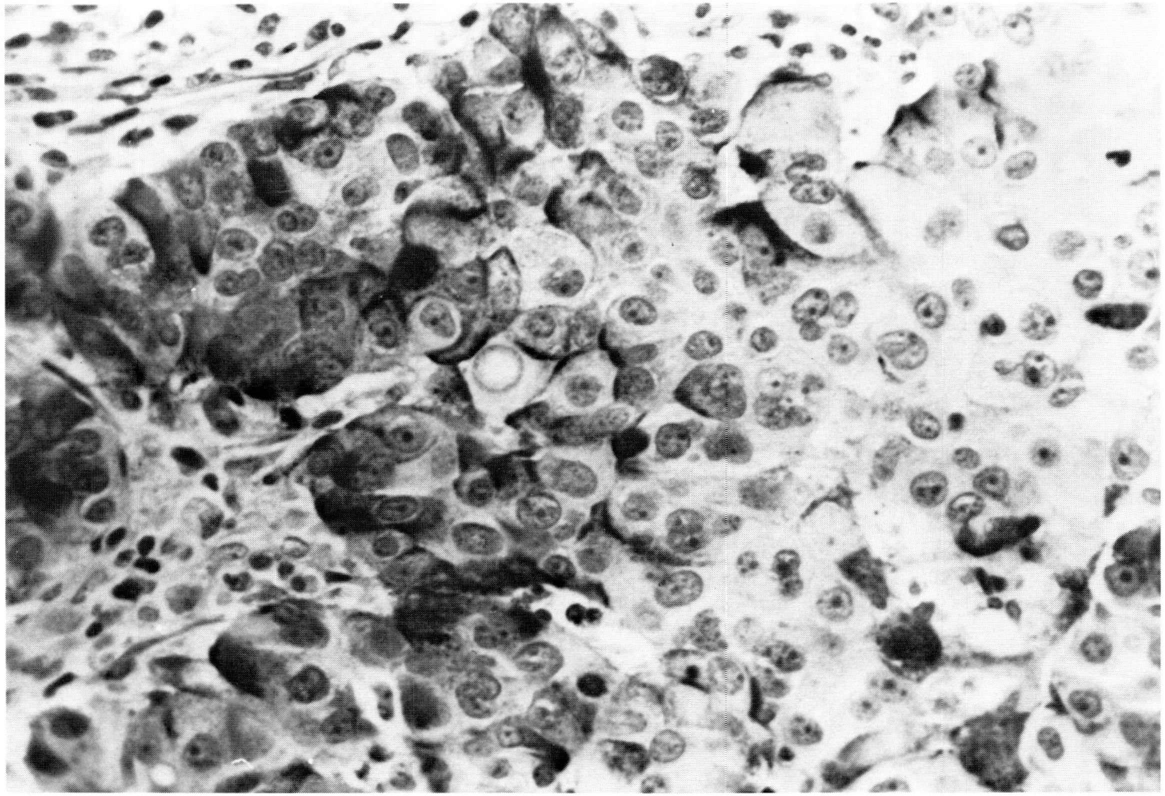

B

FIGURE 12. Heterogeneity of DF3 antigen expression by human breast carcinoma. MAb DF3 reactivity with a section of paraffin fixed infiltrating ductal breast carcinoma was evaluated with the ABC immunoperoxidase method: (A) Magnification × 2.5; (B) Higher magnification of A (Magnification × 16).

Table 8
MAb DF3 ANTIGEN DISTRIBUTION IN PRIMARY AND METASTATIC MAMMARY CARCINOMA LESIONS[a]

	% Reactive cells in tumor		
Site of tumor	**Patient #1**	**Patient #2**	**Patient #3**
Primary	60	70,100,60,80[b]	50
Metastases			
Axillary node	40	60	70,80[b]
Distant			
Bone	55	90	
Brain			50
Kidney		5	
Liver	40		
Lung	40	60,10[b]	90
Meninges		45	
Ovary		95	

[a] By immunoperoxidase staining.
[b] Different lesions.

From Kufe, D., Inghirami, G., Abe, M., Hayes, D., Justi-Wheeler, H., and Schlom, J., *Hybridoma,* 3, 223, 1984. With permission.

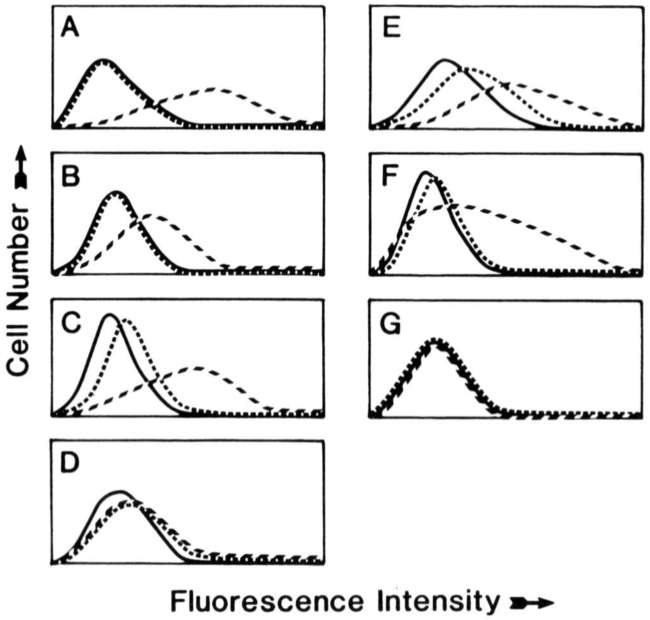

FIGURE 13. Cell surface MAb reactivity with human carcinoma cell lines. Cultured human carcinoma cell lines were incubated with MAbs DF3 (dark broken line), OC125 (light broken line), and 287 (thick, solid line), followed by fluoresceinated goat anti-mouse IgG. Fluorescence was determined by FACS: (A) breast carcinoma ZR-75-1; (B-G) ovarian carcinoma; (B) OV-A; (C) OV-D; (D) OV-M; (E) OVCAR-3; (F) OV-P; (G) OV-S. Reproduced with permission (56). (From Friedman, E. L., Hayes, D. F., and Kufe, D. W., *Cancer Res.,* 46, 5189, 1986. With permission.)

as a "cocktail", were compared to any single MAb alone. Ehrlich et al.[58] have added further support for the use of multiple MAbs. The affinity of a mixture of two MAbs, generated against different epitopes of human chorionic gonadotropin, is as much as 10-fold higher than that of either MAb alone. Thus, these studies suggest that the use of a MAb cocktail may play a significant role in future radioimmunoimaging trials.

VI. CONCLUSION

In summary, imaging of human carcinomas with labeled MAbs is a promising diagnostic modality. Sensitivity, specificity, cell membrane stability, and affinity of the TAA with which the MAb reacts may all influence the success of immunoscintigraphy. The expression of the TAA is influenced by neoplastic antigenic heterogeneity. Thus, the optimal choice of reagents may ultimately be a cocktail of MAbs generated against a variety of tumor-associated antigens.

REFERENCES

1. **Old, L. J. and Boyse, E. A.,** Immunology of experimental tumors, *Annu. Rev. Med.,* 15, 167, 1964.
2. **Klein, G.,** Experimental studies in tumor immunology, *Fed. Proc. Fed. Am. Soc. Exp. Biol.,* 28, 1739, 1969.
3. **Herbermann, R. B.,** Immunogenecity of tumor antigens, *Biochim. Biophys. Acta,* 473, 93, 1977.
4. **Sjogren, H. O., Hellstrom, I., and Klein, G.,** Resistance of polyoma virus immunized mice to transplantation of established polyoma tumors, *Exp. Cell Res.,* 23, 204, 1961.
5. **Klein, G., Sjogren, H. O., and Klein, E.,** Demonstration of host resistance against isotransplantation of lymphomas induced by the gross agent, *Cancer Res.,* 22, 955, 1962.
6. **Geering, G., Old, L. J., and Boyse, E. A.,** Antigens of leukemias induced by naturally occurring murine leukemia virus: their relation to the antigens of gross virus and other murine leukemia viruses, *J. Exp. Med.,* 124, 753, 1966.
7. **Abelev, G. I., Perova, S. D., Khramkova, N. I., Postnikova, Z. A., and Irlin, I. S.,** Production of embryonal alpha-globulin by transplantable mouse hepatomas, *Transplantation,* 1, 174, 1963.
8. **Gold, P. and Freedman, S. O.,** Demonstration of tumor-specific antigens in human colonic carcinomata by immunological tolerance and absorption techniques, *J. Exp. Med.,* 121, 439, 1965.
9. **Coggin, J. H. and Anderson, N. G.,** Cancer, differentiation and embryonic antigens: some central problems, *Adv. Cancer Res.,* 19, 105, 1974.
10. **Klein, G.,** Tumor antigens, *Annu. Rev. Microbiol.,* 20, 223, 1966.
11. **Ristow, S. and McKhann, C.,** Tumor-associated cell surface antigens, in *Mechanisms of Tumor Immunity Part I.* Green, S., Cohen, R., and McCluskey Eds., John Wiley & Sons, New York, 1977, 109.
12. **Pressman, D.,** The development and use of radiolabeled antitumor antibodies, *Cancer Res.,* 40, 2960, 1980.
13. **Spar, I. L., Bale, W. F., Marrack, D., Dewey, W. C., McCardle, R. J., and Harper, P. V.,** ^{131}I-labeled antibodies to human fibrinogen. Diagnostic studies and therapeutic trials, *Cancer (Philadelphia),* 20, 865, 1967.
14. **Bale, W. F., Spar, I. L., and Goodland, R. L.,** Experimental radiation therapy of tumors with I^{131} carrying antibodies to fibrin, *Cancer Res.,* 20, 1488, 1960.
15. **Spar, I. L., Perry, J. M., Benz, L. L., DeWeese, J. A., Mahoney, E. B., Izzo, M. J., Schwartz, S. I., and Yu, P. N.,** Detection of left atrial thrombi, *Am. Heart J.,* 78(6), 731, 1969.
16. **DeLand, F. H., Kim, E. E., Corgan, R. L., Casper, S., Primus, F. J., Spremulli, E., Estes, N., and Goldenberg, D. M.,** Axillary lymphoscintigraphy by radioimmunodetection of carcinoembryonic antigen in breast cancer, *J. Nucl. Med.,* 20, 1243, 1979.
17. **Goldenberg, D. M., DeLand, F., Kim, E., Bennett, S., Primus, F. J., van Nagell, J. R., Jr., Estes, N., DeSimone, P., and Rayburn, P.,** Use of radiolabeled antibodies to carcinoembryonic antigen for the detection and localization of diverse cancers by external photoscanning, *N. Engl. J. Med.,* 298, 1384, 1978.
18. **Goldenberg, D. M., Kim, E. E., DeLand, F. H., Bennett, S., Primus, F. J.,** Radioimmunodetection of cancer with radioactive antibodies to carcinoembryonic antigen, *Cancer Res.,* 40, 2984, 1980.

19. **Mach, J. P., Carrel, S., Forni, M., Ritschard, J., Donath, A., and Alberto, P.,** Tumor localization of radiolabeled antibodies against carcinoembryonic antigen in patients with carcinoma, *N. Engl. J. Med.*, 303, 5, 1980.
20. **Goldenberg, D. M., DeLand, F. H., Kim, E. E., and Primus, F. J.,** Xenogeneic antitumor antibodies in cancer radioimmunodetection, *Transplant. Proc.*, 12, 188, 1980.
21. **Goldenberg, D. M., Kim, E. E., DeLand, F., Spremulli, E., Nelson, M. O., Gockerman, J. P., Primus, F. J., Corgan, R. L., and Alpert, E.,** Clinical studies on the radioimmunodetection of tumors containing alpha-fetoprotein, *Cancer (Philadelphia)*, 45, 2500, 1980.
22. **Kim, E. E., DeLand, F. H., Nelson, M. O., Bennett, S., Simmons, G., Alpert, E., and Goldenberg, D. M.,** Radioimmunodetection of cancer with radiolabeled antibodies to alpha-fetoprotein, *Cancer Res.*, 40, 3008, 1980.
23. **Order, S. E., Klein, J. L., and Leichner, P. K.,** Antiferritin IgG antibody for isotopic cancer therapy, *Oncology*, 38, 154, 1981.
24. **Goldenberg, D. M., Kim, E. E., Deland, F. H., van Nagell, Jr., J. R., and Javadpour, N.,** Radioimmunodetection of cancer using radioactive antibodies to human chorionic gonadotropin, *Science*, 208, 1284, 1980.
25. **Goldenberg, D. M., Kim, E. E., and Deland, F. H.,** Human chorionic gonadotropin radioantibodies in the radioimmunodetection of cancer and for the disclosure of occult metastases, *Proc. Natl. Acad. Sci. U.S.A.*, 78, 7754, 1981.
26. **Primus, F. J. and Goldenberg, D. M.,** Immunological considerations in the use of goat antibodies to carcinoembryonic antigen for the radioimmunodetection of cancer, *Cancer Res.*, 40, 2979, 1980.
27. **Sekine, H., Ohno, T., and Kufe, D. W.,** Purification and characterization of a high molecular weight glycoprotein detectable in human milk and breast carcinomas, *J. Immunol.*, 135, 3610, 1985.
28. **Hsu, S.-M., Raine, L., and Fanger, H.,** Use of avidin-biotin-peroxidase complex (ABC) in immunoperoxidase techniques: a comparison between ABC and unlabeled antibody (PAP) procedures, *J. Histochem. Cytochem.*, 29, 577, 1981.
29. **Kabawat, S. E., Bast, R. C., Welch, W. R., Knapp, R. C., and Colvin, R. B.,** Immunopathologic characterization of a monoclonal antibody that recognizes common surface antigens of human ovarian tumors of serous, endometrioid, and clear cell types, *Am. J. Clin. Pathol.*, 79, 98, 1983.
30. **Kufe, D., Inghirami, G., Abe, M., Hayes, D., Justi-Wheeler, H., and Schlom, J.,** Differential reactivity of a novel monoclonal antibody (DF3) with human malignant versus benign breast tumors, Hybridoma 3, 223, 1984.
31. **Hayes, D. F., Zalutsky, M. R., Kaplan, W., Noska, M., Thor, A., Colcher, D., and Kufe, D. W.,** Pharmacokinetics of radiolabeled monoclonal antibody B6.2 in patients with metastatic breast cancer, *Cancer Res.*, 46, 3157, 1986.
32. **Dillman, R. O., Beauregard, J. C., Sobol, R. E., Royston, I., Bartholomew, R.-M., Hagan, P. S., and Halpern, S. E.,** Lack of radioimmunodetection and complications associated with monoclonal anticarcinoembryonic antigen antibody cross-reactivity with an antigen on circulating cells, *Cancer Res.*, 44, 2213, 1984.
33. **Colcher, D., Horan Hand, P., Nuti, M., and Schlom, J.,** A spectrum of monoclonal antibodies reactive with human mammary tumor cells, *Proc. Natl. Acad. Sci. U.S.A.*, 78, 3199, 1981.
34. **Keenan, A. M., Harbert, J. C., and Larson, S. M.,** Monoclonal antibodies in nuclear medicine, *J. Nucl. Med.*, 26, 531, 1985.
35. **Wessels, B. W. and Rogus, R. D.,** Radionuclide selection and model absorbed dose calculations for radiolabeled tumor associated antibodies, *Medical Phys.*, 11, 638, 1984.
36. **Dillman, R. O.,** Monoclonal antibodies in the treatment of cancer, *Crit. Rev. Oncol. Hematol.*, 1, 357, 1984.
37. **Meeker, T. C., Lowder, J., Maloney, D. G., Miller, R. A., Thielemans, K., Warnke, R., and Levy, R.,** A clinical trial of anti-idiotype therapy for B cell malignancy, *Blood*, 65, 1349, 1985.
38. **Sears, H. F., Herlyn, D., Steplewski, Z., and Koprowski, H.,** Phase II clinical trial of a murine monoclonal antibody cytotoxic for gastrointestinal adenocarcinoma, *Cancer Res.*, 45, 5910, 1985.
39. **Stahel, R. A., Mabry, M., Sabbath, K., Speak, J. A., Bernal, S. D.,** Selective cytotoxicity of murine monoclonal antibody LAM2 against human small-cell carcinoma in the presence of human complement: possible use for in vitro elimination of tumor cells from bone marrow, *Int. J. Cancer*, 35, 587, 1985.
40. **Kufe, D. W., Nadler, L., Sargent, L., Shapiro, H., Hand, P., Austin, F., Colcher, D., and Schlom, J.,** Biological behavior of human breast carcinoma-associated antigens expressed during cellular proliferation, *Cancer Res.*, 43, 851, 1983.
41. **Weinstein, J. N., Parker, R. J., Holton, O. D., III, Keenan, A. M., Covell, D. G., Black, C. D. V., and Sieber, S. M.,** Lymphatic delivery of monoclonal antibodies: potential for detection and treatment of lymph node metastases, *Cancer Invest.*, 3, 85, 1985.

42. **Thompson, C. H., Lichtenstein, M., Stacker, S. A., Leyden, M. J., Salehi, N., Andrews, J. T., and McKenzie, I. F. C.,** Immunoscintigraphy for detection of lymph node metastases from breast cancer, *Lancet,* 2, 1245, 1984.
43. The Hammersmith Oncology Group and the Imperial Cancer Research Fund, Antibody-guided irradiation of malignant lesions: three cases illustrating a new method of treatment, *Lancet,* 1, 1441, 1984.
44. **Abe, M. and Kufe, D.,** Identification of a distinct family of high molecular weight tumor-associated glycoproteins, *J. Immun.,* 139, 257, 1987.
45. **Hayes, D. F., Zurawski, V. R., Jr., and Kufe, D. W.,** Comparison of circulating CA15-3 and carcinoembryonic antigen levels in patients with breast cancer, *J. Clin. Oncol.,* 4, 1542, 1986.
46. **Hilkens, J., Buijs, F., Hilgers, J., Hageman, Ph., Calafat, J., Sonnenberg, A., van der Valk, M.,** Monoclonal antibodies against human milk-fat globule membranes detecting differentiation antigens of the mammary gland and its tumors, *Int. J. Cancer,* 34, 197, 1984.
47. **Welt, S., Grando, R., Mattes, M. J., Thomson, T. M., Leonard, R. W., Zanzonico, P. B., Bigler, R. E., Yeh, S., Oettgen, H. F., and Old, L. J.,** Monoclonal antibody localization to a cycloplasmic antigen of melanoma heterotransplants in nu/nu mice: imaging at 8-10 weeks, *Proc. Am. Soc. Clin. Oncol.,* 5, (Abstr.) 904, 1986.
48. **Hellstrom, I., Brown, J. P., and Hellstrom, K. E.,** Melanoma-associated antigen p97 continues to be expressed after prolonged exposure of cells to specific antibody, *Int. J. Cancer,* 31, 553, 1983.
49. **Ritz, J., Pesando, J. M., Notis-McConarty, J., and Schlossman, S. F.,** Modulation of human acute lymphoblastic leukemia antigen induced by monoclonal antibody in vitro, *J. Immunol.,* 125, 1506, 1980.
50. **Pesando, J. M., Tomaselli, K. J., Lazarus, H., and Schlossman, S. F.,** Distribution and modulation of a human leukemia-associated antigen (CALLA), *J. Immunol.,* 131, 2038, 1983.
51. **Nadler, L. M., Stashenko, P., Hardy, R., Kaplan, W. D., Dutton, L. N., Kufe, D. W., Antman, K. H., and Schlossman, S. F.,** Serotherapy of a patient with a monoclonal antibody directed against a human lymphoma-associated antigen, *Cancer Res.,* 40, 3147, 1980.
52. **Goldenberg, D. M., Kim, E. E., Bennett, S. J., Nelson, M. O., and Deland, F. H.,** Carcinoembryonic antigen radioimmunodetection in the evaluation of colorectal cancer and in the detection of occult neoplasms, *Gastroenterology,* 84, 524, 1983.
53. **Kennel, S. J., Foote, L. J., Lankford, P. K., Johnson, M., Mitchell, T., and Braslawsky, G. R.,** Direct binding of radioiodinated monoclonal antibody to tumor cells: significance of antibody purity and affinity for drug targeting or tumor imaging, *Hybridoma,* 2, 297, 1983.
54. **Haskell, C. M., Buchegger, F., Schreyer, M., Carrel, S., and Mach, J.-P.,** Monoclonal antibodies to carcinoembryonic antigen: ionic strength as a factor in the selection of antibodies for immunoscintigraphy, *Cancer Res.,* 43, 3857, 1983.
55. **Sekine, H., Hayes, D. F., Ohno, T., Keefe, K. A., Schaetzl, E., Bast, R. C., Knapp, R., and Kufe, D. W.,** Circulating DF3 and CA 125 antigen levels in serum from patients with epithelial ovarian carcinoma, *J. Clin. Oncol.,* 3, 1355, 1985.
56. **Friedman, E. L., Hayes, D. F., and Kufe, D. W.,** Reactivity of monoclonal antibody DF3 with a high molecular weight antigen expressed in human ovarian carcinomas, *Cancer Res.,* 46, 5189, 1986.
57. **Krizan, Z., Murray, J. L., Hersh, E. M., Rosenblum, M. G., Glenn, H. J., Gschwind, C. R., and Carlo, D. J.,** Increased labeling of human melanoma cells in vitro using combinations of monoclonal antibodies recognizing separate cell surface antigenic determinants, *Cancer Res.,* 45, 4904, 1985.
58. **Ehrlich, P. H., Moyle, W. R., Moustafa, Z. A., and Canfield, R. E.,** Mixing two monoclonal antibodies yields enhanced affinity for antigen, *J. Immunol.,* 128, 2709, 1982.
59. **Kufe, D. W., Hayes, D. F., Abe, M., Ohno, T., Lundy, J., and Schlom, J.,** Monoclonal antibody assays for breast cancer, in *Cancer Diagnosis In Vitro Using Monoclonal Antibodies,* Kupchik, H. Z., Ed., Marcel Dekker, New York, 1988, 67.
60. **Hayes, D. F., Noska, M., Kufe, D. W., and Zalutsky, M. R.,** Effect of radioiodination on the binding of monoclonal antibody DF3 to breast carcinoma cells, *Nucl. Med. Biol.,* 15, 235, 1988.

Chapter 5

RADIOCHEMISTRY OF HALOGENATED ANTIBODIES

Janet F. Eary, Kenneth A. Krohn, Raj Kishore, and Wil B. Nelp

TABLE OF CONTENTS

I. INTRODUCTION

The most authentic radiolabeled antibody is probably one prepared as a natural product grown in a medium containing ^{35}S or ^{75}Se labeled methionine or another amino acid labeled with ^{3}H or ^{14}C. These labels are completely impractical for radioimmunoscintigraphy or radioimmunotherapy because of the nuclear characteristics of the radioisotopes and/or their low specific activities. As a practical alternative, two general schemes of introducing heteroatomic labels into antibodies have been developed: covalent labels with radiohalogens and bifunctional chelate complexes with radioactive metals. The purpose of this chapter is to review the state of the art in radiohalogenated antibodies and to suggest future research directions.

In preparation of this review, a computerized literature search was performed to survey the current trends in antibody iodination methodology. The search was constrained in three ways, requiring that the reference include ''antibodies'' and ''isotope labeling'' and ''iodine, iodine isotopes, or iodination''. The search yielded 63 references that have been reviewed and will be selectively cited. Equal numbers of these papers used the chloramine-T and the Iodogen methods, with only three referring to lactoperoxidase and one referring to the electrolytic methods.

The relative merit of chelation labels vs. halogen labels remains the subject of controversy in the antibody radiopharmaceutical literature. In this chapter, several criteria are accepted in choosing an appropriate label for an antibody. Ideally, the investigator strives to find an optimum balance between each of these criteria; any study that emphasizes one aspect with total neglect of the others has been viewed with skepticism in our review of the literature. The criteria we use in selecting an appropriate antibody label are as follows:

1. The labeling procedure should preserve the biological activity of the antibody molecule.
2. The radioisotope should remain bound to the antibody in vivo, and remain at the site where it is delivered.
3. The isotope should have acceptable nuclear properties, including half-life, gamma energies, and particle emissions. This criteria will be different if the goal is radioimmunoscintigraphy or radioimmunotherapy.
4. Convenience and cost should not be considerations in selecting a label until the overall value of radiolabeled antibodies has been demonstrated.

II. CHEMISTRY AND RADIOCHEMISTRY OF HALOGENS FOR ANTIBODY LABELING

A. Iodine

Historically, antibodies have been radiolabeled with iodine isotopes because of the availability of ^{125}I and ^{131}I and the ease of performing iodine conjugations to various amino acid residues of protein molecules. Iodine-125 is a convenient isotope for in vitro work because of its low principal photon energy (28 KeV). With a 60.2-day half-life ($T_{1/2}$), it is suitable for experimental systems in which a number of observations over weeks are required. Since the low energy photons are easily attenuated, care must be taken to count samples in identical geometries. Iodine-131 with beta particle emission, a 364 KeV principal gamma photon and a $T_{1/2}$ of 8.04 days (Table 1), is the most widely used radiohalogen for in vivo imaging studies. It has been used for years in the treatment of thyroid cancer and is now being used in Curie quantities for radioiodination of antibodies for radioimmunotherapy.[1]

Iodine-123, with no beta particle emission, a 159-KeV principal gamma photon and a $T_{1/2}$ of 13.3 hr, remains the most attractive radiohalogen for imaging because its half-life is convenient and its photon energy is compatible with scintillation cameras. In the past,

Table 1
SPECIFIC ACTIVITIES AVAILABLE FOR RADIOHALOGENS

Isotope	$T_{1/2}$ (days)	Specific activity (Ci/mmol)	Dilution factor[a]	Ref.
^{125}I	60.1	2.13×10^3	1.02	Catalog
^{131}I	8.04	1.6×10^3—3.3×10^3	5.0—10.3	Catalog
^{123}I	0.54	2.4×10^4—1.6×10^5	1.5—10.0	Manuel Lagunas-Solar
^{77}Br	2.33	2.0×10^3—4.5×10^3	12.4—28.0	Los Alamos
^{18}F	0.076	2.5×10^4—9.5×10^4	18.0—68.4	Fowler JNM 1985
^{211}At	0.30	4.35×10^5	Diluted with iodine	Dick Lambrecht

[a] Total atoms/radioactive atoms.

availability of high grade ^{123}I for radiopharmaceutical use has been limited and it has been relatively costly. This situation is improving slowly. There are a few reports of ^{123}I-labeled antibodies used with SPECT imaging.[2] Because of its short $T_{1/2}$, ^{123}I may be unsuitable for radioimmunoimaging with whole antibodies where imaging as late as 48 to 72 hr following administration is desirable, but its importance will increase as the use of antibody fragments gains wider acceptance and imaging intervals are shortened.

B. Bromine and Fluorine

C–Br bonds are 10 to 15 Kcal stronger than comparable C–I bonds, but bromine isotopes are not often used in protein labeling procedures. A further advantage of bromine over iodine for in vivo studies is that there is no uptake of the ion by thyroid tissue; bromide ion equilibrates in the extracellular space.[3] Bromine-77 has a half-life of 56 hr and 239-KeV (30%) and 521-KeV (21%) gamma emissions. One can use ^{77}Br for imaging, however, these energies are not optimal for gamma cameras. Isotopes 74, 75, and 76 of bromine all have half-lives which are short in relation to the serum half-life of antibodies and their fragments. Perhaps the most promising is ^{76}Br, which has a half-life of 16.2 hr and decays by positron emission (57%), but we are unaware of any attempts to label MAbs with this isotope.

The longest-lived fluorine isotope, ^{18}F, is a positron emitter, but also has a short half-life, 110 min. The C–F bond has a high dissociation energy, with probably good in vivo stability, but direct fluorinations are difficult and often harsh. Reactions involving fluorination of prosthetic groups and subsequent syntheses have been developed.[4] Methyl 3-[^{18}F]-fluoro-5-nitrobenzimidate and 4-[^{18}F]-fluorophenacyl bromide have been prepared in 30 to 50% yields within 50 to 70 min after production of ^{18}F by cyclotron barbardment. Both have been coupled to immunoglobulins in 95% yield and can be rapidly purified by chromatography, but the immunointegrity of the products has not been critically evaluated. The advantages of positron-emitting isotopes for quantitative tomographic imaging and the ease of producing large amounts of ^{18}F make this a likely subject for future research.

C. Astatine

^{211}At, an isotope with a 7.21-hr half-life, has been considered for applications where alpha particle-emitting therapeutic agents are desired. ^{211}At decays by electron capture (58.1%) and the emission of alphas (41.9%) at 5.866 MeV. Astatination of MAbs is described in Chapter 2 of this volume and deserves extensive additional research effort.

III. CHEMISTRY OF PROTEIN IODINATION

Iodine exists in oxidation states of +1, +5, and +7, in addition to −1, which is the most stable state for halogens in aqueous solution. The −1 oxidation state (iodide ion) does

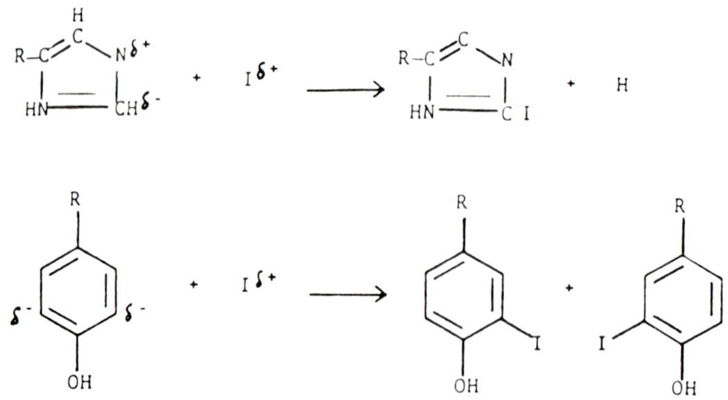

FIGURE 1. Iodination.

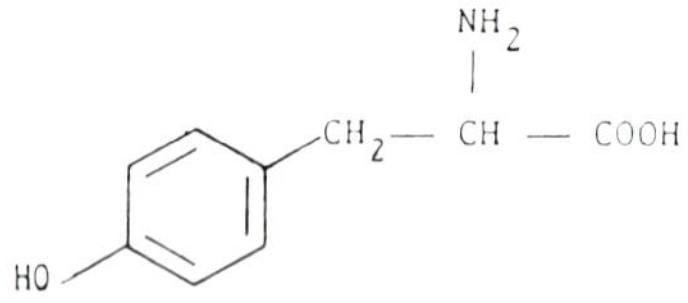

FIGURE 2. Tyrosine.

not react with protein molecules. Most iodination methods (Figure 1) involve the conversion of chemically stable I^- ion to quasi-stable I^+ before substitution for hydrogen in aromatic amino acid residues. The substitutions take place at atomic sites which are the most electronegative.

A. Sites of Iodination

The iodination of an immunoglobulin can take place on several amino acids — tyrosine (tyr), histidine (his), cysteine (cys), methionine (met), phenylalanine (phe), and tryptophan (trp). Under normal conditions, most of the iodination takes place at tyrosine residues, but under some conditions histidine and phenylalanine are labeled.

1. Tyrosine (Figure 2)

The hydroxyl group on the tyrosyl residue is an electron-donating substituent which delocalizes the negative charge into the benzene ring. The positions ortho to it are electronegative and attractive for substitution by electrophiles. Reactivity of the tyrosyl residues in a protein can be altered by steric factors related to the conformation of the protein or chemical blockage of the residues. Steric blockage takes place when the large iodine atom is not able to approach the negatively charged ortho sites on the tyrosyl ring. Chemical blockage of the iodination sites results from substitution of the ortho positions or chemical modification of the hydroxyl groups. Substitutions in the benzene ring of tyrosine can also increase its reactivity toward electrophilic substitutions. The pK value of tyrosine, 10.2, is lowered to 8.2 by monoiodination and to 6.4 by diiodination.[5] The practical result of this pK change is that the second step in diiodination of tyrosine takes place faster than monoiodination.

2. Histidine (Figure 3)

Histidine contains an imidazole ring which reacts with electrophilic iodinating agents, though less readily than tyrosine. The site of monoiodination is adjacent to the side chain. Diiodination at the other ring carbon position also occurs.[5,6]

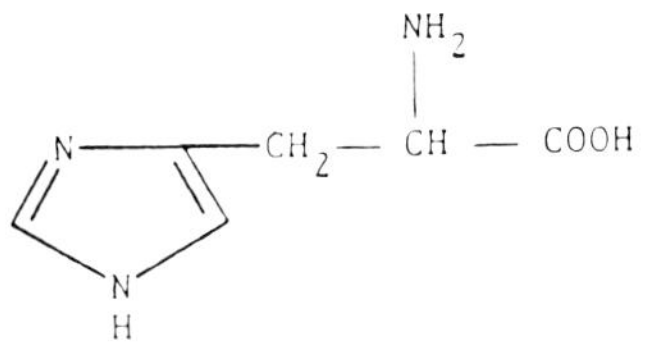

FIGURE 3. Histidine.

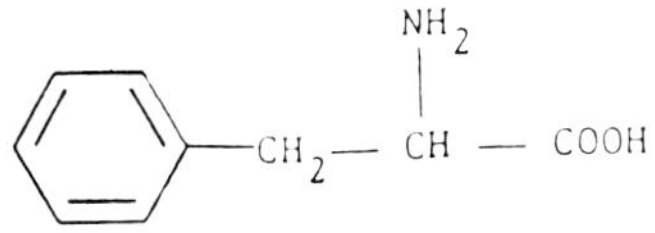

FIGURE 4. Phenylalanine.

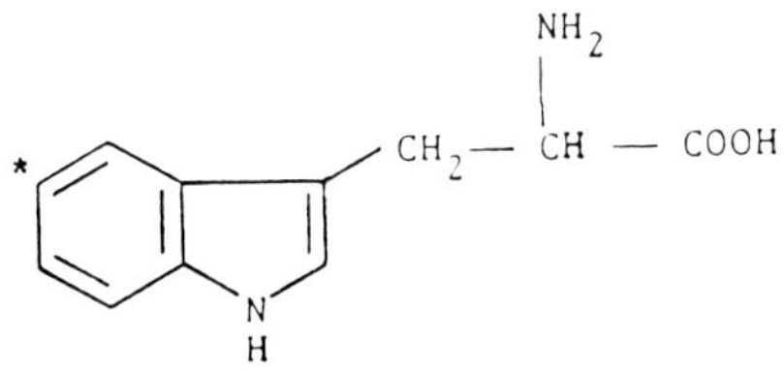

FIGURE 5. Tryptophan.

3. Phenylalanine (Figure 4)

Phenylalanine lacks the activating phenolic group of the tyrosine residue and is, therefore, much less reactive towards electrophilic iodination. However, iodination has been reported at the para position in very highly iodinated proteins[7] and the potential for iodination of phenylalanine is discussed in more detail in Section VI.A of this chapter.

4. Cysteine and Methionine

Cysteine contains a highly reactive sulfhydryl group which dimerizes under mildly oxidizing conditions. Under acidic conditions the substitution of the sulfhydryl proton by I also occurs, to yield sulfenyl iodide. The RS–I bond is not very stable and dissociates spontaneously with time. Further oxidation yields sulfenyl periodide, RSI_3, which is even more unstable. Methionine reacts readily with iodine in neutral and alkaline solutions to form CH_3-S(I)-$(CH_2)_2$-CH(NH_2)COOH. Depending on their location in the protein molecule, methionine residues vary in their susceptibility to iodination.

5. Tryptophan (Figure 5)

Tryptophan can be iodinated at the position para to the indole nitrogen at high pH with I_2, as well as with other electrophilic iodinating agents. Reaction of iodine with tryptophan residues does not appear to be a significant factor in protein iodination.[5]

B. Electrophilic Methods of Iodination

Almost all methods of radioiodination involve the use of oxidizing agents to convert iodide ion, I^-, to a positive oxidation state or the use of iodine in a partially electropositive oxidation state, such as in ICl. The various electrophilic radioiodination methods which have been used for antibody labeling are summarized in this section.

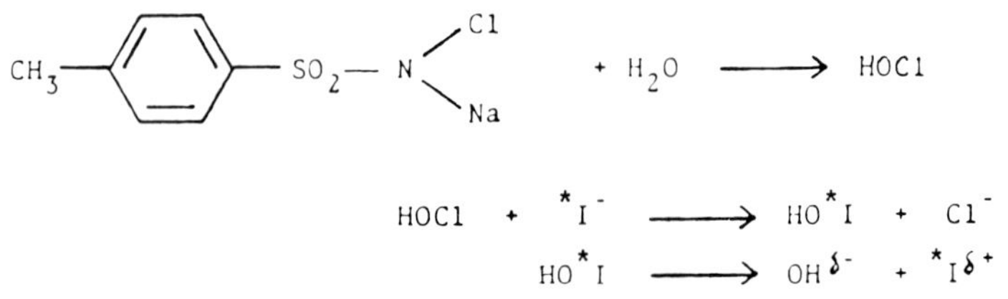

FIGURE 6. Chloramine-T Iodination.

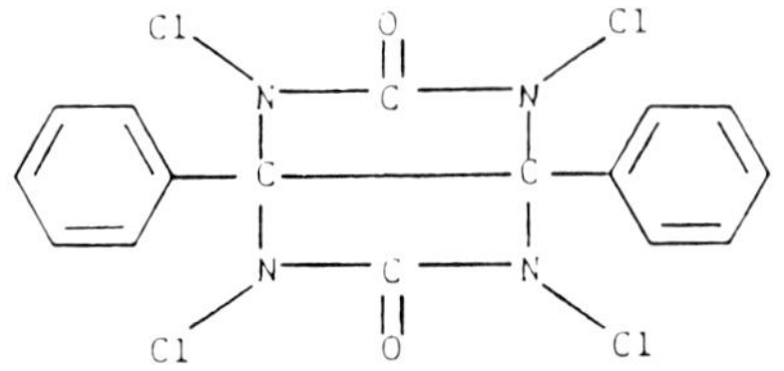

FIGURE 7. Iodogen.

1. Chloramine-T Method

Chloramine-T (N-chloro-4-methylbenzenesulfonamide sodium salt) (Figure 6) is an oxidizing agent that was first used for protein iodination by Hunter and Greenwood.[8,9] They recommended the use of 50 to 100 μg chloramine-T for iodination in volumes of 100 to 200 μℓ and reaction times of 30 to 50 sec. The reaction can be terminated by addition of $NaHSO_3$ or $Na_2S_2O_3$, followed by carrier NaI.

Our laboratory has used 22.8 μg of chloramine-T per mg of antibody in volumes of 1 to 2 mℓ with good MAb iodination yields.[1] Under these conditions the reaction time is increased to 5 to 10 min. Chloramine-T is a potent oxidizing agent and is capable of denaturing labile immunoglobulins by breaking peptide bonds.[10,11] Because of this, the amount of chloramine-T and the reaction time should be optimized for both labeling efficiency and retention of immunoreactivity for each antibody. The best labeling efficiency is obtained at pH 7.2. However, NaI containing radioiodine undergoes oxidation at this pH to IO_3^- and other unidentified forms of iodine,[7] resulting in lower iodination yields. It is best to store radioiodine in 0.1 *N* NaOH solution and to adjust the pH to 7.2 just before iodination by the addition of a suitable buffer, such as 0.5 *M* phosphate buffered saline (PBS).

Markwell[12] has described a method in which chloramine-T is immobilized on polystyrene beads. These modified polystyrene beads are now available under the trade name "Iodobeads" (Pierce Chemical Company, Rockford, Ill.). Each bead has an oxidative capacity of 0.55 μmol. Iodination can be performed by adding the required number of Iodobeads to a mixture of radioactive iodide and immunoglobulin in 0.1 to 1 mℓ. The reaction is allowed to proceed for about 15 min and is terminated by physical separation of the reaction mixture from the beads. The technique has the advantage of convenience and simplicity, as well as the freedom from chemical contaminations which are introduced in the standard chloramine-T procedure.

2. Iodogen Method

Fraker and Speck[13] first described the use of 1,3,4,6-tetrachloro-3α,6α-diphenylglycouril (Iodogen) as a reagent for the iodination of proteins (Figure 7). The chief advantage of Iodogen is its insolubility in water. Procedurally, Iodogen is dissolved in chloroform or methylene chloride and then evaporated on the inside walls of a reaction vial. It can be stored in this form in a dessicator. The iodination mixture, containing the immunoglobulin and Na*I in the appropriate buffer, is added to the Iodogen-coated reaction vial. The reaction is allowed to proceed for 10 to 15 min and is terminated by the transfer of the reaction mixture to a noncoated tube.

3. Lactoperoxidase Method

Marchalonis[14] first described an iodination method using enzymes to iodinate proteins and Thorell and Johansson[15] modified the procedure to its present form. Lactoperoxidase is obtained from bovine milk and, in the presence of H_2O_2, catalyzes the oxidation of iodide to a reactive species which results in the iodination of immunoglobulins and other proteins. Typically, the reaction is carried out in a small volume (50 to 100 $\mu\ell$) in the presence of 1 to 5 μg lactoperoxidase and 5 to 10 $\mu\ell$ H_2O_2. The reaction is allowed to run for 15 to 30 min and is terminated by the addition of cysteine or by a tenfold dilution. The disadvantages of this technique are the low iodination efficiency and the need to separate iodinated MAb from iodinated lactoperoxidase. The advantages lie in the mildness of the reaction conditions and complete specificity for exposed tyrosyl residues.

Enzymobead reagent (Bio-Rad Laboratories, Richmond, Calif.) consists of both glucose oxidase and lactoperoxidase enzymes covalently bound to small hydrophilic polyacrylamide beads.[16,17] In the presence of glucose, glucose oxidase produces a small but continuous amount of hydrogen peroxide. The reaction is started by adding glucose to a suspension of Enzymobeads, immunoglobulin, and Na*I. After 15 to 25 min the reaction is terminated by either centrifugation or gel filtration. This method combines the advantages of enzymatic iodination with the solid phase separation of the Iodobead and Iodogen techniques.

4. Electrolytic Method

Rosa et al.[18] first described a method for electrolytic iodination and applied it to the labeling of fibrinogen. A platinum crucible containing protein in phosphate buffer at pH 7.5 serves as the anode. Platinum foil encased in a glass tube with a dialysis membrane on the lower end serves as the cathode. After the addition of Na*I, a 1 mA current is passed for 30 to 90 min. Iodination takes place at the surface of the anode. This method does not utilize chemical oxidizing agents or enzymes and is capable of producing very pure uniformly iodinated preparations. The procedure is done with addition of carrier NaI and, hence, has not been widely used for antibody labeling.

C. Conjugation Methods

Even though most antibodies can be labeled with iodine using the techniques described above, these methods may not result in suitable products under any one of the following conditions:

1. If the amino acid residue most easily iodinated is located within the antigen binding site, iodination could result in loss of immunoreactivity.
2. When iodinatable residues are sterically inaccessible, the protein is refractory to iodination. This is more likely to be the case with Fab and $F(ab')_2$ fragments where the Fc position, which has a high proportion of tyrosine residues, is absent.
3. The presence of multiple free sulfhydryl (SH) groups causes a reducing environment and blocks electrophilic iodination.

When any of the above conditions are present, the iodination of the antibody may still be successfully achieved by conjugating a preiodinated molecule to the antibody. This section discusses examples of conjugation reactions.

1. Bolton-Hunter Reagent

The N-hydroxysuccinimide ester of p-hydroxyphenylpropionic acid (SHPP) (Figure 8)

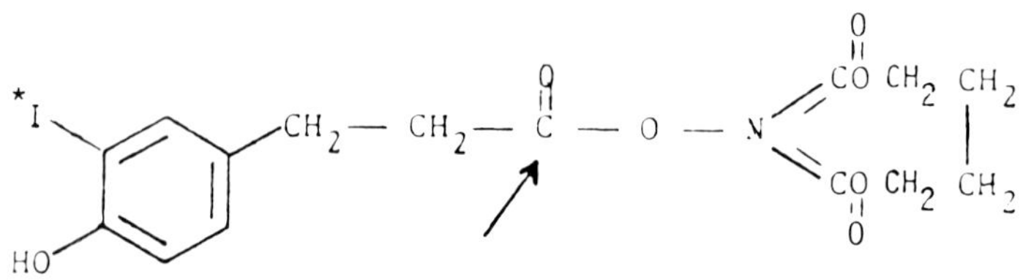

FIGURE 8. Bolton-Hunter Reagent.

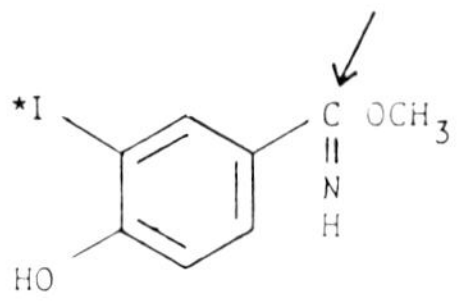

FIGURE 9. Wood's Reagent.

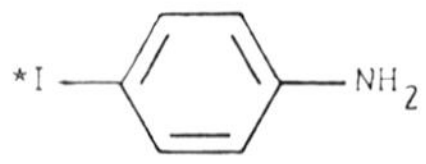

FIGURE 10. p-Iodoanaline.

can be iodinated using the chloramine-T method. This technique was first described by Bolton and Hunter.[19] Iodinated SHPP conjugates with proteins to form amide bonds with the terminal group of lysine at the position indicated in Figure 8 by the arrow. The location of iodine in SHPP is analagous to that in iodinated tyrosine. One of the major drawbacks of this method is the susceptibility of SHPP to hydrolysis during iodination and conjugation. Water competes with the terminal — NH_2 groups of the MAb and results in a lowering of yield. There is also a possibility of antibody denaturation with the organic solvents used for SHPP.

2. Wood's Reagent

The use of methyl p-hydroxylbenzimidate for protein iodination was first described by Wood et al[20] (Figure 9). This reagent can also be iodinated using chloramine-T and the compound is stable in aqueous solutions. When the iodoimidoester is incubated with protein, it couples with the terminal amino group of a lysine at the location marked in Figure 9 with the arrow. The advantage of this method is its resistance to hydrolysis compared to the Bolton-Hunter reagent. The disadvantage is that conjugation frequently requires hours compared to seconds for SHPP. This reaction is similar to the method for introducing ^{18}F that was described in Section II.B above.

3. p-Iodoaniline

This procedure was described by Hayes and Goldstein[21] specifically for iodination of lectins and papain. In this method an aniline (Figure 10) is first iodinated, again using the chloramine-T method. The presence of an amino group on the benzene ring activates it to iodination, very much like a phenolic group, although the NH_2 is less effective. Iodination takes place at the para and ortho positions and the resulting iodoaniline can be diazotized for coupling to the protein. This technique merits further evaluation since iodoaniline structures may not be enzymatically deiodinated as easily as tyrosine.

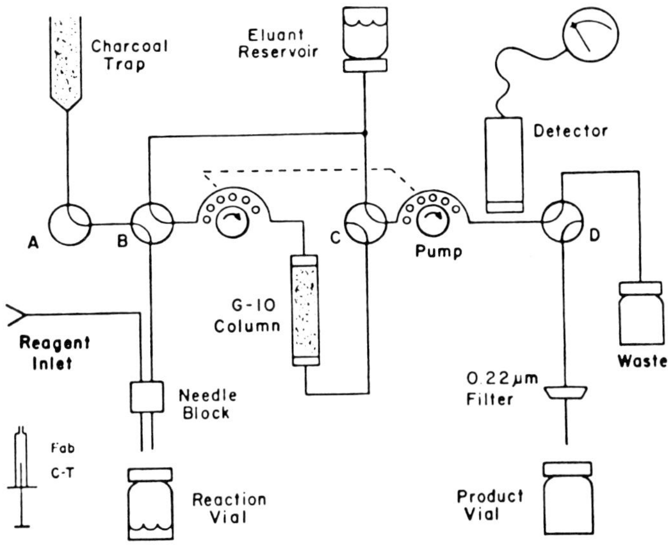

FIGURE 11. Schematic of Iodination Reactor. (From Ferens, J. M. et al., *J. Nucl. Med.*, 25, 367, 1984. With permission.)

4. Photoaffinity Methods

Heterobifunctional reagents which can be photoactivated can be used for conjugation to antibodies. Several such reagents have been described by Ji and Ji[22] and by Tejedor and Ballista.[23] The N-hydroxysuccinimide ester of 4-azidosalicylic acid (NHS-ASA) is commercially available as an ^{125}I derivative or it can be synthesized the using the procedure described by Ji and Ji.[22] Photolabeling of the protein is carried out by mixing it with the bifunctional reagent and irradiating the mixture with UV light. These methods have primarily been used for labeling surface membrane proteins, but they may be effective for some specialized applications of antibody labeling.

D. Special Techniques for High-Level Labeling

In our laboratory, the chloramine-T method is preferred over other methods for high-level iodinations for several reasons.[1] The iodine monochloride method requires addition of carrier iodine which reduces specific activity. The lactoperoxidase method introduces foreign protein which complicates the subsequent purification of the radioiodinated monoclonal antibody prior to human administration. Iodogen requires the potentially hazardous transfer of large amounts of volatile radioiodine from the shipping vial to a precoated labeling vial. For reasons of radiation safety, this method is avoided in high activity labelings, although it is satisfactory and often advantageous at lower activity levels.[24] Iodinations using the chloramine-T method can be carried out in the original shipping vial and do not require the addition of carrier iodine. The product can be easily purified by gel chromatography and overcomes the objections to each of the other techniques.

With our high level chloramine-T method, approximately 2000 to 4000 times as much protein is labeled as in the classical method[8,9] and about 125 times as much radioactive iodine is utilized. However, the molar ratios of chloramine-T to both protein and iodine in the reaction mixture are held considerably lower, being about 0.3% and 1%, respectively, of the classical levels. The various components of our remote radioiodination apparatus (Figure 11) include the shipping vial which becomes the reaction vial, a needle block carrying

Table 2
RADIATION DOSE (mREM) TO CHEMIST FROM LABELING WITH 4200 mCi OF ^{131}I

Organ	Total (mREM)	Annual limit (mREM)	Annual limit (%)
Hand	880	75,000	1.2
Body	210	5,000	4.2
Thyroid	220	30,000	0.7

two stainless steel spinal needles, a charcoal trap which is vented to atmosphere inside a fume hood, an eluant reservoir filled with 0.05 *M* phosphate-buffered saline suitable for human injection, a Sephadex® G-10 preparative column, a two-channel peristaltic pump, a radiation detector, a series of four, electrically driven teflon valves, and a 0.22 μm filter for product sterilization.

The entire apparatus is shielded with 3 in. of leaded glass and 4 in. of lead bricks inside a fume hood. Remote controls for the valves and pumps are located outside the hood. The reaction takes place in the shipping vial, which contains reductant-free high specific activity ^{131}I. The chloramine-T labeling reagents are introduced into the shipping vial through stainless-steel needles connected to the reagent inlet line. After mechanical agitation, the reaction is terminated by addition of the $Na_2S_2O_3$ quenching mixture through the same needle. Iodine vapors that develop during agitation are vented through the charcoal trap.

Purification of the reaction mixture over a Sephadex® G-10 column occurs when the inlet valves are rotated and a peristaltic pump transfers the mixture from the vial to the top of the column. After the transfer is complete, valves are rotated once more to direct sterile eluant from the reservoir to the column which empties into a waste vial. The fractions eluting from the column that contain product are detected by a radiation monitor and can be collected by rotating a valve to direct the eluent through a sterilization filter into the radiopharmaceutical vial. After the elution of the waste products from the column, the entire system is eluted with buffer, then filled with 0.1% sodium azide in normal saline. The system has remained sterile and pyrogen free for more than six months.

This remotely operated system gives radiochemical yields of almost 100% and we collect as much as 90% of the initial activity as labeled product suitable for injection. The molar ratio of iodine to protein in preparations for radioimmunoscintigraphy is about 1/10th of that reported by Hunter and Greenwood[8] an average of about 0.25 atoms of iodine per molecule of protein. The immunoreactivity of the iodinated fragments, as measured by a cell-binding assay, was usually at least 80% of the baseline value in diagnostic labelings and decreased as the molar ratio of iodine to Fab fragment increased.

The radiation exposure associated with labeling was approximately 210 mrem to the whole body and 880 mrem to hands for an entire year in which 4.2 Curies of ^{131}I was handled in this apparatus (Table 2). These doses compare favorably with those received by a technician when performing open vial chloramine-T labelings with only a few mCi of ^{125}I in the fume hood. The apparatus could be modified to perform iodogen, lactoperoxidase, and bead labeling methods.[1]

IV. ANALYTICAL MEASUREMENTS OF ANTIBODY RADIOPHARMACEUTICALS

The various methods employed for antibody radiolabeling have numerous effects on the structure and function of the product. An ideal method will yield a product in which all of the label is attached to the protein and the antibody retains its full chemical and immunologic properties. The extent of departure from this ideal must be evaluated for each labeled product, whether it is intended for in vitro, animal, or human use.

It is no longer adequate to simply measure the fraction of free isotope in a radiopharmaceutical preparation. Techniques now exist for detecting, quantitating, and hopefully eliminating much more subtle chemical impurities. Any radioanalytical procedure for a protein must be applied before labeling as well as after, to detect any changes in the chemical properties of the molecule being traced. The investigator should consider chromatographic methods and electrophoresis as well as receptor binding assays. These measurements must also be correlated with the in vivo behavior of the antibody tracer.

A. Chromatographic and Electrophoretic Methods

Radiochemical composition dictates the time course of biodistribution of any radiotracer. The interpreter of a MAb imaging study must have confidence that any deviation from a normal distribution pattern is a result of pathology within the patient, rather than batch-to-batch variations in the radiochemical composition of the injected tracer.

Sodium dodecyl sulfate-polyacrylamide gel electrophoresis, SDS-PAGE,[25] is the method generally accepted for careful evaluation of a radiolabeled antibody product. This procedure can be used to analyze the product for purity and location of radiolabel on the various proteins in the product. Modifications, such as the use of slab gels, give similar information.

The technique involves dissolution of the radiolabeled antibody in SDS and application of this product solution to a gel which may contain a range of polyacrylamide concentrations (10 to 25%) for separation of proteins ranging from 4000 to 150,000 daltons. Electrophoresis can be performed with or without the use of 2-mercaptoethanol to separate the heavy and light chains of the gamma globulins. At the completion of electrophoresis, the separated protein bands are stained with Coomassie brilliant blue, dried and analyzed by placing the whole gel on autoradiographic film or by slicing the gel and counting each slice for radioactivity. In this way the type and concentration of the proteins in the product can be assessed and compared with a series of protein standards of known molecular weights, to identify the molecular size of protein fractions that were radiolabeled.

Thin layer electrophoresis is a less complicated procedure which yields valuable, but less detailed, information on the quality of the product. Using cellulose acetate or agarose strips as the solid phase, the radiolabeled antibody is separated from the unbound ionic radioactive species, yielding a percentage of total activity that is protein bound. The product is spotted at the cationic end of the strip, and allowed to electrophorese in a pH adjusted buffer system, usually Na barbital. Requiring approximately 15 min as compared to 7 to 8 hr for SDS-PAGE, this procedure is a quick, simple way to evaluate the product for free activity. An alternative procedure, isoelectric focusing, combines the resolution advantages of PAGE with the speed of thin layer techniques and may emerge as one of the most useful techniques for measuring the radiochemical composition of antibody radiopharmaceuticals.

High-pressure liquid chromatography (HPLC) is the fastest, most efficient method for qualitative and quantitative analysis of proteins. The best separations result from small bore columns packed with small, uniformly sized particles. Under these conditions, high pressures and high flow rates can be maintained throughout the entire column bed. The sensitivity for detection of proteins by optical density at 254 or 280 nm is in the picomole to nanomole range with good resolution.

In choosing an HPLC system for protein analysis, a number of aspects about the analysis must be considered. For instance, is it necessary that the biologic activity of the analyte be retained during the analysis? What is the nature of the separation desired? Many choices are available, including separation of proteins by size or apparent molecular weight, the use of ion exchange materials, hydrophobic extraction, and reverse phase chromatography. This review is restricted to size exclusion chromatography and ion exchange resins.

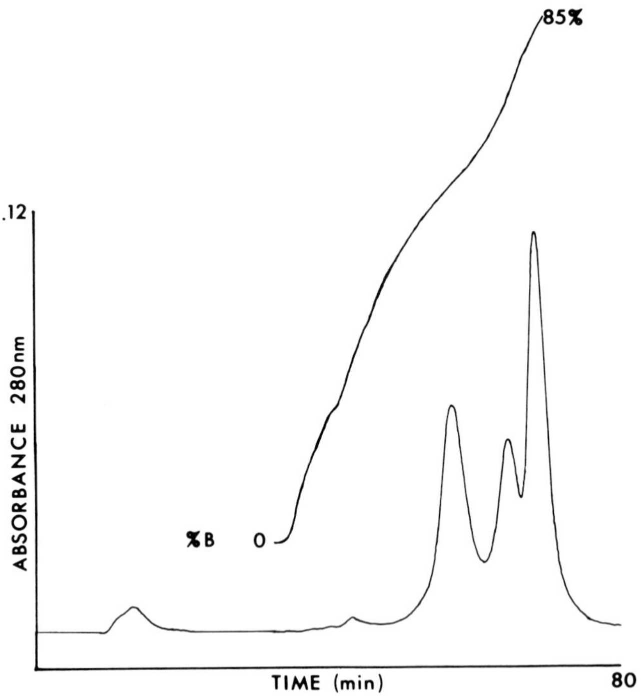

FIGURE 12. Chromatogram of ion exchange purified 96.5 on high-performance hydroxylapatite. Conditions were as follows: columns, 100 × 7.8 mm hydroxylapatite with 50 × 4.0 mm hydrophobic polymerguard (Bio-Rad); sample g anion exchange purified at 96.5; flow rate, 0.4 mℓ/min. Buffer A: 0.01 *M* sodium phosphate, 10 *M* $CaCl_2$, pH 6.8. Buffer B: 0.3 *M* sodium phosphate, 10 *M* $CaCl_2$, pH 6.8. Gradient: 40 min linear gradient of 0 to 60% B, 7 min linear gradient of 60 to 85% B, 2 min isocratic gradient at 85% B, 1.2 min linear gradient of 85 to 100% B.

In size-exclusion chromatography (SEC), separation of compounds is based on the apparent molecular size of molecules and the pore size of the gel. During column flow, the smaller molecules in the solution are able to penetrate gel pores, while the larger molecules are not. As a result large molecules elute first; very small molecules such as unbound I^- are retained the longest. In a size-exclusion separation, the biologic activity of proteins is maintained within specified pH ranges so that this technique is applicable to both preparative and analytical separations. A number of compressible solid phase materials have been widely available for SEC, but the introduction of hard, noncompressible permeable beads such as the TSK series (Bio-Rad Laboratories) permit faster and higher resolution size exclusion chromatography of MAbs.

Ion-exchange columns of hydroxyapatite are showing promise in the separation of immunoglobulins. These weak anion exchange columns work well at neutral pH without organic modifiers and enable good recovery of the antibody product. Like size-exclusion systems, preservation of antibody reactivity is maintained and is even improved when nonimmunoreactive molecules are removed. It has been shown to be useful in separation of immunoglobulins by class, and in the removal of denatured immunoglobulins from labeled preparations (Figure 12).

B. Immunoreactivity Assays

When chemically pure antigen is available, classical radioimmunoassay (RIA) techniques[27] can be used to evaluate the capacity of a radiolabeled antibody for binding to an antigen.

Table 3
LITERATURE MEASUREMENTS OF IMMUNOLOGIC INTEGRITY

None	12%
Refer to previous report	41%
Qualitative result	18%
Quantitative assay	27%
Scatchard analysis	2%

This method is probably the most accurate one for assessing antibody immunoreactivity. In RIA, the labeled antibody product is incubated with unlabeled antibody and antigen. Separation of the bound antibody from free antibody is achieved by precipitation procedures and centrifugation or by chromatography.

The Scatchard plot,[28] constructed by plotting bound/free antibody vs. amount of bound antigen yields the antibody affinity constant (slope) and maximum binding capacity (y-intercept). This method is a reliable means for directly comparing the immunoreactivity of one product to another. It gives quantitative indications of quality in units that can be compared between laboratories.

In some cases, however, antigen is not available in sufficient quantity to allow the use of RIA procedures. This has led to the development of assays in which the antigen is available on intact cell culture lines, cell membrane extracts from similar lines, or from freshly harvested tissues. Assuming no changes in antigen expression in succeeding generations of cell culture lines, these binding assays are simple means of evaluating radiolabeled antibody immunoreactivity with the tumor cells in question directly. A number of assay procedures have been developed in which the labeled antibody, diluted in bovine serum albumin or fetal calf serum, is incubated directly with a suspension of tumor cells. After washing the centrifuged cell pellet several times in phosphate buffered saline, the percentage of total activity bound in the pellet gives an estimation of antibody immunoreactivity. In cases where the antigen is on the cell surface, a suspension of formalin-fixed cells has an indefinite storage life[29] and, therefore, more reproducible assays over several weeks or months can be performed. We feel very strongly that when an antibody is in developmental stages, the immunoreactivity by Scatchard analysis should be determined. We also feel that each labeled batch of antibody should be tested for immunoreactivity as a part of the quality control procedures before administration to the patient. Unfortunately, this type of evaluation is not often performed; a recent review of the antibody literature revealed that 26 of 63 papers did not report immunoreactivity in the relevant group of labelings, but referred to previously reported values (Table 3). Eight didn't address immunoreactivity at all and 11 papers reported results qualitatively, most frequently by titration methods that are not acceptable as product quality control evaluations. Titration or single-condition assays can be set up to give falsely high results even when an extensive amount of damaged protein is present. Labeled antibody investigations should include the development of a critical and quantitative assay for immunointegrity.

C. Pharmaceutical Quality

When radiolabeled antibody products are intended for human use, sterility is essential. Although most laboratories culture labeled products for bacterial and fungal growth in the clinical microbiology laboratory, results on product sterility are usually not available before the radiopharmaceutical product has been used. A 0.22 μm filter removes bacterial contamination present in the product, but does not eliminate possible contamination with pyrogens.

A pyrogen test using the limulus amebolysate coagulates in the presence of threshold levels of pyrogens. Kits can be purchased with various threshold levels. The product sample is tested against a known negative control and an endotoxin positive sample in a 1 hr incubation at 37°C. If a positive result is obtained in the sample, repeated assays on serial dilutions of the sample will allow calculation of the levels of endotoxin present. By definition 1 ng endotoxin equals 5 endotoxin units[30] and ≤2.5 endotoxin units (or 0.5 ng) may be injected per kilogram patient body weight.

The FDA has proposed an extensive series of biological tests that are prerequisite to in vivo use of monoclonal antibodies.[31] These relate entirely to the safety of the antibody preparation and are performed before the MAb is labeled and thus will not be detailed in this review.

D. In Vivo Correlations of Radiochemical Analyses

Incorporation of a ^{11}C or ^{18}F atom into a small biochemical metabolite or a ^{99m}Tc or ^{111}In ion into a simple ligand often results in a uniquely definable molecular structure. In contrast, a radioactive heteroatomic substitution into a large polypeptide or an antibody results in labeling at many sites. An average antibody molecule will have approximately one reactive site per 4000 daltons. Some of these binding sites will result in a more firm attachment of the label to the protein than others; and some sites, when labeled, will have a greater impact on the biological activity of the molecule than others. These principles apply equally to halogenation at aromatic residues and to bifunctional chelation, which generally occurs at lysines and terminal amino groups.

In addition to direct chemical modification caused by the radiolabel that has been introduced, the labeling procedure may cause nonspecific side reactions on the protein molecule that result in a spectrum of labeled products that can behave differently in vivo. A protein radiopharmaceutical will consist of a distribution of molecules, each with an integer number of tracer atoms incorporated per protein molecule. That is, a product may average 0.5 mol of isotopic label per mole of protein, but the product spectrum will only contain molecules with zero, one, or two atoms incorporated per molecule. The product mixture's composition can be approximated by the binomial probability distribution for n tracer atoms distributed among m potential labeling sites per molecule. The labeling sites are generally sufficiently far apart that probabilities per site are independent of the number of atoms that have already been attached per molecule.

Even within the subgroup of molecules having one atom substituted per protein molecule, a spectrum of biological properties may result because some labeling sites can be more critically involved in the in vivo behavior of the protein than others. The assignment for the radioanalytical chemist is to develop assays that will distinguish between those molecules in which the radioactive tracer has caused an unacceptable effect on the protein molecule and those in which it has not. If such an analytical method also allows for preparative scale purification, it will be even more valuable.

Chemical alterations caused by other reagents used in the labeling process can have an even broader spectrum of consequences. For example, chloramine-T is used for electrophilic halogenation, but it is also capable of breaking peptide bonds[10,11] and forming aldehydes which are potential protein cross linking structures. The number of molecules of nonradioactive chemical reactant used in labeling will be much larger than the number of molecules of radioactive tracer; and, therefore, the potential for chemical degradation is higher than that for loss of protein function by the radioactive substituent.

After a radiolabeled antibody product has been developed, and passed tests of pharmaceutical quality and performance, in vivo testing is required. Because many tumors can be grown as subcutaneous implants in athymic animals, the majority of preliminary biodistribution experiments are performed with nude mice. The distribution of intravenously injected radiolabeled antibody is followed in the blood and tissues by sacrificing groups of similarly treated animals at selected time points. Comparison of retained activity in the blood, tumor, and other organs can be made in the data analysis. Nude rats and guinea pigs are also available and may be especially useful for dosimetric studies where larger interorgan distances are desired.

Otsuka et al.[32] have published a possible alternative to implanted tumors. Tumor antigens chemically coupled to agarose beads were injected intravenously into a mouse or rat for creation of an artificial tumor. The beads are trapped in the pulmonary arterial vascular bed where they simulate a tumor. This technique presents some limitations, but it also offers several distinct advantages over implanted tumors. A known amount of tumor antigen is attached to the beads, which have a known surface volume. The antigen is evenly dispersed, and has a consistent and adequate blood flow. When the animal is sacrificed, the amount of radioactivity retained allows for very accurate calculations of antibody-antigen binding. The system depends on availability of purified antigen for coupling to the beads.

During in vivo testing of an antibody radiopharmaceutical, it is important to carefully characterize the organ, blood and tumor concentrations as a function of time. Since nonspecific binding of gamma globulin may occur in tumor or other tissues, it is most valuable to compare the biokinetic behavior of the labeled antibody of interest with that of a nonspecific (control) antibody of the same class. This can be done conveniently by coadministering the two antibodies intravenously using ^{125}I and ^{131}I for labeling the control and specific antibodies, respectively.

Regardless of the biological assay system used, several aspects of antibody behavior in vivo need to be quantitated. Examination of the sites of nonspecific and specific binding, as well as ratios of activities in tissues, are important parameters in biodistribution. The calculation of biologic $T_{1/2}$ for each organ, tumor, and blood is also critical. These data are often represented as target-to-background ratios calculated from raw data. The Localization Index (LI)[33,34] has been used extensively as a means for examining the specificity of tumor uptake of antibody in dual isotope (specific and control) labeled antibody experiments. LI factors out the blood activity to facilitate comparisons.

$$LI = \frac{\dfrac{\%\text{ injected specific MAb/g tumor}}{\%\text{ injected MAb/g blood}}}{\dfrac{\%\text{ injected control MAb/g tumor}}{\%\text{ injected control MAb/g blood}}}$$

In addition to numerical data, many authors use gamma camera images of tumor bearing animals to document the localization of antibody to tumor. One such example[34] published an antibody biodistribution study with numerical data plus images of tumor-bearing and nontumor-bearing animals.

V. DEHALOGENATION REACTIONS

The principal disadvantage of iodinated proteins has generally been described as ''deiodination,'' a phenomenon that derives from two causes, one thermodynamic, the other enzymatic.

A. Hydrolysis

Hydrolytic deiodination may occur via a reaction with water molecules in a step that is the microscopic reversal of the labeling reaction (Figure 13). The I-aryl bond strength for iodobenzene is about 60 kcal/mol, but the hydroxyl substituent reduces it to 54, a value smaller than most covalent bonds.[35]

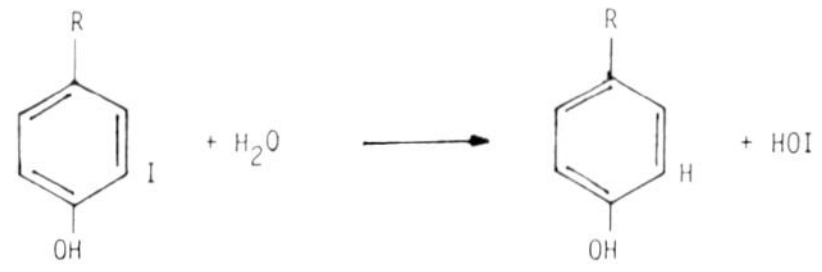

FIGURE 13. Hydrolytic Deiodination.

Iodinated proteins deiodinate both in vitro[36] and in vivo. The *in vitro* deiodination is dependent on the extent of iodination,[37] as well as the concentration and linear energy transfer of radiation in a sample. For radioiodine it also depends on the internal radiation dose delivered by the sample[38] and the storage time. Yallow and Berson[39] interpreted the slow release of iodine from radioiodinated preparations to be a result of the decay catastrophe which is a consequence of the recoil of the atom following a radioactive decay. This effect is enhanced in cases of multiple radioiodine substitutions per protein molecule. The autoradiolysis of the protein by radiation is also responsible for deiodination in aqueous solutions of iodinated proteins. This effect is dependent on the radiation dose and is observed more with ^{131}I-labeled proteins than with ^{125}I-labeled proteins. Autoradiolysis can be reduced either by dilution of the preparation with water, especially with addition of protein, such as albumin, or by the addition of free radical quenchers such as ethanol.[38]

B. Enzymatic Decomposition

In vivo enzymatic deiodination of thyroxine to triiodothyronine, the thyroid hormone which has considerably more biologic activity, is a well-recognized model system for studying dehalogenation. Deiodination of MAbs is pronounced in molecules which have structures similar to thyroid hormones. The most studied enzyme, T_4 5′-deiodinase, exists principally in the plasmalemma.[40] Investigators have speculated that its role is as an enzymatic barrier, leading to the predominantly extracellular distribution of thyroxine with a mechanism to insure that the hormone reaching the nucleus is thyronine.[40]

The enzymatic pathways for degradation of thyroid hormones solely involves monodeiodination.[41] Detailed studies using L-monoiodotyrosine as substrate show that enzymatic deiodination requires triphosphopyridine nucleotide but not oxygen.[42] Deiodination of diiodotyrosine is mechanistically similar to that of monoiodotyrosine, but the rate is slower. Maximum enzymatic activity occurs at pH 6.3 to 7.4 and is enhanced by thiols.[43-45] Evidence for a pH optimum determined by the pKa of the phenolic OH is contradictory.[44,45] Deiodinase enzymes are most abundant in thyroid, kidney, and liver, but they also appear peripherally, including in adipose tissue and CNS.[44] Deiodination is increased in disease states associated with enhanced leukocyte phagocytic activity.[46] The mechanism is uncertain, but the effect is accelerated T_4 turnover.

The available literature on deiodinase enzymology may lead to better iodination antibody radiopharmaceuticals. For example, it is known that thyroxine analogues, modified at the aliphatic side chains, are substrates for the same deiodinase system as the authentic thyroid hormone.[44] A 170 kdalton antibody is admittedly a large aliphatic side chain, but if the principle holds, then a vast literature on enzymatic deiodination becomes useful to the investigation of antibody dehalogenation. In fact, computer graphic modeling of deiodinase enzymes and inhibitions is now sufficiently sophisticated that investigators are beginning to suggest the possibility of specific iodinated ligands which could modulate peripheral thyroid hormones metabolism and act as antithyroid drugs. This same modeling strategy might be expected to lead also to more resistant iodination labels for MAbs.

We have predicted that deiodination will be reduced in preparations where iodine is located in the para position with respect to the side chain. This position is occupied by the hydroxyl group in tyrosine and suggests that methods which iodinate phenylalanine selectively should be explored further.

VI. PROSPECTS FOR IMPROVED HALOGENATED ANTIBODIES

A. Iodophenylalanine Derivatives

There are several problems that need to be solved in order to obtain better preparations of halogenated MAbs than those currently available. The most serious problem is that of deiodination secondary to catabolism of the radiolabeled antibody or fragment. For example, it has been found that heavy iodination of one antibody can result in substantial loss of biological activity, while this is not seen with another antibody. This difference might be due to iodination of a tyrosine residue in the binding pocket of the first antibody. One approach to solving the deiodination problem will be to introduce new aromatic residues into the antibody at other amino acid sites.

The most common method for iodination of proteins is at tyrosine residues. Electrophilic iodine replaces a hydrogen atom at a position ortho to the hydroxyl and meta to the alanine substituent. Alternatively, phenylalanine can be labeled,[7] particularly in polypeptides where it is the only aromatic amino acid present. Iodination of non-tyrosine containing polypeptides is achieved by labeling a tyrosine analogue, such as the Bolton-Hunter reagent, and then secondarily attaching the pre-iodinated analogue to the peptide. A similar labeling scheme is needed for introducing new phenylalanine groups into antibodies.

There are several factors that suggest the advantage of p-iodophenylalanine labels. The 4-iodophenyl C-I bond is stronger than the 3-iodo-4-hydroxyphenyl-bond by about 5 kcal/mol.[35] Deiodination enzymes recognize the I atom ortho to OH as a thyroid hormone and can cause deiodination, whereas they may not recognize the phenyl-I bond in the absence of the ortho-OH substituent. Furthermore, 3-iodo-4-hydroxyphenyl structures are degraded to I^- and the radioactive iodide subsequently goes to gut, thyroid, urine, and bladder. In contrast, 4-iodophenyl groups are degraded by enzymes principally to iodophenyl benzoates which conjugate with glycine to give hippuric acid, resulting in rapid renal excretion. This latter argument is the basis for the successful use of p-iodophenylpentadecanoic acid for myocardial imaging.[47] Each of these three factors (bond strength, susceptibility to enzymic dehalogenation, and pharmacokinetic fate of degradation products) favors para iodination.

Perhaps the best method for radioiodination of deactivated aromatic rings utilizes replacement reactions at trimethylsilyl (TMS) derivatives. The TMS group can be attached to the phenyl ring by the method used by Wilbur et al.[48] The derivatized ring is then labeled by adding radioiodine, in glacial acetic acid, in molar ratio of 1:1; a stoichiometric amount of N-chlorosuccinimide can then be used to oxidize the iodine. A similar chemistry could be used to radioiodinate triazene derivatives. The details of this labeling chemistry have been developed as they apply to phenylalkylamines. Tri-n-butyltin derivatives have been used to prepare antibodies radiolabeled through nonactivated aromatic rings.[49] The immunoreactivity of the antibody was retained and the biodistribution in mice showed no increase in thyroid radioactivity from 2 to 72 hr after administration, evidence that in vivo deiodination is not occurring.

Chemical bridges between proteins and substituted phenyl rings are available that are specific for several amino acids.[50] For the most part, this technology comes from the laboratories of molecular biologists developing bifunctional cross-linking reagents as tools for basic protein and nucleic acid research and for introducing chromophores for biochemical analyses. The common chemical characteristics of these groups are threefold: a benzene ring, a group that prepares the aromatic ring for secondary chemistry, and a group that reacts with some specific chemical structure in the glycopolypeptide that has been selected to be modified and/or labeled. The succinimide and imidate structures described in Sections III.C.1 and III.C.2 are the best developed chemistries and result in substitution at lysine, usually quite acceptable in retaining biologic activity of the MAb.

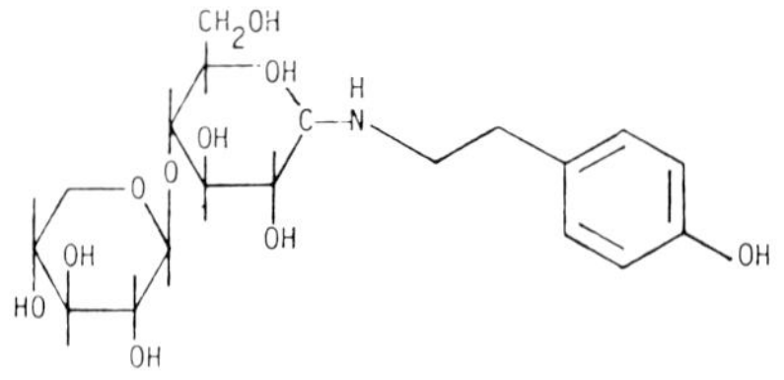

FIGURE 14. Tyramine-Cellobiose Adduct.

B. Saccharide Bridges Between Halogens and Proteins

Another approach to antibody labeling which attempts to minimize the effects of free I^- from protein catabolism is addition of an iodinated tyramine cellobiose adduct to an antibody. The method, suggested by the work of Pittman et al.[51] was described as providing a means of localizing intracellularly trapped radiolabeled lipoprotein in specific sites of catabolism. They observed that the sugar portion of the molecule did not alter the biodistribution and metabolism of the protein, but kept the radioligand trapped within cells following lysosomal catabolism (Figure 14).

The tyramine-cellobiose adduct was synthesized by reductive amination with sodium cyanoborohydride. After removal of free tyramine by silicic acid chromatography, the adduct was radioiodinated by the Iodogen method as described in Section III.B.2. Linkage of the iodinated adduct to the protein was performed with cyanuric chloride. This chemistry could also be accomplished with phenethylamine rather than tyramine, to give the advantages of the 4-iodophenyl structure described above.

Pittman et al. found that low density lipoprotein could be labeled by this method and that the label stayed at the site where the molecule was catabolized. An antibody radiolabel of this type might also be retained at its site of catabolism, for example in the tumor cell following antigenic modulation. Target-to-background levels may be improved if treatment of the antibody by cyanuric chloride does not result in unacceptable denaturation. This would give iodinated MAbs one of the most advantageous properties of indium-labeled MAbs, namely that radioactive label that localizes intracellularly is retained rather than being rapidly excreted.

REFERENCES

1. **Ferens, J. M., Krohn, K. A., Beaumier, P. L., Link, J. M., Brown, F. P., Hellstrom, I., Hellstrom, K. E., Carrasquillo, J. A., and Larson, S. M.,** High level iodination of monoclonal antibody fragments for radiotherapy, *J. Nucl. Med.*, 25, 367, 1984.
2. **Larson, S. M., Carrasquillo, J. A., Krohn, K. A., McGuffin, R. W., Williams, D. L., Hellstrom, I., and Hellstrom, K. E.,** Diagnostic imaging of malignant melanoma with radiolabeled antitumor antibodies, *J. Am. Med. Assoc.*, 249, 811, 1983.
3. **Stocklin, G.,** Bromine-77 and iodine-123 radiopharmaceuticals, *Int. J. Appl. Radiat. Iso.*, 28, 131, 1977.
4. **Kilbourn, M. R., Dence, C. S., Welch, M. J., and Mathias, C. J.,** Fluorine-18 labeling of proteins, *J. Nucl. Med.*, 28, 462, 1987.
5. **Regoeczi, E.,** *Iodine-labeled Plasma Proteins*, Vol. 1, CRC Press, Boca Raton, Fla., 1984.
6. **Wolff, J. and Covelli, I.,** Factors in the iodination of histidine in proteins, *Eur. J. Biochem.*, 9, 371, 1969.
7. **Krohn, K. A., Knight, L. C., Harwig, J. F., and Welch, M. J.,** Differences in the sites of iodination of proteins following four methods of radioiodination, *Biochim. Biophys. Acta*, 430, 497, 1977.
8. **Hunter, W. M. and Greenwood, F. C.,** Preparation of ^{131}I labeled human growth hormone of high specific activity, *Nature (London)*, 194, 495, 1962.
9. **Greenwood, F. C., Hunter, W. M., and Glover, J. S.,** The preparation of ^{131}I labeled human growth hormone of high specific radioactivity, *Biochem. J.*, 89, 119, 1963.

10. **Feigl, F.,** *Spot Tests in Organic Analysis,* Elsevier, New York, 1960, 292.
11. **Krohn, K. A., Sherman, L., and Welch, M.,** Physicochemical properties of the IC1, chloramine-T, and electrolytic reaction products, *Biochim. Biophys. Acta,* 285, 404, 1972.
12. **Markwell, M. A. K.,** A new solid state reagent to iodinate proteins, *Anal. Biochem.,* 125, 427, 1982.
13. **Fraker, P. J. and Speck, J. C.,** Protein and cell membrane iodination with a sparingly soluble chloramide, 1,3,4,6-tetrachloro-3a,6a-diphenylglycouril, *Biochem. Biophys. Res. Commun.,* 80, 849, 1978.
14. **Marchalonis, J. J.,** An enzymatic method for the trace iodination of immunoglobulins and other proteins, *Biochem. J.,* 113, 299, 1969.
15. **Thorell, J. I. and Johansson, B. G.,** Enzymatic iodination of polypeptides with ^{125}I to high specific activity, *Biochim. Biophys. Acta,* 251, 363, 1971.
16. **David, G. S.,** Solid state lactoperoxidase: a highly stable enzyme for simple gentle iodination of proteins, *Biochem. Biophys. Res. Commun.,* 48, 464, 1972.
17. **David, G. S. and Reisfeld, R. A.,** Protein iodination with solid state lactoperoxidase, *Biochemistry,* 13, 1014, 1974.
18. **Rosa, V., Scansselati, G. A., Bennisi, F., Riccioni, N., Giagnoni, P., and Giordani, R.,** Labeling of human fibrinogen with ^{131}I by electrolytic iodination, *Biochim. Biophys. Acta,* 86, 519, 1964.
19. **Bolton, A. E. and Hunter, W. M.,** The labeling of proteins to high specific radioactivities by conjugation to ^{125}I containing acylating agent, *Biochem. J.,* 133, 529, 1973.
20. **Wood, T. F., Wu, M. M., and Gerhart, J. C.,** The radioactive labeling of proteins with an iodinated aminidation reagent, *Anal. Biochem.,* 69, 339, 1975.
21. **Hayes, C. E. and Goldstein, I. J.,** Radioiodination of sulfhydryl sensitive proteins, *Anal. Biochem.,* 67, 580, 1975.
22. **Ji, T. H. and Ji, I.,** Macromolecular photoaffinity labeling with radioactive photoactivable heterobifunctional reagents, *Anal. Biochem.,* 121, 286, 1982.
23. **Tejedor, F. and Ballista, J. P. G.,** Iodination of p-nitrophenyl ethers used as photolabels, *Anal. Biochem.,* 128, 115, 1983.
24. **Badger, C. C., Krohn, K. A., Peterson, A. V., Shulman, H., and Bernstein, I. D.,** Experimental radiotherapy of murine lymphoma with I-131 labeled anti-thy 1.1 monoclonal antibody, *Cancer Res.,* 45, 1536, 1985.
25. **Laemmili, U. K.,** Analysis of bacteriophage-T early RNA's and proteins on slab gels, *J. Mol. Biol.,* 79, 237, 1973.
26. **Hochschwender, S., Bartholomew, R., Sanchez, N., Vasquez, P., Wollert, R., and Carlo, D. J.,** Immunoreactivity of the monoclonal antibody (MAB) 96.5 against the P97 melanoma associated antigen is directly related to production of inactive variants, *J. Nucl. Med.,* 27, 958, 1986.
27. **Thorell, J. I. and Larson, S. M.,** *Radioimmunoassay and Related Techniques: Methodology and Clinical Applications,* C. V. Mosby, St. Louis, 1978.
28. **Scatchard, G.,** The attraction of proteins for small molecules and ions, *Ann. N.Y. Acad. Sci.,* 51, 660, 1949.
29. **Beaumier, P. L., Neuzil, D. F., Yang, H. M., Noll, E. A., Krohn, K. A., Hellstrom, I., Hellstrom, K. E., and Nelp, W. B.,** Formaldehyde fixed cells compared with live cells for antibody immunoreactivity assay, *J. Nucl. Med.,* 26(Abstr.), 826, 1985.
30. **Reinhold, R. B. and Fine, J.,** A technique for quantitative measurement of endotoxin in human plasma, *Proc. Soc. Exp. Biol. Med.,* 137, 334, 1971.
31. **Merchant, B.,** Points to Consider in the Manufacture of Monoclonal Antibody Products for Human Use, Office of Biologics, National Center for Drugs and Biologics, Food and Drug Administration, Rockville, Md., 1987.
32. **Otsuka, F. L., Welch, M. J., McElvany, K. D., Nicolotti, R. T., and Fleischman, J. B.,** Development of a model system to evaluate methods for radiolabeling monoclonal antibodies, *J. Nucl. Med.,* 25, 1343, 1984.
33. **Moshakis, V., McKinney, R., Raghauen, D., and Neville, A. M.,** Localization of human tumor xenografts after IV administration of radiolabeled monoclonal antibodies, *Br. J. Cancer,* 44, 91, 1981.
34. **Beaumier, P. L., Krohn, K. A., Carasquillo, J. A., Eary, J. F., Hellstrom, K. E., Hellstrom, I., Nelp, W. B., and Larson, S. M.,** Melanoma localization in nude mice with monoclonal Fab against p97, *J. Nucl. Med.,* 26, 1172, 1985.
35. **Vedeneyev, V. I., Gurvich, L. V., Kondrat'yev, V. A., Medvedev, V. A., and Frankevich, Y. L.,** *Bond Energies, Ionization Potentials, and Electron Affinities,* Edward Arnold, London, 1966.
36. **McFarlane, A. S.,** Efficient trace labeling of proteins with iodine, *Nature (London),* 182, 53, 1958.
37. **Ceska, M., Berglund, A., Lundkirst, V., and Grossmuller, F.,** Influence of the degree of iodination and storage time on the immunological activity of ^{125}I-IgE, *Immunochemistry,* 9, 565, 1972.

38. **Kishore, R., Eary, J. F., Krohn, K. A., Nelp, W. B., Menard, T. W., Beumier, P. L., Hellstrom, K. E., and Hellstrom, I.**, Autoradiolysis of iodinated monoclonal antibody preparations. Symposium on Radionuclide-Labeled Monoclonal Antibodies: Techniques and Applications, American Chemical Society, Miami Beach, Fla., 1985.
39. **Yallow, R. S. and Berson, S. A.**, Symposium on In Vitro Procedures with Radioisotopes in Clinical Medicine and Research, Vienna, 1969.
40. **Leonard, J. L. and Rosenberg, I. N.**, Subcellular distribution of thyroxine 5'-deiodinase in the rat kidney: a plasma membrane location, *Endocrinology*, 103, 274, 1978.
41. **Smallridge, R. C. and Whorton, N. E.**, 3'-Monoiodothyronine degradation in rat liver homogenate: enzyme characteristics and documentation of deiodination by high-pressure liquid chromatography, *65th Annual Meeting Endocrine Society*, San Antonio, Texas, 1983.
42. **Stanbury, J. B. and Morris, M. L.**, Deiodination of diiodotyrosine by cell-free systems, *J. Biol. Chem.*, 233, 106, 1958.
43. **Smallridge, R. C., Burman, K. D., Ward, K. E., Wartofsky, L., Dimond, R. C., Wright, F. D., and Latham, K. R.**, 3'5'-diiodothyronine to 3'-monoiodothyronine conversion in the fed and fasted rat, *Endocrinology*, 108, 2336, 1981.
44. **Koehrle, J., Auf'mkolk, M., Hartmut, R., Hesch, R. -D., and Cody, V.**, Rat liver iodothyronine monodeiodinase. Evaluation of the iodothyronine ligand binding site, *J. Biol. Chem.*, 261, 11613, 1986.
45. **Ientile, R., Macaione, S., Russo, P., Pugliese, G., and DiGiorgio, R.**, Phenolic and tyrosyl ring deiodination in thyronine from rat retina during postnatal development, *Eur. J. Biochem.*, 142, 15, 1984.
46. **Engler, D. and Burger, A. G.**, The deiodination of the iodothyronines and of their derivatives in man, *Endocrine Rev.*, 5, 151, 1984.
47. **Machulla, H. J.**, Radioactive labeling of fatty acids for metabolic studies, in *Applications of Nuclear and Radiochemistry*, Lambrecht, R. and Marcos, N., Eds., Pergamon Press, 1982.
48. **Wilbur, D. S., Stone, W. E., and Anderson, K. W.**, Regiospecific incorporation of bromine and iodine into phenols using trimethylsilylphenol derivatives, *J. Org. Chem.*, 48, 1542, 1983.
49. **Wilbur, D. S., Jones, D. S., Fritzberg, A. R., and Morgan, A. C.**, Radioiodination of monoclonal antibodies. Labeling with *para*-iodophenyl (PIP) derivatives for in vivo stability of the radioiodine label, *J. Nucl. Med.*, 27(Abstr.), 959, 1986.
50. **Lundblad, R. L. and Noyes, C. M.**, *Chemical Reagents for Protein Modification*, CRC Press, Boca Raton, Fla., 1984.
51. **Pittman, R. C., Carew, T. E., Glass, C. K., Green, S. R., Taylor, C. A., Jr., and Attie, A. D.**, Radioiodinated, intracellularly trapped ligand for determining the sites of plasma protein degradation in vivo, *Biochem. J.*, 212, 791, 1983.

Chapter 6

LABELING ANTIBODIES WITH METALS USING BIFUNCTIONAL CHELATES

W. C. Eckelman and C. H. Paik

TABLE OF CONTENTS

I. INTRODUCTION

A. History of Protein and Antibody Radiolabeling

Soon after the discovery of ^{131}I in a tellurium target bombarded in the Berkeley cyclotron, Hamilton and Soley used this radionuclide in its simplest chemical form to study iodine metabolism.[1] In the following years, other molecules were radioiodinated; the ability to iodinate proteins at high specific activity was a major factor in the development of the insulin radioimmunoassay by Yalow and Berson.[2] Antibodies were also first radiolabeled using ^{131}I.[3,4] As early as 1957, Pressman et al.[5] were able to localize tumors by scanning using radioiodinated antibodies. Beierwaltes reported in 1971 that human cancer growing in the cheekpouch of the hamster could be localized.[6] In addition, Beierwaltes had used radioimmunotherapy to successfully treat one patient in 1951. This was reported in the *University of Michigan Medical Bulletin* in 1956. Since that time a number of antibodies have been radioiodinated and used for clinical studies.[7]

Historically, most iodinated radiopharmaceuticals used in nuclear medicine have eventually been replaced by ones labeled with a metallic radionuclide such as ^{99m}Tc, ^{111}In, or ^{67}Ga. The reasons for this are usually the inferior nuclear properties of ^{131}I and the chemical instability of ^{131}I labeled compounds compared to those labeled with ^{99m}Tc and other metallic radionuclides. On the surface, this should apply to antibodies just as it has applied to other radiolabeled compounds used for in vivo diagnosis. But on inspection of the potential clinical uses of radiolabeled antibodies, this same logic is not as applicable. As in most in vivo studies using radionuclides, the tracer principle is usually invoked in describing radiolabeled antibody studies. What is being traced is another matter. If tracing the distribution of the antibody per se is of primary concern, the radiolabel that most accurately gives that information is the most useful. This then would depend on the nuclear and chemical properties; a decay scheme suited to external imaging and a stable chemical bond would be most important. If, on the other hand, tracing the distribution of a therapeutic antibody is the primary concern, the considerations change. If ^{131}I-labeled antibodies are being used for therapy, it seems best to use ^{131}I (or ^{123}I) labeled antibodies radiolabeled at the same specific activity to carry out the diagnostic study. In this case, a more stable radiolabel used in the diagnostic study would not trace the therapeutic drug. The rate of deiodination, the effect of the specific activity on the binding to targets, and the pharmacokinetics are better traced using ^{131}I rather than ^{99m}Tc or ^{111}In as a radiolabel.

B. Choice of Radionuclide

The choice of radionuclide usually begins with an examination of the nuclear properties of the atom. If the radionuclide is intended for diagnosis, the match between the gamma-ray energy and the imaging device is of primary concern. Because gamma-ray imaging is often information-density poor, the absorbed radiation dose to the patient is also important. The absorbed radiation dose limits the quantity that can be injected, which in turn limits the quality of the image. For therapeutic radionuclides, the absorbed radiation dose is the most important characteristic in the opposite sense: the higher the absorbed radiation dose to the target, the more useful the radiotracer is. If gamma rays for imaging are present, that adds to the attractiveness of the therapeutic nuclide. The range of the radiation as measured by the linear energy transfer (LET) is also important as is the spatial relationship between the decaying radionuclide and the nucleus of the cell. Table 1 contains the major emissions from the radionuclides most often suggested for diagnostic imaging. Of these, ^{123}I and ^{99m}Tc have the best decay characteristics given their balance between absorbed radiation dose and abundance of gamma rays useful for imaging. However, ^{123}I is a cyclotron product and, therefore, is much less available than the convenient generator product ^{99m}Tc. In fact, greater than 90% of the studies carried out in clinical, diagnostic nuclear medicine use ^{99m}Tc.

Table 1
MAJOR EMISSIONS AND ABSORBED RADIATION DOSE FOR DIAGNOSTIC RADIONUCLIDES

Radionuclide ($T_{1/2}$)	Emission	Ni⁺	Ei	Δi
^{67}Ga (78 hr)	Gamma	0.38	0.093	0.075
	K-I.C.E.	0.28	0.084	0.050
	Gamma	0.24	0.185[a]	0.094
	Gamma	0.02	0.209	0.011
	Gamma	0.16	0.300	0.103
	Gamma	0.04	0.394	0.036
				0.369
^{99m}Tc (6 hr)	Gamma	0.88	0.140[a]	0.263
	K-I.C.E.	0.09	0.119	0.023
				0.286
^{111}In (2.8 days)	Gamma	0.89	0.172[a]	0.33
	K-I.C.E.	0.09	0.145	0.03
	Gamma	0.94	0.247[a]	0.49
	K-I.C.E.	0.05	0.220	0.02
	K-X-ray	0.47	0.023	0.02
	K-X-ray	0.24	0.023	0.01
				0.900
^{123}I (13 hr)	Gamma	0.83	0.159[a]	0.283
	K-I.C.E.	0.13	0.127	0.036
	K-X-ray	0.47	0.027	0.027
	K-X-ray	0.24	0.027	0.014
	K-X-ray	0.13	0.031	0.008
	Auger elec.	2.19	0.001	0.004
				0.365
^{131}I (8 days)	Beta	0.07	0.096	0.01
	Beta	0.90	0.192	0.37
	Gamma	0.06	0.284	0.03
	Gamma	0.82	0.364[a]	0.64
	K-I.C.E.	0.01	0.330	0.01
	Gamma	0.06	0.637	0.09
	Gamma	0.02	0.723	0.03
				1.22

Note: ⁺Ni, mean number per disintegration; Ei, mean energy in MeV per particle; Δ, equilibrium absorbed dose in g·rad/uCi·hr.

[a] Gamma ray used for imaging.

Technetium-99m became popular not only because of its ideal nuclear properties for imaging with the Anger gamma camera, but more importantly, because of its ready availability from the ^{99}Mo generator system.[8]

In Table 2, the major emissions of some potential therapeutic radionuclides are given based on an excellent review by Jungerman et al.[9] They demonstrate that ^{131}I and ^{123}I can be used for both diagnosis and therapy. Antimony-119 delivers 90% of its energy in only 6.5 μm and, therefore, is probably not useful for cell surface antigen labeling because of the short range. This radionuclide would have to be delivered to the nucleus. The other radionuclides have energy-deposition ranges of 5 to 77 cell diameters. An additional nuclide

Table 2
MAJOR EMISSIONS AND ABSORBED RADIATION DOSE FOR THERAPEUTIC RADIONUCLIDES

Radionuclide ($T_{1/2}$)	Emission	Ni+	$\bar{E}$	X_{90} (μm)
^{67}Cu (2.6 days)[a]	Beta	0.20	0.192	762
	Beta	0.35	0.161	562
	Beta	0.45	0.132	461
	Imaging gamma ray	0.47	0.184	—
^{97}Ru (2.9 days)[b]	Auger	0.96	0.002	0.18
	Auger	0.16	0.015	3.8
	Auger	0.05	0.018	5.5
	I.C.E.	0.03	0.194	374
	Imaging gamma ray	0.86	0.216	—
^{100}Pd (3.6 days)[c]	Auger	0.91	0.002	0.185
	Auger	0.14	0.017	4.5
	Auger	0.04	0.019	4.5
	Auger	0.008	0.022	7.5
	I.C.E.	0.02	0.071	58.6
	I.C.E.	0.04	0.081	36.5
	I.C.E.	0.16	0.052	43.3
	I.C.E	0.31	0.061	0.42
	Imaging gamma ray	.57	.084	—
^{119}Sb (1.6 days)[d]	Auger	0.88	0.004	0.42
	I.C.E.	0.86	0.019	6.2
	Auger	0.14	0.021	7.0
	X-ray	0.86	0.026	—
	Imaging gamma ray	None		—
^{101m}Rh (4.3 days)[e]	Auger	0.92	0.002	0.19
	Auger	0.14	0.016	4.1
	Auger	0.05	0.019	6.9
	Auger	0.008	0.021	7.0
	Imaging gamma ray	0.87	0.307	—
^{123}I (0.55 days)[f]	Auger	0.95	0.003	0.29
	Auger	0.12	0.023	7.52
	I.C.E.	0.11	0.127	151
	Imaging gamma ray	0.83	0.159	—
^{131}I (8 days)[g]	Beta	1.00	0.183	822
	Imaging gamma ray	0.81	0.364	—
^{197}Hg (2.7 days)[h]	Auger	0.50	0.012	2.5
	Auger	0.04	0.052	33
	I.C.E.	0.65	0.064	48
	I.C.E.	0.15	0.071	62
	Imaging gamma ray	.96	.071	—

Note: +Ni, mean number per disintegration; $\bar{E}$ (beta), average energy in MeV; X_{90} (μm), the distance in μm from the decay that represents a space containing 90% of the deposited dose.

[a] 50% of the energy deposited in 180 μm Rad/μCi/sec at 180 μm = 0.36.
[b] 50% of the energy deposited in 120 μm Rad/μCi/sec at 120 μm = .054.

Table 2 (continued)
MAJOR EMISSIONS AND ABSORBED RADIATION DOSE FOR THERAPEUTIC RADIONUCLIDES

[c] 50% of the energy deposited in 25.6 μm Rad/μCi/sec at 25.6 μm = 52.2.
[d] 50% of the dose deposited in 3.5 μm Rad/μCi/sec at 3.5 μm = 11720.
[e] 50% of the energy deposited in 4.8 μm Rad/μCi/sec at 4.8 μm = 1156.
[f] 50% of the energy deposited in 82.7 μm Rad/μCi/sec at 82.7 μm = .558.
[g] 50% of the energy deposited in 263 μm Rad/μCi/sec at 263 μm = .165.
[h] 50% of the energy deposited in 31.1 μm Rad/μCi/sec 31.1 μm = 52.9.

Table 3
POSITRON EMITTING RADIOTRACERS FOR ANTIBODY LABELING

Nuclide	$T_{1/2}$(hr)	Positron energy (MeV)	Photons (MeV)
^{72}As[a]	26	2.49 (77%)	0.630 (8%)
^{89}Zr	78	0.897 (22%)	0.909 (99%)
^{68}Ga[b]	1.1	1.89 (90%)	1.077 (37%)
^{64}Cu	12.7	0.657 (19%)	—

[a] Generator system ^{72}Se → ^{72}As.
[b] Generator system ^{68}Ge → ^{68}Ga.

of interest for therapeutic applications is ^{90}Y, a 2.7-day half-life beta emitter (maximum energy 2.29 MeV). All except ^{119}Sb and ^{90}Y have gamma rays of sufficient energy to be detected by external imaging. The short half-life of ^{123}I and the high abundance of low energy Auger-electrons make it better suited as an intracellularly localized radiolabel to be used as ^{125}I has been in iododeoxyuridine.[10]

Alpha-emitting radionuclides have also been suggested as radiolabels for therapeutic applications of antibodies. Astatine-211 has a 7 hr half life, emits alpha particles, and follows many of the chemical reactions proposed for iodine.[11] It is produced in a cyclotron with high-energy alpha particles at relatively low yields. It has been linked to various small molecules and colloids.[12] Harrison and Royle have proposed an improved method for radiolabeling IgG with ^{211}At.[13] In their procedure, iodine is not used as a carrier for ^{211}At and the para-^{211}At-astatobenzoic acid is purified before being conjugated to IgG by the mixed anhydride method. The labeling efficiency is greater than 30% and the radiolabeled complex has slow blood clearance suggesting a stable chemical bond.

More readily available alpha emitters are ^{212}Pb and ^{212}Bi which are eluted from a ^{228}Th generator. One microcurie of ^{212}Pb and daughters will yield an integrated dose of 232 rads of high LET radiation and 25 rads of low LET radiation in a 1 g tumor.[14] These radionuclides have been used to label colloid and are presently being investigated as antibody labels.[15]

Finally, Table 3 contains positron-emitting metallic radionuclides suggested by O'Brien as possible labels for antibodies.[16] These have not been studied in detail nor have antibodies been labeled with metallic radionuclides for positron-emission tomography.

C. Ideal Properties of the Radioligand

The ideal properties must be considered in light of the process being "traced"; that is, the ideal properties in one situation may be less than ideal in another situation. Certainly,

Table 4
PHARMACOKINETICS OF METABOLIC PRODUCTS

		% Administered dose			
Compound	**Organ**	**1 hr**	**6 hr**	**24 hr**	**20 days**
Iodide	Whole body	92.1	62.4	23.9	12.9
	Liver	1.4	0.9	0.2	—
	Intestine	15.4	9.4	1.6	—
	Blood	14.7	9.0	1.6	0.2
	Stomach	13.6	8.3	1.4	—
	Thyroid	1.5	6.9	13.8	12.2
Compound	**Organ**	**$T_{1/2}$ (hr)**	**Component (%)**	**$T_{1/2}$ (hr)**	**Component (%)**
^{99m}TcDTPA	Whole body	1.0	58	9.2	42
	Kidneys	.24	57	16.0	1
Compound	**Organ**				
$^{111}InCl_3$[a]	Liver	$\gg$physical $T_{1/2}$ (33%)			
	Bone marrow	$\gg$physical $T_{1/2}$ (33%)			
	Whole body	$\gg$physical $T_{1/2}$ (33%)			

[a] Urine 11% in 10 days, feces 4% in 10 days.

the metabolism of iodinated radiotracers can present a problem because of the high dose to the thyroid due to iodide uptake. But, if the diagnostic radioiodinated antibody is being used to measure the distribution of the therapeutic iodinated antibody, the rate of metabolism in a particular patient will be known and, therefore, the iodinated protein is the best tracer. In most cases, antibodies labeled with metallic radionuclides are being used for diagnosis and, therefore, the radiolabel should remain with the antibody and not affect the antibody immunochemistry for the duration of the study. However, the clinical use of an antibody radiolabeled with a metallic radionuclide is still not well defined. These radiolabeled antibodies are competing with other imaging modalities with much higher information density to establish the size, shape, and position of a tumor. If the general location of the tumor or the metastases can be specified, CAT scanning or perhaps MRI would be superior in detecting small tumors. High tumor to nontumor ratios and high count rates are necessary to detect even 1 cm^2 tumors at depths of 1 to 5 cm using the Anger camera.[17] In the very important case where the metastases are extensive and a whole-body survey is indicated, the radiodiagnostic technique has an advantage. Larson et al.[18] have also suggested staging and monitoring therapeutic response as important goals of cancer diagnosis with radionuclides. Radioiodinated antibodies and metallic-containing radiolabeled antibodies are, thus, not in the competitive situation they are thought to be. Often in publications describing the metal-containing bifunctional chelates, the distribution of the respective metabolites is put forth as the reason for choosing metallic radionuclides over iodine. If iodide is released, the whole body excretion is slow and the thyroid receives a substantial dose, whereas if the bifunctional chelate is metabolized, the labeled chelate would be excreted rapidly by the kidneys (Table 4). However, there is little evidence that the chelates are released as such by hydrolysis of a relatively stable amide bond, but rather metallic radionuclides are released by ligand exchange. For example, for ^{111}In this results in ^{111}In transferrin formation at a rate of 10% per day.[19,20] Indium-111-transferrin has a long biological half-life (Table 4). When the biodistribution of iodine-labeled antibodies are compared with ^{111}In-labeled antibodies, the

Table 5
CONJUGATION OF CHELATORS TO ANTIBODIES

Antibody	Concentration mg/mℓ	Chelator	Ratio[a]	Volume mℓ	pH	Number of Chelator[b]	Ref.
Antimyosin (Fab)	5.0	mDTPAA[c]	NA	1.0	8.0	NA	77
103A	5.0	mDTPAA	250	NA	7.5	0.5	26
Anti HSA	0.3	mDTPAA	870	1.0	8.3	0.2	35
Anti CEA	15	CDTPAA[d]	1.0	0.02	7.0	0.7	29
IgG	15	CDTPAA	1.0	0.02	7.0	0.7	60
17-1A	0.3	CDTPAA	5.0	1.0	8.2	1.3	39
Anti HSA	0.3	CDTPAA	100	1.0	8.2	1.7	39
Anti HSA	8.7	CDTPAA	5.0	0.1	8.2	1.5	47
Anti HSA	11.4	CDTPAA	3.0	0.1	8.2	1.5	47
103A	5.0	cmbEDTA[e]	250	NA	5.0	0.9	26
AntiTf Receptor	29	BABE[f]	10	0.115	9.0	3.5	78

[a] Chealtor/antibody molar ratio.
[b] Number of chelators conjugated per antibody.
[c] DTPA carboxycarbonic mixed anhydride.
[d] Cyclic DTPA dianhydride.
[e] 1-(p-carboxymethoxybenzyl)EDTA, a carbodiimide was used as a coupling agent.
[f] (S)-N-4-(2,3-bis[bis(carboxymethyl)amino]propylbromoacetamide.

iodine-labeled antibodies have a higher blood activity and lower normal tissue activities than the corresponding ^{111}In labeled antibodies.

The use of ^{99m}Tc labeled antibody diagnostically as a tracer for a therapeutic radioiodinated antibody is one example where a relatively stable molecule is not the appropriate control for the therapy. Another example is a protein that is altered to produce rapid blood clearance. Proteins in general are cleared from the blood slowly so that when a radioactive protein is the substrate, the detection of the target radioactivity is difficult. However, for a substrate to be useful as an imaging agent, strict adherence to the requirement that all properties be identical to the parent structure may not be necessary, since an accelerated blood clearance would be a desirable feature for obtaining a high target to background ratio at an early interval after injection. In many individual instances, selected criteria, such as those given in the preceding examples, are preferred and, in particular, this deviation from a perfect biological tracer is an important strategy in the design of radiolabeled antibodies for tumor detection. Alteration of blood clearance by chemical modification or the use of antibody fragments is another important example of this, as is the use of heavily iodinated fibrinogen.[21]

II. BIFUNCTIONAL CHELATES

A. Synthesis

There are three methods for radiolabeling antibodies with metallic radionuclides. The antibody can be directly labeled with a metallic radionuclide but this approach suffers from two weaknesses: the native functional groups may not bind the metal with sufficient affinity to produce an inert radiolabel and these functional groups may be needed to interact with the antigen. Should the radiolabel interfere with this, the normal behavior of the molecule will be altered. The antibody can also be labeled indirectly using either a relatively easily synthesized bifunctional chelate, such as an anhydride, or more complicated molecules with functional groups that are more selective in reacting with the amino residues of antibodies. Some of the reaction conditions used to conjugate chelators to antibodies and other proteins are outlined in Tables 5 and 6.

Table 6
CONJUGATION OF CHELATORS TO OTHER PROTEINS

Protein	Concentration mg/mℓ	Chelator	Ratio[a]	Volume mℓ	pH	Number of Chelators[b]	Ref.
HSA	6.7	dφEDTA[c]	10	NA	7—10	2.0	62
HSA	12.5	mDTPAA[d]	NA	20	7—8	NA	34
Fibrinogen	10	mDTPAA	NA	5.0	8.0	NA	71
Lysosome	20	cDTPAA[e]	NA		7.0	0.6	69
HSA	18.8	cDTPAA	1	NA	7.0	0.6	38
HSA	?	Deferoxamine	?	Variable	7.4	0.8	79

[a] Chelator/antibody molar ratio.
[b] Number of chelators conjugated per antibody.
[c] 1-(p-benzenediazonium)-(ethylenedinitrilo)tetraacetic acid.
[d] DTPA carboxycarbonic mixed anhydride.
[e] Cyclic DTPA dianhydride.

1. De Novo Synthesis

These bifunctional chelates are prepared starting with simple molecules so that the metal chelating portion and the protein-linking group can be placed appropriately. One of the first compounds prepared was 1-(p-benzenediazonium)-ethylenediamine-N,N,N′,N′-tetraacetic acid (azo EDTA).

The first synthetic method involved a multi-step synthesis starting with 1-phenylglycinonitrile to obtain the azo EDTA.[22] One of the major problems with the synthesis of multifunctional molecules is the purification of the intermediates and the final product. Yeh et al.[23] later developed a shorter procedure using amino acid derivatives to produce the azo EDTA.

The same research group also produced another bifunctional chelate that reacted with sulfhydryl groups. This molecule 1-(p-bromoacetamidophenyl) ethylenedinitrilotetraacetic acid[24] has been used to label bleomycin and proteins with ^{111}In. Numerous alternatives are available using this chelate (Figure 1).

Paik et al.[25] prepared the N′-(p-benzenediazonium)-N,N,N″,N″-diethylenetriaminetetraacetic acid (DTTA) on the basis that the DTPA derivative might be more inert than the EDTA derivative of Sundberg.[22] However, extensive work with a model system showed that the diazonium reaction was quite nonspecific. The azo coupling yields of p-methylbenzenediazonium ion with tyrosine and histidine increase as a function of pH.[25] This indicates that the reactive species is the anion and not the neutral molecule. At high pH, selective modification cannot be achieved by the azo coupling reaction if the amino acid residues are in the same concentration. As a result, the diazonium derivative of DTTA was reacted with methyl p-hydroxybenzimidate hydrochloride to give the imidate because the imidate is thought to be selective for the lysine moiety.[19] The reaction is carried out at a pH greater than 8.5. Because they believed that these reaction conditions cause loss of immunologic activity of the antibody, Gansow et al.[26] used a modification of the procedure of Yeh et al.[23] to prepare a carboxymethoxybenzyl derivative of EDTA. This chelating agent was linked to proteins at pH 5 using the carbodimide procedure. The de novo synthetic method has not been popular in conjugating chelating agents to antibodies mainly because of the many synthetic steps.

The initial work on de novo synthesis of EDTA and DTPA analogues was to label proteins with ^{111}In. The recent interest in radiolabeling with ^{67}Cu and ^{212}Bi for therapy, however, has led to the synthesis of new bifunctional chelators. Moi et al.[27] synthesized 6-(p-bromoacetamidobenzyl) 1, 4, 8, 11-tetraazacyclotetradecane-N,N′,N″, N‴-tetraacetic acid via

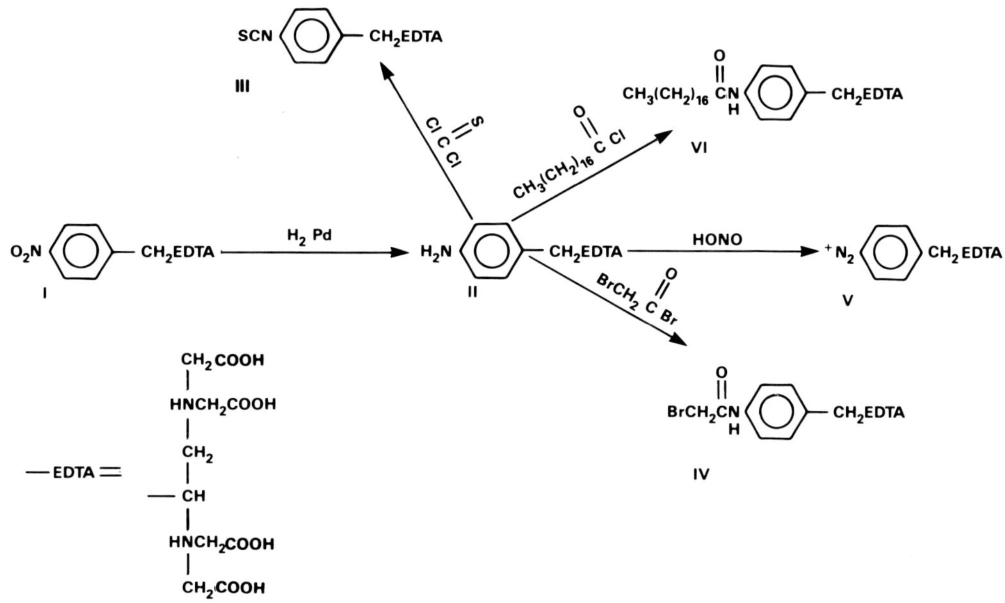

FIGURE 1. Examples of various bifunctional chelating agents (From Wensel, T. G. and Meares, C. F., *Radioimmunoimaging and Radioimmunotherapy*, Burchiel, S. W. and Rhodes, B. A., Eds., Elsevier, Amsterdam, 1983, 185. With permission.)

a six-step synthesis. This macrocyclic compound was reported to form an inert complex with ^{67}Cu. Copper-67 complexes of noncyclic EDTA and DTPA derivatives were reported to decompose very rapidly in serum. Brechbiel et al.[28] reported the synthesis of 1-(p-isothiocyanatobenzyl) diethylenetriamine-pentaacetic acid. The bifunctional chelator was then conjugated to antibody at the amino group of lysine residues. Bismuth and ^{111}In complexes of this antibody-DTPA-conjugate were reported to be inert in vitro. Antibodies labeled with ^{111}In using this method were also reported to give a lower liver concentration (9% injected dose [ID]/g) at 24 hr postinjection in mice than with ^{111}In labeled antibody DTPA conjugates produced via the cyclic DTPA dianhydride method (16% ID/g) and the DTPA carboxycarbonic mixed anhydride method (11% ID/g). The authors stated that the low liver activity was an indicator of the stability of the ^{111}In complex of their antibody DTPA conjugate. However, the authors did not report a statistical analysis of their in vivo data. The liver activity of ^{111}In after injection of the antibody-DTPA conjugates derived from the acylation reactions are much higher than those reported by Hnatowich et al.[29] and Khaw et al.[30] (5.5% and 7.8%, respectively). It is not known whether this discrepancy was caused by differences in specific binding of different antibodies to the liver or differences in non-specific binding caused by a different degree of antibody denaturation.

An important aspect of de novo synthesis is the possibility of a site-directed reaction. Alvarez et al.[31] have linked DTPA molecules via an acylation reaction to an amino group of phenylenediamine and a tripeptide containing glycine-tyrosine-lysine. The second amino group was then conjugated to aldehyde groups derived from oxidation of carbohydrate moieties in the Fc region of antibody. Quadri et al.[32] and Brown et al.[33] also reported the conjugation of DTPA derivatives containing a primary alkylamine to the carbohydrate moieties. The advantage of the site-directed reaction is that it allows the conjugation of a large number of DTPA molecules to the antibody without altering the immunoreactivity of antibody. It also appears that the carbohydrate modified antibody-DTPA-^{111}In shows a lower liver activity than antibody-DTPA-^{111}In prepared using an acylation reaction.[31,32]

2. Acylating Agents

a. Anhydride Method

The anhydrides are, in general, easier to synthesize because DTPA itself is used as the starting material. There are two anhydride methods for conjugating DTPA to antibodies. Krejcarek and Tucker[34] adapted the mixed anhydride technique commonly used in peptide synthesis to radiolabel antibodies. The anhydride was prepared by combining DTPA and isobutylchloroformate. The resulting mixed carboxycarbonic anhydride of DTPA was then used without purification. Paik et al.[35] reinvestigated this technique and found that the mixed anhydride was unstable and, therefore, needed to be analyzed for anhydride concentration immediately before use. Two methods of analysis were developed; one, a spectroscopic method using excess benzylamine, and the other, a gravimetric method using $Ba(OH)_2$ to trap the released carbon dioxide. Large differences between the theoretical and actual concentration of anhydride were observed.

The second method is to use the dianhydride prepared by mixing DTPA with acetic anhydride in the presence of pyridine. This compound was first prepared to produce bifunctional chelates of biochemicals[36,37] but has been used more recently first by Hnatowich et al.[38] and then by Paik et al.[39] to label proteins including antibodies. Presumably, DTPA is conjugated to the lysine moieties in the antibody. This method is preferable to the mixed anhydride method mainly because the cyclic dianhydride is more stable and, consequently, the quality control is easier. The dianhydride method, however, has the possibility of causing inter-and intramolecular cross linking of antibody, but the extent of the cross linking is reported to be negligible when the number of DTPA molecules conjugated per antibody is less than one.[39,40]

b. Carbodiimide Method

A water soluble carbodiimide, 1-ethyl-3(3-dimethylaminopropyl)carbodiimide (EDC) is a very common agent for the conjugation of amino compounds to the carboxy groups of protein in hapten synthesis[41] and enzyme modification.[42] Mechanistic studies suggest that the carboxy groups of protein react first with the carbodiimide to produce a reactive intermediate, O-acylisourea. This intermediate then reacts with nucleophiles such as amino and hydroxy groups. This method was used by DeNardo et al.[43] to conjugate ^{14}C-glycine ethylester to the carboxy group of a coagulation protein, factor VIII. They reported the conjugation of 600 glycine ethylester molecules (MW 136) per factor VIII (MW 3×10^6) without altering its biologic activity. Janoki et al.[44] conjugated the amino groups of desferrioxamine to the carboxy groups of human serum albumin using a carbodiimide coupling method at pH 4.7. They did not report the number of desferrioxamine molecules conjugated per HSA. The HSA-desferrioxamine conjugate has also been radiolabeled[45] with ^{67}Ga. The experimental simplicity involving a one-pot synthesis is the advantage of this method. The disadvantage is that the reaction mechanism, as a whole, is very complex. The formation as well as the disappearance of the O-acylisourea is pH dependent. Therefore, the maintenance of a constant pH is very important for a reproducible conjugation of nucleophiles to proteins. Secondly, the concentration of nucleophiles to be conjugated has to be much higher than the concentration of the amino groups in the protein in order to prevent an inter- or intramolecular cross linking between the carboxy groups and amino groups in the protein. Consequently, the conjugation yield is very low. The carbodiimide method can also be used for the conjugation of a carboxy group of DTPA to the amino groups of an antibody.[46] In a reaction containing a molar excess of DTPA, the carbodiimide first can react with DTPA to form an O-acylisourea of DTPA. This intermediate reacts with the amino groups of an antibody to conjugate DTPA or reacts with water to form free DPTA. Quadri et al.[32] varied the DTPA/antibody ratio and the EDC/DTPA ratio in order to optimize the conjugation of DTPA to antibody. The conjugation reactions at a DTPA/antibody molar ratio of 1000 and

EDC/DTPA molar ratio from two to four gave rise to about 0.8 DTPA molecules conjugated per antibody when the reaction was carried out at pH 6.3. The conjugation increased to 3.4 DTPA molecules per protein when the DTPA/antibody and EDC/DTPA ratios were increased to 3000 and four, respectively. The same reaction gave rise to 0.6 DTPA molecules when the pH of the reaction was 5.0. The conjugation of 0.8 DTPA and 3.4 DTPA molecules reduced the immunoreactivity of the antibody from 90% for the unconjugated control antibody to 67% and 47%, respectively. The extent of deactivation is somewhat higher for the carbodiimide method than the cyclic DTPA dianhydride reaction. The cyclic DTPA dianhydride method gave rise to two DTPA molecules conjugated per antibody without causing a deactivation of immunoreactivity.[47]

c. N-Hydroxysuccinimide Method

Najafi et al.[48] synthesized a penetaester of DTPA by reacting cyclic DTPA dianhydride with N-hydroxysuccinimide. The pentaester was reported to be more stable than cyclic DTPA dianhydride and, consequently, gave rise to a higher DPTA conjugation yield than the dianhydride. However, the DTPA conjugation using the pentaester caused a higher degree of dimers and polymer formation. Najafi and Hutchinson[49] recently have reported that a diester of DTPA reduced the degree of polymerization to that of cyclic DTPA dianhydride. Indium-lll-labeled antibody-DTPA prepared via the ester was reported to be less stable than that prepared via the dianhydride.

3. Aldehyde and Other Coupling Agents

Other less complicated procedures using glutaraldehyde to form a Schiff base between a chelating agent such as penicillamine and the lysine groups on a protein have also been suggested.[50] Glutaraldehyde is relatively nonspecific, causing cross linking and protein polymers. As a result, Ternynck and Aurameas[51] proposed that benzophenone could be reacted with one substrate at pH 6, the conjugate could be purified, and then the second substrate could be coupled at higher pH. This prevents the problems associated with the glutaraldehyde coupling. This same problem can also be avoided by reaction of deferoxamine with one carbonyl group of the glutaraldehyde first, followed by reaction of the protein through the other carbonyl group.[52] Various bis-imidates[53] and bis-(hydroxy succinimide) esters[54] have been used as protein coupling agents. However, these bifunctional coupling agents have not been reported for conjugating chelating agents to antibodies.

B. Chelate-to-Antibody Ratio

1. Reaction Conditions and Effect on Immunologic Activity

Increasing the number of chelating groups per antibody produces opposing effects. On one hand, increasing the number of chelating agents per antibody increases the chelate concentration for a given protein concentration. This is important because the protein concentration is low as is the DTPA concentration and, therefore, the radiochemical yields are generally not quantitative. As a comparison, the standard ^{99m}Tc DTPA kit used in the clinic contains about 2 mg/mℓ DTPA which is orders of magnitude greater than that usually found in bifunctional chelate preparations of antibodies. Higher specific activity is also attainable with increased chelating agents per antibody, but this has become a moot point since lower injected amounts of labeled antibody produce lower target to nontarget ratios rather than higher, as one would predict from saturable binding processes.[55] This latter point is interesting because in most studies with the mathematically similar, receptor binding application, the trend is to produce higher specific activity radioligands rather than lower specific activity ligands. The rationale for higher specific activity is based on the Scatchard rearrangement of the law of mass action. The bound-to-free ratio (B/F) is equal to the product of the affinity constant (K_a) and the receptor concentration (R_o) minus the product of the affinity constant and the bound concentration.

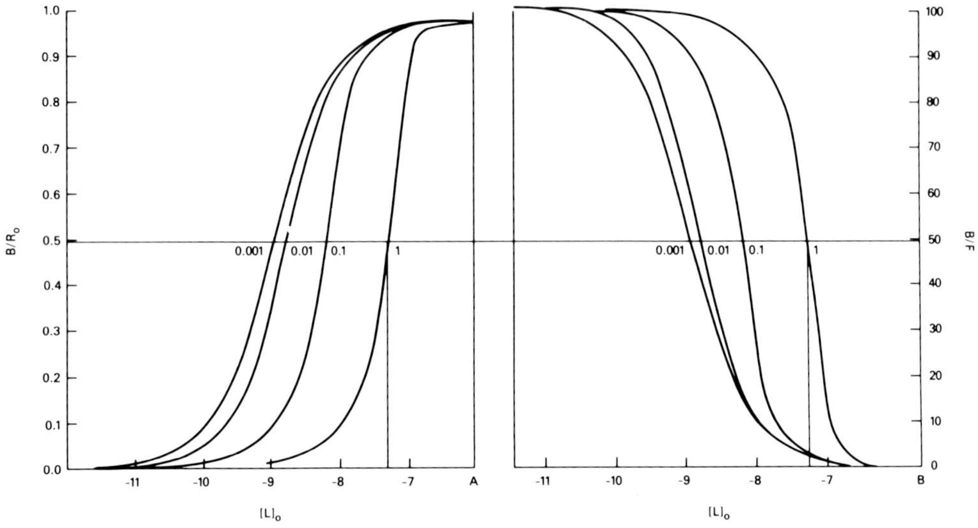

FIGURE 2. Theoretical curves showing the bound (B) to free (F) ratio and the B to total receptor (R_o) as a function of free L_o. The ratio of the volume of the target tissue to the total volume of distribution is given for each line. The ratio of one is the usual test tube experiment. A K_a of 10^9 per mole and R_o of 10^{-9} *M* were used.

$$B/F = K_aR_o - K_aB$$

Therefore, as the concentration of ligand is decreased, the second term, $-K_AB$, becomes negligible and the B/F ratio approaches a maximum. Selikson et al.[56] have shown that the B/F ratio is maximal as a function of total ligand added (L_o) until the fractional saturation of the receptor is about 10% and then drops rapidly as the receptor is further saturated as the Scatchard equation would predict (Figure 2). From this simple example, it would appear that high specific activity receptor-binding ligands and high specific activity antibodies would be superior for external imaging because they represent the highest possible target-to-non-target ratio. In an equilibrium situation with a single ligand and a single receptor or antibody-antigen site this is true. But in vivo there is more than one site competing for the receptor-binding ligand or antibody and, therefore, this conclusion derived for a single target tissue must be reconsidered. The change in the bound concentration as a function of the total receptor concentration gives a different picture. If there is a high concentration of receptor or antigen in the target tissue, but a lower concentration of receptor or antigen in another part of the body, maximum contrast between the two sites is obtained by a complicated mathematical formula relating the relative receptor concentration and the total ligand concentration. In Figure 3 we can see that using a ligand concentration of 10^{-9} *M* and Ka of 12.9×10^9 per mole the greatest discrimination in binding for two receptor concentrations would occur between 10^{-10} and 10^{-9} *M* of total receptor or antigen. This is calculated based on an equilibrium situation where all reagents are contained in the same volume, for example, a test tube. For the in vivo situation, the relationships would be more complicated and a titration of the optimal receptor-binding ligand or antibody concentration would be most efficient if receptor or antigen is at high concentration. Larson et al.[57] have shown an increased specificity index (that is target-to-nontarget ratio or B/F) as a function of increased antigen present in human melanoma. At 48 hr after injection the specificity index ranges from one to six as the tumor concentration of p97 antigen increases from approximately 15 to 20 ng/mg of tumor. Increasing the antibody dose has a complementary effect in that increasing antibody dose favors the higher concentration of antigen and, therefore, there is a higher amount of radioactivity in the tumor compared to sites of lower concentration of antigen

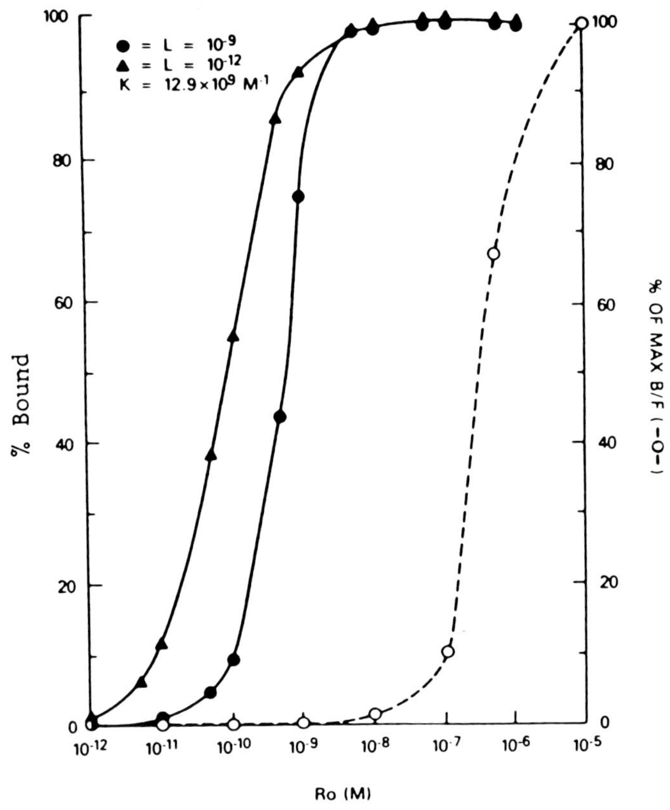

FIGURE 3. The percent of bound (% bound) and the percent of maximum bound to free (% max B/F) as a function of total receptor concentration.

such as the liver. In conclusion there are two effects that must be balanced. Maximum discrimination between two sites containing different antigen or receptor concentration occurs at saturation values between 10 and 90%, but because of the competitive binding between the radiolabeled ligand and the nonradioactive ligand, the amount of radioactivity in the target tissue will generally be less. Therefore, there will be a lower percent of dose/g of target tissue, but the difference in percent of dose/g between two sites will be greater under the optimal conditions. As a result, the specific activity requirements for diagnostic applications of monoclonal antibodies will probably not be great.

The requirement for high specific activity will be necessary for therapeutic applications of monoclonal antibodies. Humm[58] has calculated the weight of labeled IgG for a tumor dose of 80 Gy (8000 rads) using several radionuclides (Table 7).

Certainly, 8000 rads may not be necessary in all cases and many assumptions must be made about the interaction between the emissions and the cells, but the order of magnitude antibody per cell calculated suggests that high specific activity is a necessity. Recently, Eckelman et al. reviewed the use of Gd labeled antibodies to enhance nuclear magnetic resonance (NMR) imaging of tumors.[59] Many of the same arguments apply to the therapeutic use of radiolabeled antibodies. In the practical case 0.1%/g of the injected human dose of 50 mg of MoAb is bound to the tumor; the molarity of Gd (again assuming a 1:1 labeling) is about 3.1×10^{-7} *M*.[59] This represents about 1.9×10^{6} MoAb per cell, a number that exceeds the number of most cell surface antigens per cell. If there are fewer than 10^{6} antigens per cell, then the percent of saturation must be high according to the data in Table 7. High percentage of saturation has not been achieved with receptor binding radiotracers.[59] On the

Table 7
ESTIMATES OF THE AMOUNT OF RADIONUCLIDE NECESSARY TO DELIVER TO 80 GY.

Isotope	Wt of labeled IgG for tumor dose of 80 Gy (μg/g tumor)	MoAb/g tumor (× 10 [10] molecules)	MoAb/Cell[a] (molecules)
^{111}At	0.0043	1.6	160
^{90}Y	0.22	82.8	8280
^{77}As	0.70	263.5	26350
^{131}I	2.40	903.4	90340

[a] Assuming 10^8 cells/g; this equals radionuclides per cell assuming 1:1 labeling.

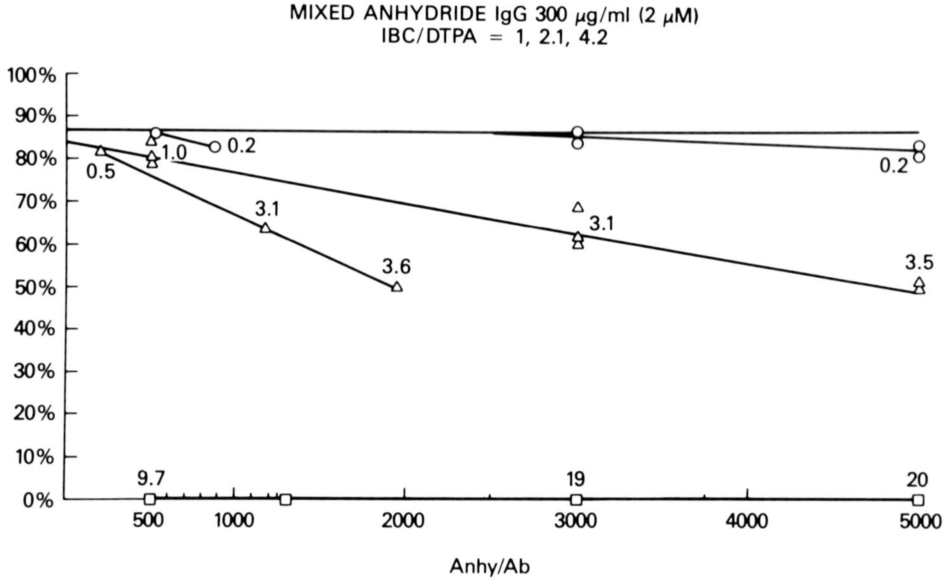

FIGURE 4. The immunologic activity as a function of the molar ratio of added mixed anhydride to antibody ratio. The numbers on the curves are the measured DTPA molecules per antibody. (From the work of Paik et al.[35])

other hand, if the MoAbs are not bound to cell surface antigens, but rather trapped non-specifically, then the dosimetry changes drastically, particularly for short range radiations. Very seldom has the concentration of radioactivity in the tumor been shown to be bound specifically as it has for receptor-binding radiotracers. The approaches used to increase the number of Gd atoms per antibody will be equally effective for therapeutic antibodies, although in both cases a decrease in immunologic activity is a very undesirable side effect.[59]

The major problem with increasing the number of chelating groups per antibody is that it decreases the immunologic activity. This is an important concern because it decreases the specificity of antibody-mediated diagnosis or therapy. Studies on the effects of the number of chelating groups per antibody have been carried out for DTPA labeled antibodies (Figures 4 to 10). The effect of the mixed anhydride on the immunologic activity of the antibody has been studied in detail by Paik et al.[35] The key to this study was the development of analytic methods to measure the actual concentration of mixed anhydride available for reaction. If the anhydride-to-antibody ratios are plotted against immunologic activity, one can see a difference in values that produces a specific decrease in immunologic activity for

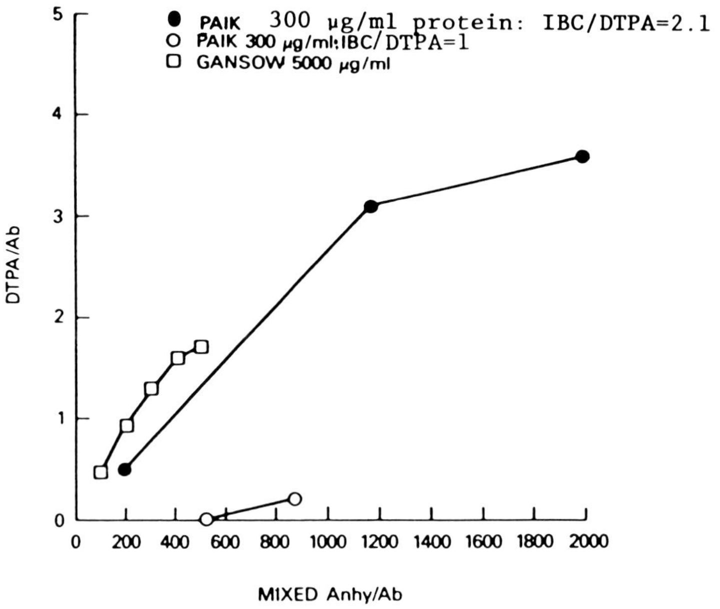

FIGURE 5. The measured DTPA molecules per antibody as a function of the mixed anhydride to antibody ratio. (From the work of Paik et al.[35] and Gansow et al.[14])

both the number of chelating agents per antibody and the ratio of anhydride to antibody. It appears that an anhydride-to-antibody ratio of 1173 at a protein concentration of 300 μg/mℓ introduces 3.1 DTPA molecules per antibody as measured by ^{111}In titration. The immunologic activity is decreased from 87.4 to 63.6%, a 27% decrease (Figure 4). Another study by Gansow et al.[14] related the anhydride-to-antibody ratio to the number of chelating groups incorporated by using ^{14}C labeled DTPA, but did not comment on the resulting immunologic activities (Figure 5).

Similar studies have been carried out using the cyclic dianhydride (cDTPAA) at various protein concentrations (Figures 8 and 9). Hnatowich et al.[60] worked at high protein concentrations and, therefore, the coupling of DTPA was more efficient than that found at the lower protein concentration used by Paik et al.[39] Paik et al. also looked at the effect of chelate concentration on the immunoreactivity of different antibodies. The difference in sensitivity between an antibody to HSA and a colorectal antibody 17-1A was remarkable. It appears that conjugation techniques will not be generally applicable and that each antibody will have to be studied in detail. This is also evident for different fragments because the ratio of variable region to constant region will be lower, increasing the chance of destroying the immunologic activity of a small fragment such as Fab compared to the intact IgG. In addition, the number of lysine groups in each antibody domain is not known for many of the antibodies, and since that is the target group for the DTPA anhydride, the sensitivity to the number of chelating groups for antibody fragments could be different.

Wong et al.[61] analyzed both the moles of cyclic DTPA anhydride incorporated as a function of the moles added and the decrease in immunologic binding as measured by cell binding for a number of cell types. The incorporation of DTPA was similar for the two antibodies studied as was the decrease in cell binding as a function of DTPA incorporation (Figures 6 and 7).

Brechbiel et al.[28] recently reported a comparison of four bifunctional chelates in vitro and in vivo (Figure 10). The cyclic anhydride of DTPA and the isothiocyanatobenzyl derivative

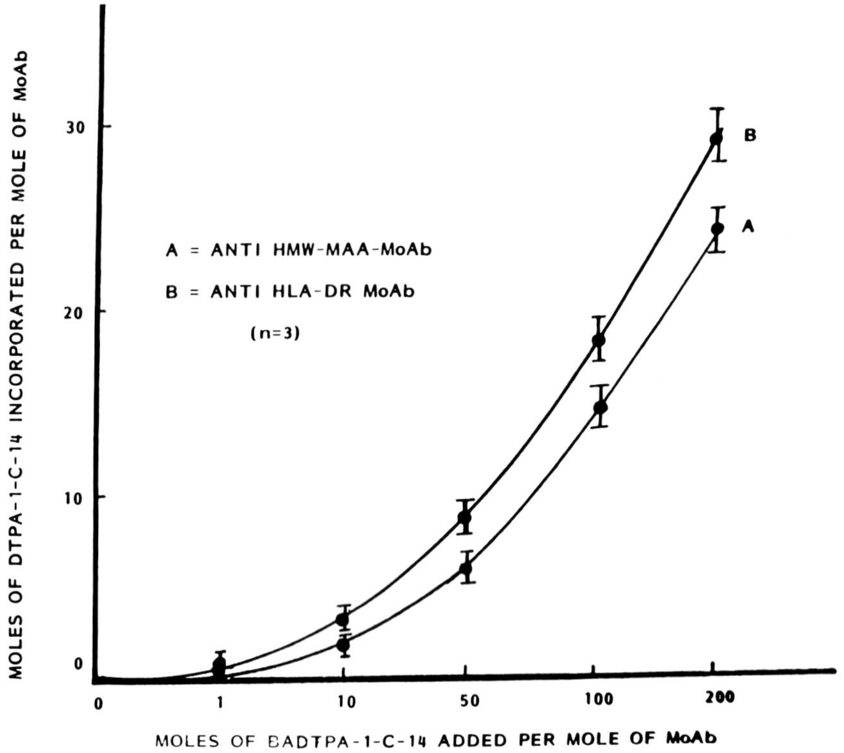

FIGURE 6. The molar ratios of ^{14}C-DTPA incorporated per mole of antibody using the bicyclic anhydride of DTPA (BADTPA) with anti-human melanoma associated antigen (HMW-MAA) and anti-human class II major histocompatibility complex antigen (HLA-DR). (Reprinted with permission from *Appl. Radiat. Isot.*, 38, Wang, T. S. T., Ng, A. K., Alsedairy, S., Fawwaz, R. A., Hardy, M. A., and Alderson, P. O., A method for direct quantification of the amount of DTPA In-111 monoclonal antibody preparations, Copyright 1987, Pergamon Press plc.)

of EDTA showed the sharpest drop in immunologic activity as a function of chelates per antibody. The compound that appeared to cause the least damage was the isothiocyanatobenzyl derivative of DTPA. These studies were carried out using monoclonal antibody B72.3. The images of tumors in nude mice reflected the relative immunoreactivities even though all antibodies were purified by a two column technique. Apparently, loosely bound or kinetically labile radiolabel is the cause of the distribution differences.

The difference between immunologically active antibody and immunologically inactive antibody is not a result of the difference in chelating agents per antibody, but most likely, the position of the chelating agent. Paik et al.[47] have shown that immunologically active and inactive antibody contain the same number of chealting groups per antibody as measured by ^{111}In titration, thus the site of addition of the chelating group, for example, in the variable binding region is likely to be the key factor influencing immunoreactivity.

2. *Measurement of Chelate-to-Antibody Ratio*

The number of chelating agents per antibody molecule has been determined by a number of processes. Sundberg et al.[22] use ^{14}C-labeled azo-Φ-EDTA to determine the EDTA incorporated. This was compared with the number of chelating groups available for indium binding. The binding of indium was monitored by perturbed angular correlation of the ^{111}In emissions, which is strongly affected by the interaction of the ^{111}In with macromolecules permitting the fraction of ^{111}In bound to protein to be determined. Using this technique, about 40% of the chelating groups could be detected. This result was confirmed by terbium

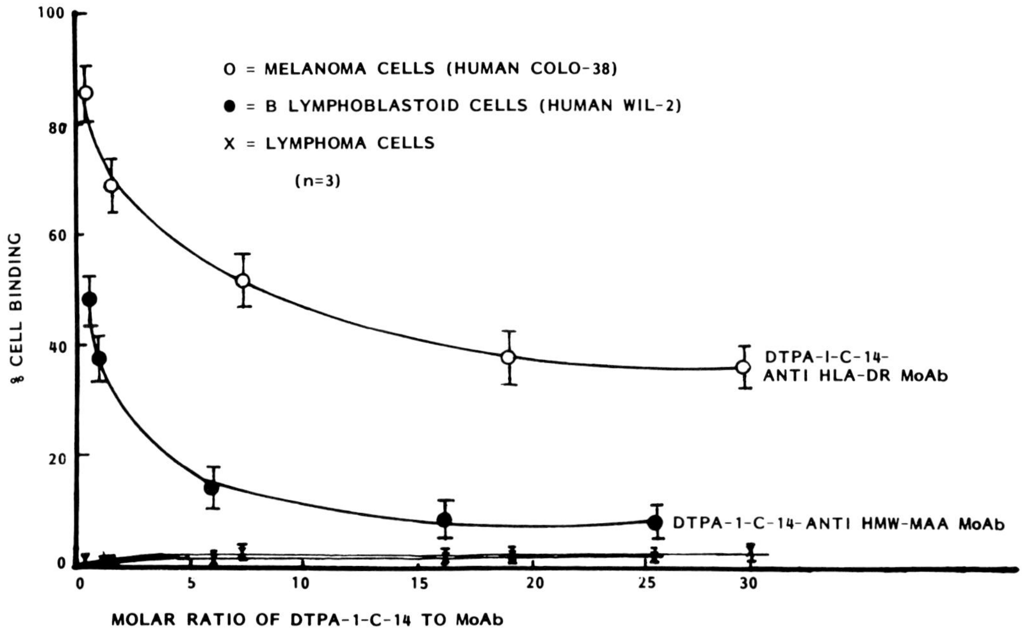

FIGURE 7. Cell-binding assay of ^{14}C-DTPA-anti HMW-MAA MoAb and ^{14}C-DTPA-anti HLA-DR MoAb. (Reprinted with permission from *Appl. Radiat. Isot.*, 38, Wang, T. S. T., Ng, A. K., Alsedairy, S., Fawwaz, R. A., Hardy, M. A., and Alderson, P. O., A method for direct quantification of the amount of DTPA In-111 monoclonal antibody preparations, Copyright 1987, Pergamon Press plc.)

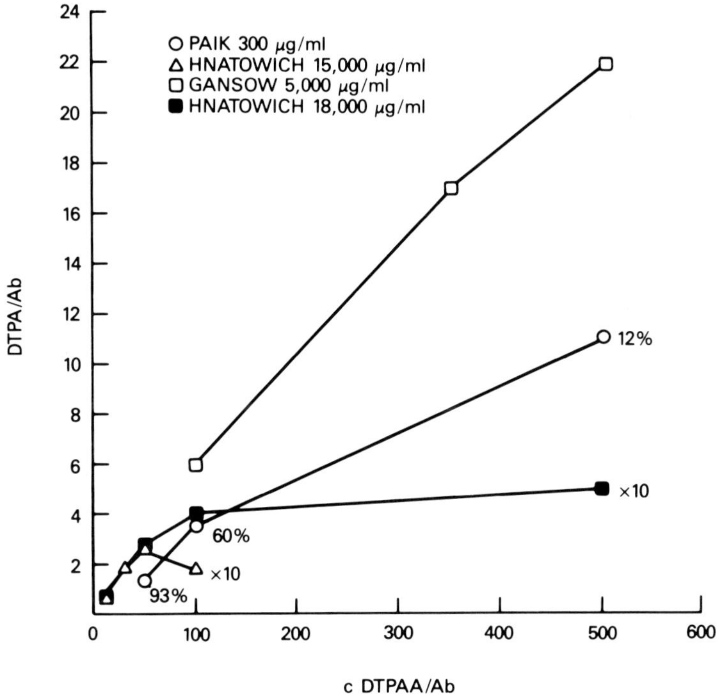

FIGURE 8. The measured DTPA molecules per antibody as a function of the molar ratio of added cyclic anhydride. (From the work of Paik et al.,[39] Hnatowich et al.,[60] Gansow et al.,[14] and Hnatowich et al.[38] The % on the curve from Paik et al. is the resulting immunoactivity.

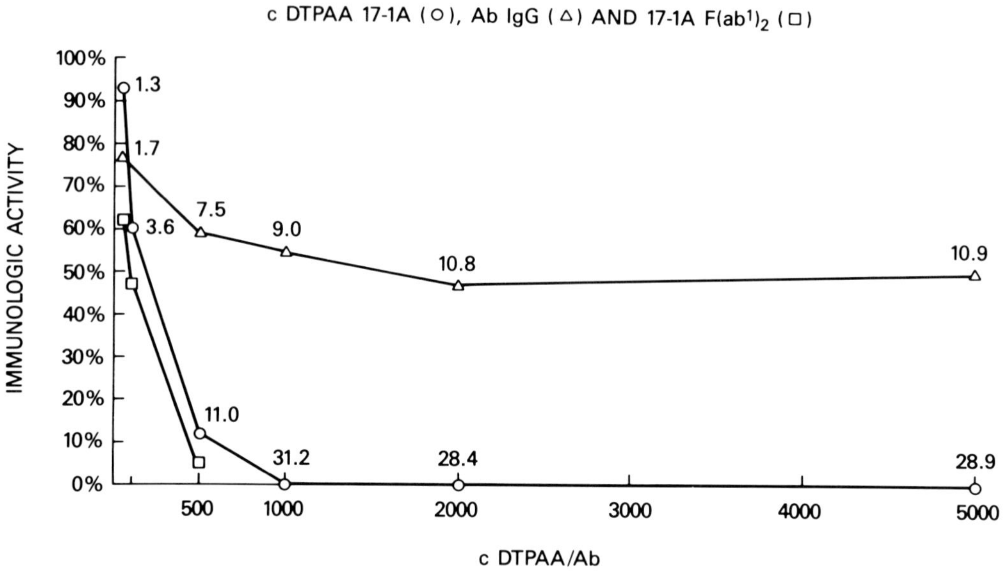

FIGURE 9. The immunologic activity as a function of the added cyclic DTPA antibody for three antibodies. The numbers on the curves represent the number of measured DTPA per antibody. (Based on Paik, C. H., Ebbert, M. A., Murphy, P. R., Lassman, C. R., Reba, R. C., Eckelman, W. C., Pak, K. Y., Powe, J., Steplewski, Z., and Kaprowski, H., *J. Nucl. Med.*, 24, 1158, 1983; Powe, J., Pak, K. Y., Paik, C. H., Steplewski, Z., Ebbert, M. A., Herlyn, D., Ernst, C., Alavi, A., Eckelman, W. C., Rebo, R. C., and Koprowski, H., *Cancer Drug Delivery*, 1, 125, 1984.)

titration monitored by fluorescence spectroscopy. A control experiment using hydrolyzed protein confirmed the correct total number of ligands.

Other groups have followed their lead and used ^{14}C-labeled chelating groups and titration of the chelating groups with indium. No-carrier-added ^{111}In can be used if the starting-DTPA-to-protein ratio is small so that the fraction of protein-bound ^{111}In is a statistically valid number. Two assumptions are associated with this measurement: the binding parameters for the conjugated DTPA and free DTPA must be the same, and the direct (adventitious) binding of ^{111}In to protein must be negligible. Meares et al.[62] indicated that labeling with ^{111}In at neutral pH resulted in direct binding of ^{111}In to HSA. In addition, metal contamination plays a large part in all tracer chemistry and in this case it must either be nonexistent or at least nonpreferential, that is, the bound DTPA and the free DTPA must be either not contaminated or contaminated to the same extent. In cases where the starting DTPA-to-protein ratio is large, a molar excess of carrier indium to DTPA must be used for the titration of protein-bound DTPA. This does not carry the same assumptions as the no carrier added ^{111}In procedure because carrier indium saturates both the free DTPA and the bound DTPA. Indium-111 ion is used as a tracer for the cold indium.

III. RADIOLABELING

A. Reaction Conditions

The reaction conditions depend on the radionuclide, the concentration of chelating agent, and the specific activity required. The most detailed radiolabeling studies have been carried out with ^{111}In (Table 8). Less detailed work has appeared for ^{99m}Tc and other radionuclides (Table 9). The key in most metallic radiolabeling procedures is to keep the metal ion in solution using a high concentration of a weak complexing agent, such as acetate or citrate, and then add that complex to the derivatized antibody to radiolabel the bifunctional chelate by ligand exchange.

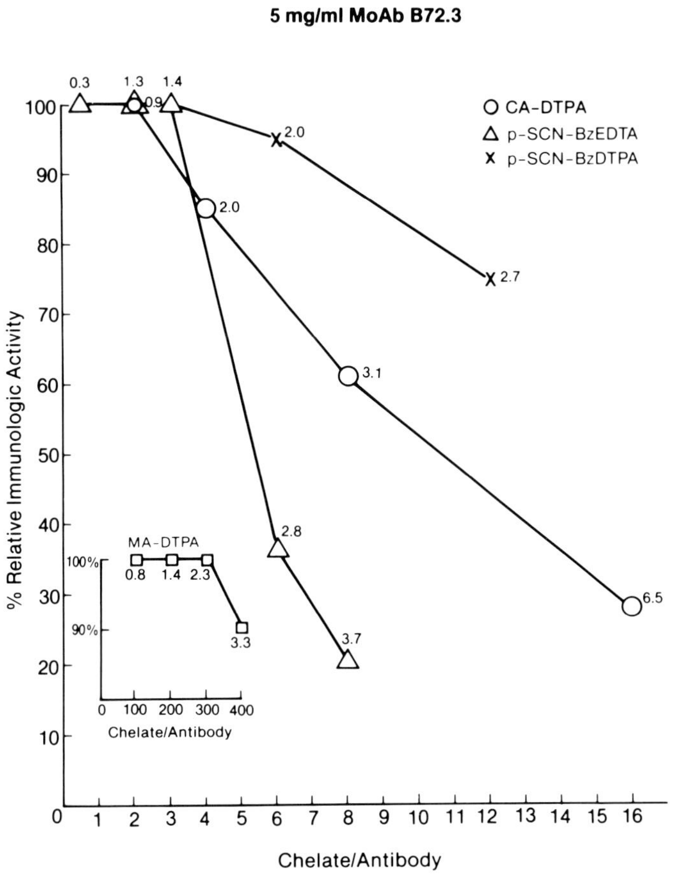

FIGURE 10. The percentage relative immunologic activity as a function of chelates per antibody for four conjugation techniques: cyclic dianhydride (CA-DTPA), the mixed anhydride (MA-DTPA), the isothiocyanato derivative of EDTA (p-SCN-BzEDTA), and the isothocyanato derivative of DTPA (p-SCN-BzDTPA).

B. Labeling Yield and Specific Activity

1. Radiolabeling with ^{111}In

The radiochemical yield depends indirectly on the protein concentration, but more directly on the chelating agent concentration. The theoretical specific activity of ^{111}In-labeled antibody conjugates containing 1 DTPA molecule per Ab is 324 uCi ^{111}In per μg of IgG (MW = 150,000) assuming the formation of a 1:1 complex of ^{111}In and DTPA. At the highest protein concentration of 20 mg/mℓ of IgG and a 1:1 DTPA/Ab ratio, the concentration of DTPA will be $1.3 \times 10^{-4}M$ or 52 μg DTPA/mℓ. At the lowest concentration of protein suggested, 300 μg/mℓ of IgG, the concentration of DTPA will be 2×10^{-6} M or 0.79 μg DTPA/mℓ. this is more than three orders of magnitude lower than the DTPA concentration used in clinical ^{111}In-DTPA or ^{99m}Tc-DTPA kits.

The experimentally obtainable specific activity is of the order of 1% of the theoretical specific activity, especially when the mass of antibody and, thus that of DTPA, is very small. This is mainly because DTPA is blocked by metallic contaminants and, thus, the effective concentration of DTPA is very low. It is important to appreciate that each experimental step, such as Sephadex® G-50 column chromatography to separate antibody-DTPA from free DTPA, increases the possibility of contaminating antibody-DTPA solution with

Table 8
^{111}IN RADIOLABELING CONDITIONS

Chelate	Time (hr)	T(°C)	pH	Ref.
0.1 *M* Glycine	0.25	25	3.5	77
0.05 *M* Citrate	NA	r.t.	3.6	26
0.5 *M* Citrate	0.25	37	6.0	80
0.5 *M* Acetate	NA	r.t.	5.5—6.0	38
0.5 *M* Acetate	NA	r.t.	6.0	29
0.02 *M* Citrate	0.5	4	4.8	39
0.02 *M* Citrate	0.5	4	4.8	47
0.03 *M* Citrate	0.1—1.25	r.t.	5.0	78
0.3 *M* Acetate	12	4	6—6.5	81
0.1 *M* Glycine	?	?	3.5	82

Table 9
RADIOLABELING CONDITIONS

Radiolabel	Buffer	Time (hr)	T(°C)	pH	Ref.
^{99m}Tc	0.3 *M* Phosphate	NA	r.t.	8.0	71
^{46}Sc	0.5 *M* Citrate	0.25	37	6.0	80
^{67}Ga	0.5 *M* Citrate	0.25	37	6.0	
^{99m}Tc	0.1 *M* Acetate	0.17	r.t.	6	69
^{90}Y	0.5 *M* Acetate		r.t.	5	20
^{99m}Tc	0.1 *M* Acetate	0.25	r.t.	4.5	70
^{109}Pd	HEPES-HCl		r.t.	5—6	84
^{67}Ga	0.01 NHCl	0.25	r.t.	?	79

metallic ions. When the mass of antibody is of the order of 100 μg, the contamination by even minute amounts of metallic impurities can cause an adverse effect on the radiolabeling of antibody-DTPA with metallic radionuclides. The best procedure for radiolabeling a small amount of antibody is to use a concentrated antibody solution for the DTPA conjugation reaction, in order to increase the conjugation yield. The antibody-DTPA conjugate is then radiolabeled without separating free DTPA molecules. Antibody DTPA-^{111}In can be easily separated from DTPA-^{111}In by Sephadex® G-50 molecular permeation chromatography. Paik, et al.[47] reported that the reactivities toward ^{111}In ions of free DTPA, immunoreactive antibody-DTPA, and nonimmunoreactive antibody-DTPA from the same conjugation reaction are about the same. Therefore, the radiochemical yield of immunoreactive antibody-DTPA is determined by the relative concentration of each DTPA species.

2. Radiolabeling with ^{99m}Tc

a. Direct Labeling

Direct labeling, that is, using the amino acids of the antibody to complex the metal, may result in a labile chemical bond because of the stereochemistry of the functional groups in the tertiary structure of the antibody. Only when the protein is known to bind the metal with high affinity is direct labeling useful. Even in those cases, the protein is usually labeled by injecting a soluble salt that exchanges with the protein. The injection of ^{67}Ga-citrate and ^{111}In-chloride are examples of direct labeling of proteins in vivo. It appears that neither ^{111}In nor ^{67}Ga have been labeled directly to antibodies. On the other hand, ^{99m}Tc has been directly labeled to proteins, and particularly to antibodies,[63-66] but the stability and inertness of the bond are in question. Although the investigators utilized different buffer systems, pH, and incubation times, a common feature is the use of stannous ion as a reducing agent. The advantage of direct labeling is the experimental simplicity. However, in at least one case, the resulting antibody complex with ^{99m}Tc has been reported to be unstable. This necessitated the use of an elaborate molecular permeation chromatographic system to purify the ^{99m}Tc-labeled antibodies.[65] This is consistent with the observation of Eckelman et al.[67] who had published in 1971 that albumin binding of ^{99m}Tc is so weak that multiple chromatographic purifications resulted in further radiochemical impurities as a result of dissociation. The competitive binding of ^{99m}Tc by stannous oxide also was a source of radiochemical impurities. Since then, other reviews have documented the same instabilities. Steigman et al.[68] suggested that the mechanism of binding was related to sulfhydryl groups, but Lanteigne and Hnatowich[69] recently proposed the importance of a helix structure. Paik et al.[70] suggested that ^{99m}Tc is bound by both a high affinity, low capacity site and by a low affinity, high capacity site. Their study suggests that the high affinity site is indeed related to the presence of sulfhydryl groups. However, the extent of high affinity site binding is not quantitative and depends on the antibody fragment used. For IgG and $F(ab')_2$ which contain disulfide bridges between the heavy chains, a high titer of reduced disulfide groups are detected in the presence of stannous ion. For Fab, which does not have a disulfide bridge between the heavy chains, very few sulfhydryl groups could be detected. This trend parallels the percentage binding of ^{99m}Tc when binding to the low affinity sites is prevented by the presence of excess DTPA. For IgG, about 24% of the ^{99m}Tc binds to high affinity sites whereas for $F(ab')_2$ only 16% of the ^{99m}Tc is bound to the high affinity sites. Very little ^{99m}Tc is bound to Fab with high affinity.

These results are useful in interpreting other data. For instance, Rhodes et al.[65] probably increase the high affinity binding by long incubation of antibodies with stannous ion. Khaw et al.[71] probably have a small percentage of directly bound antibody because they use Fab fragments, whereas Lonteigne and Hnatowich[69] show binding via DTPA and directly to IgG. The best solution to the problem of low affinity binding of ^{99m}Tc has been put forth by Paik et al.[70] They suggest that all radiolabeling with ^{99m}Tc or with ^{111}In should be done in the presence of excess DTPA. Even though that may decrease the radiochemical yield, it guarantees an inert chemical bond either directly to the protein through the high affinity sites for ^{99m}Tc, or through the bifunctional chelate for Tc and In.

b. Indirect Labeling

The indirect labeling methods have mostly involved the use of DTPA bound to the protein. The labeling parameters are reviewed in Tables 8 and 9. The complications of labeling at low concentration of DTPA have been outlined in the previous section. Other chelating agents, derivatives of dimercaptoacetamide[72] and bis N-methylthiosemicarbazone[73] and metallothionein[74] have been conjugated to antibodies for ^{99m}Tc labeling. Although ^{99m}Tc labeling conditions and biodistribution studies of the labeled products were reported, a systematic investigation of the effectiveness of these chelators for complexing ^{99m}Tc in competition with antibody has not been reported.

IV. CONCLUSION

Many uncertainties remain in the use of antibodies labeled with metallic radionuclides. The role of those intended for diagnostic use is not well defined and those intended for therapeutic use are largely untested. Two considerations have arisen from the many radiolabeling studies. One is that the amount of direct binding of metals to protein, especially ^{99m}Tc, which would be thought to be small, is quite significant mainly because the concentration of chelating agent is small. This direct binding must be avoided because directly bound radionuclide is usually labile in vivo and detracts from the localization specificity. The second consideration is the sensitivity of antibody immunoreactivity to the number of chelating groups conjugated. However, there is an inverse relationship between the number of DTPA molecules conjugated per antibody and antibody immunoreactivity. One has to optimize the balance between the above two factors. The maintenance of immunoreactivity appears to be a more important factor because there is no appropriate purification method to separate all monoclonal antitumor antibody from deactivated antibody.

The quality of radioimmunoimaging of tumors depends on a relative term, a tumor-to-blood or a tumor-to-normal-tissue ratio. This term is influenced by variables such as specificity of antibody, immunological purity, the mode of radiolabeling, affinity constant, the concentration of antibody injectate, the concentration of antigen or the size of tumor, antigen modulation, circulating antigen, host antibody, physiological half life of antibody, and blood flow. For a given antibody specificity and tumor model system, one of the major factors contributing to a high background activity is deactivated antibody or irrelevant antibody contaminated in antibody injectate. This necessitates delayed imaging due to the time required for a clearance of impure antibodies from background. Although the results vary from one study to another, perhaps due to variations in blood flow and differences in antibody and tumor system, generally it takes 1 to 2 days to achieve maximum tumor uptake. Suitable images are, however, possible 2 to 7 days after injection despite the persistence of significant ıckground activity. Immunological purity is, thus, as important as specificity for radioimmunoimaging of tumors at a short interval after injection, especially when an intact antibody ıs used because of its long physiological half life. Nevertheless, the importance of the immunological purity has not been widely recognized. A measurement of the percentage of immunoreactive antibody in injectate has been neglected in many papers reporting in vivo distribution of radiolabeled antibody. It is, therefore, very difficult to compare data from each research group to gain quantitative information on the effect of immunological impurity on tumor-to-blood ratio. Our preliminary studies indicate that the major factor contributing to high blood and normal tissue activities is a high percentage of contaminating radiolabeled, deactivated or immunologically irrelevant antibodies in the antibody injectate.[75]

A specific method for antibody purification is affinity chromatography. However, appropriate affinity columns for purification of monoclonal antitumor antibodies are not readily available because tumor antigens are either prohibitively expensive or not yet isolated. The best method appears to be high-performance liquid chromatography (HPLC). This method is the most advanced nonspecific method of purifying compounds because of its high number of theoretical plates in a given column.

A HPLC method was used by Hnatowich et al. to separate native antibody from cross-linked polymerized antibodies.[29] We also have used a 7.5 × 600 mm Bio-Sil® 250 column to separate modified antibodies based on their molecular size. The retention times (using 0.02 *M* NaH_2PO_4 at pH 7.4 and a flow rate of 1 mℓ/min) were 11 min for the first high molecular weight antibody component, 13.5 min for the second high molecular weight antibody component, and 16.5 min for monomeric anti-CEA monoclonal antibody. The intensity of high molecular weight antibody peaks increased to 10% and 25% of the total when the number of DTPA molecules conjugated per antibody was increased to 2.5 and 6, respectively. The formation of high molecular weight antibodies was caused by intermolecular cross linking of antibodies because cyclic DTPA dianhydride was used as a conjugating agent.

Juarez-Salinas et al.[76] separated immunoreactive antibody from inactive antibodies, caused by modification in their light-chain composition, by using a HPHT hydroxyapatite HPLC column. A Protein-PAK-DEAE 5PW column was also used to purify a monoclonal antibody of IgG_1 class to 95% immunoreactive antibody.[85] Although different monoclonal antibodies might behave somewhat differently in these columns, the combination of these columns appears to be very useful to purify antibodies before and after structural modifications. An improvement of purification methods will contribute substantially to the reduction of background activities and, thus, to the achievement of higher tumor-to-background ratios.

Compared with ^{131}I labeled antibodies, ^{111}In and ^{99m}Tc labeled antibodies generally give higher localization in normal tissue, especially liver and spleen, and lower activity in blood. This might reflect the chemical stability of ^{111}In and ^{99m}Tc-labeled antibodies as compared to ^{131}I labeled antibodies. For faster blood clearance, ^{111}In or ^{99m}Tc-labled $F(ab')_2$ fragments are theoretically preferable. However, a high kidney uptake of the ^{111}In or ^{99m}Tc labeled fragments appears to be a limiting factor discouraging the use of the labeled fragments as imaging agents for tumors in close proximity to kidneys. The level of kidney and liver uptake could be lowered if the bond linking DTPA and antibody was somewhat less stable than a peptide bond, permitting ^{111}In-DTPA to be cleaved from the antibody fragments.

In conclusion, there are three important considerations for radiolabeling antibodies with metallic radionuclides for radioimmunoimaging:

1. The binding of the radionuclides to weak sites of antibodies should be prevented using free DTPA as a competing ligand. This is especially important for ^{99m}Tc labeling.
2. The balance between the number of chelating agents conjugated per antibody and the altered antibody immunoreactivity should be optimized.
3. Analytical methods to purify immunoreactive monoclonal antibodies from deactivated or irrelevant antibodies must be developed.

REFERENCES

1. **Hamilton, J. G. and Soley, M. H.,** Studies in iodine metabolism by the use of a new radioactive isotope of iodine, *Am. J. Physiol.*, 127, 557, 1939.
2. **Berson, S., Yalow, R. S., Bauman, A., Rothschild, M., and Newerly, K.,** ^{131}I metabolism in human subject: demonstration of insulin binding globulin in the circulation of insulin treated subjects, *J. Clin. Invest.*, 35, 170, 1956.
3. **Pressman, D. and Eisen, H. N.,** The zone of localization of antibodies V. An attempt to saturate antibody-binding sites in mouse kidney, *J. Immunol.*, 64, 273, 1950.
4. **Pressman, D.,** Radiolabeled antibodies, *Ann. N.Y. Acad. Sci.*, 69, 664, 1957.
5. **Pressman, D., Day, E.D., and Blau, M.,** The use of paired labeling in the determination of tumor localizing antibodies, *Cancer Res.*, 17, 845, 1957.
6. **Quinones, J., Mizejewski, G., and Beierwaltes, W. H.,** Choriocarcinoma scanning using radiolabeled antibody to chorionic gonadotrophin, *J. Nucl. Med.*, 12, 69, 1971.
7. **Goldenberg, D. M., DeLand, F., Kim, E., Bennett, S., Primus, F. J., VanNaegell, J. R., Estes, N., Desimone, P., and Rayburn, P.,** Use of radiolabeled antibodies to carcinoembryonic antigen for the detection and localization of diverse cancers by external photoscanning, *N. Engl. J. Med.*, 298, 1384, 1978.
8. **Richards, P., Tucker, W. D., and Srivastava, S. C.,** Technetium-99m: an historical perspective, *Int. J. Appl. Radiat. Isot.*, 33, 793, 1982.
9. **Jungerman, J. A., Yu, K.-HP., and Zanelli, C. I.,** Radiation absorbed dose estimates at the cellular level for some electron-emitting radionuclides for radioimmunotherapy, *Int. J. Appl. Radiat. Isot.*, 35, 883, 1984.
10. **Chan, P. C., Lisco, E., Lisco, H., and Adelstein, S. J.,** The radiotoxicity of Iodine-125 in mammalian cells. II. A comparative study on cell survival and cytogenetic responses to $^{125}IUdR$, $^{131}HTdR$, *Radiat. Res.*, 67, 332, 1976.
11. **Smit, J. A., Myburgh, J. A., and Neirinckx, R. D.,** Specific inactivation of sensitized lymphocytes in vitro using antigen labeled with ^{211}At, *Clin. Exp. Immunol.*, 14, 107, 1973.
12. **Bloomer, W. D., McLaughlin, W. H., Neirinckx, R. D., Adelstein, S. J., Gordon, P. R., Ruth, T. J., and Wolf, A. P.,** Astatine-211-tellurium radiocolloid cures experimental malignant ascites, *Science*, 212, 340, 1981.
13. **Harrison, A., and Royle, L.,** Preparation of a ^{211}At-IgG conjugate which is stable in vivo, *Int. J. Appl. Radiat. Isot.*, 35, 1005, 1984.

14. **Gansow, O. A., Atcher, R. W., Link, D. C., Friedman, A. M., Seevers, R. H., Anderson, W., Scheinberg, D. A., and Strand, M.,** Generator-produced Bi-212 chelated to chemically modified monoclonal antibody for use in radiotherapy, in *ACS Symposium Series No. 241 Radionuclide Generators: New System for Nuclear Medicine Applications,* Knapp., F. F., Jr. and Butler, T. A., Eds., American Chemical Society, Washington, D. C., 1984, 215.
15. **Kozak, R. W., Atcher, R. W., Gansow, O. A., Friedman, A. M., Hines, J. J., and Waldmann, T. A.,** Bismuth-212-labeled anti-Tac monoclonal antibodies — particle-emitting radionuclides as modalities for radioimmunotherapy, *Proc. Natl. Acad. Sci. U.S.A.,* 83, 474, 1986.
16. **O'Brien, H. A.,** Overview of radionuclides useful for radioimmunoimaging and radioimmunotherapy and current status of preparing radiolabeled antibodies, in *Radioimmunoimaging and Radioimmunotherapy,* Burchiel, S., Ward, R., and Rhodes, B. A., Eds., Elsevier, Amsterdam, 1983, 161.
17. **Rockoff, S. D., Goodenough, D. J., and McIntire, K. R.,** Theoretical limitations in the immunodiagnostic imaging of cancer with computed tomography and nuclear scanning, *Cancer Res.,* 40, 3054, 1980.
18. **Larson, S. M., Carrasquillo, J. A., and Reynolds, J. C.,** Radioimmunodetection and radioimmunotherapy, *Cancer Invest.,* 2, 363, 1984.
19. **Paik, C. H., Herman, D. E., Eckelman, W. C., and Reba, R. C.,** Blood clearance and in vitro stability of proteins containing a conjugated indium-111 chelate, *J. Radioanal. Chem.,* 57, 553, 1980.
20. **Hnatowich, D. J., Virzi, V., and Doherty, P. W.,** DTPA-coupled antibodies labeled with ^{90}Y, *J. Nucl. Med.,* 26, 503, 1985.
21. **Harwig, J. F., Coleman, R. E., Harwig, S. S. L., Sherman, L. A., Siegel, B. A., and Welch, M. J.,** Highly iodinated fibrinogen: a new thrombus-localizing agent, *J. Nucl. Med.,* 16, 756, 1975.
22. **Sundberg, M. W., Meares, C. F., Goodwin, D. A., and Diamonti, C. I.,** Selective binding of metal ions to macromolecules using bifunctional analogs of EDTA, *J. Med. Chem.,* 17, 1304, 1974.
23. **Yeh, S. M., Sherman, D. G., and Meares, C. F.,** A new route to bifunctional chelating agents: conversion of amino acids to analogs of ethylenedinitrilotetraacetic acid, *Anal. Biochem.,* 100, 152, 1979.
24. **DeReimer, L. H., Meares, C. F., Goodwin, D. A., and Diamanti, C. I.,** BLEDTA: tumor localization by a bleomycin analogue containing metal-chelating group, *J. Med. Chem.,* 22, 1019, 1979.
25. **Paik, C. H., Eckelman, W. C., and Reba, R. C.,** Reactivity of amino acids in the azo coupling reaction. I. Dependence of their reactivity on pH, *Bioorg. Chem.,* 8, 25, 1979.
26. **Scheinberg, D. A., Strand, M., and Gansow, O. A.,** Tumor imaging with radioactive metal chelates conjugated to monoclonal antibodies, *Science,* 215, 1511, 1982.
27. **Moi, M. K., Meares, C. F., McCall, M. J., Cole, W. C., and DeNardo, S. J.,** Copper chelates as probes of biological systems: stable copper complexes with a macrocyclic bifunctional chelating agent, *Anal. Biochem.,* 148, 249, 1985.
28. **Brechbiel, M. W., Gansow, O. A., Atcher, R. W., Schlom, J., Esteban, J., Simpson, D. E., and Colcher, D.,** Synthesis of 1-(p-isothiocyanatobenzyl) derivatives of DTPA and EDTA. Antibody labeling and tumor-imaging studies, *Inorg. Chem.,* 25, 2772, 1986.
29. **Hnatowich, D. J., Layne, W. W., Childs, R. L., Lanteigne, D., and Davis, M. A.,** Radioactive labeling of antibody: a simple and efficient method, *Science,* 220, 613, 1983.
30. **Khaw, B. A., Strauss, H. W., Cahill, S. L., Soule, H. R., Edgington, T., and Cooney, J.,** Sequential imaging of indium-111-labeled monoclonal antibody in human mammary tumors hosted in nude mice, *J. Nucl. Med.,* 25, 592, 1984.
31. **Alvarez, V. L., Wen, M.-L., Lee, C., Lopes, A. D., Rodwell, J. D., and McKearn, T. J.,** Site-specifically modified ^{111}In labelled antibodies give low liver backgrounds and improved radioimmunoscintigraphy, *Nucl. Med. Biol.,* 13, 347, 1986.
32. **Quadri, S. M., Paik, C. H., Yokoyama, K., and Reba, R. C.,** Synthesis and in vivo comparison of antibody DTPA conjugates with different chemical bonds, Proc. 6th Int. Symp. on Radiopharmaceutical Chemistry, Boston, June 29—July 3, 1986, 266.
33. **Brown, B. A., Dearborn, C. B., Neacy, W. P., Sands, H., and Gallagher, B. M.,** Comparison of carbohydrate directed versus amine directed attachment of DTPA to murine monoclonal antibodies, Proc. 6th Int. Symp. on Radiopharmaceutical Chemistry, Boston, June 29—30, 1986, 263.
34. **Krejcarek, G. E. and Tucker, K. L.,** Covalent attachment of chelating groups to macromolecules, *Biochem. Biophys. Res. Commun.,* 77, 581, 1977.
35. **Paik, C. H., Murphy, P. R., Eckelman, W. C., Volkert, W. A., and Reba, R. C.,** Optimization of the DTPA mixed-anhydride reaction with antibodies at low concentration, *J. Nucl. Med.,* 24, 932, 1983.
36. **Eckelman, W. C., Karesh, S. M., and Reba, R. C.,** New compounds: fatty acid and long chain hydrocarbon derivatives containing a strong chelating agent, *J. Pharm. Sci.,* 64, 704, 1975.
37. **Karesh, S. M., Eckelman, W. C., and Reba, R. C.,** Biological distribution of chemical analogs of fatty acids and long chain hydrocarbons containing a strong chelating agent, *J. Pharm. Sci.,* 66, 225, 1977.
38. **Hnatowich, D. J., Layne, W. W., and Childs, R. L.,** The preparation and labeling of DTPA-coupled albumin, *J. Appl. Radiat. Isot.,* 33, 327, 1982.

39. **Paik, C. H., Ebbert, M. A., Murphy, P. R., Lassman, C. R., Reba, R. C., Eckelman, W. C., Pak, K. Y., Powe, J., Steplewski, Z., and Kaprowski, H.,** Factors influencing DTPA conjugation with antibodies by cyclic DTPA anhydride, *J. Nucl. Med.*, 24, 1158, 1983.
40. **Hnatowich, D. J., Childs, R. L., Lanteigne, D., and Najafi, A.,** The preparation of DTPA-coupled antibodies radiolabeled with metallic radionuclides: an improved method, *J. Nucl. Med.*, 65, 147, 1983.
41. **Bauminger, S., and Wilchek, M.,** The use of carbodiimides in the preparation of immunizing conjugates, in *Methods in Enzymology*, Part A, Vol. 70, Vunakis, H. V., and Langone, J. J., Eds., Academic Press, New York, 1980, 151.
42. **Swaisgood, H., and Natake, M.,** Effect of carboxyl group modification on some of the enzymatic properties of L-glutamate dehydrogenase, *J. Biochem.*, 74, 77, 1973.
43. **DeNardo, S. J., Hershgold, E. J., DeNardo, G. L., Krohn, K. A., and Godin, D. R.,** Radioactive labeling of protein carboxyl groups on Factor VIII: use of carbodiimides for nuclear medicine, *J. Nucl. Med.*, 18, 472, 1977.
44. **Janoki, G. A., Harwig, J. F., Chanachai, W., and Wolf, W.,** ^{67}GaDesferrioxamine-HSA: synthesis of chelate protein conjugates using carbodiimide as a coupling agent, *Int. J. Appl. Radiat. Isot.*, 34, 871, 1983.
45. **Yokoyama, A., Ohmomo, Y., Horiuchi, K., Saji, H., Taneka, H., Yamamoto, K., Ishii, Y., and Torizuka, K.,** Deferoximine, a promising bifunctional chelating agent for labeling proteins with gallium. Ga-67 DF-HSA: concise communication, *J. Nucl. Med.*, 23, 909, 1982.
46. **Paik, C. H., Lassman, C. R., Murphy, P. R., Ebbert, M. A., Eckelman, W. C., and Reba, R. C.,** A carbodiimide method for DTPA conjugation to antibody, *Hybridoma*, 2, 248, 1983.
47. **Paik, C. H., Hong, J. J., Ebbert, M. A., Heald, S. C., Reba, R. C., and Eckelman, W. C.,** Relative reactivity of DTPA, immunoreactive antibody-DTPA conjugates and nonimmunoreactive antibody-DTPA conjugate toward ^{111}In, *J. Nucl. Med.*, 26, 482, 1985.
48. **Najafi, A., Childs, R. L., and Hnatowich, D. J.,** Coupling antibody with DTPA: an alternative to the cyclic anhydride, *Int. J. Appl. Radiat. Isot.*, 35, 554, 1984.
49. **Najafi, A., and Hutchison, N.,** The use of DTPA diactivated ester in coupling DTPA to proteins, *Int. J. Appl. Radiat. Isot.*, 37, 548, 1986.
50. **Pritchard, J. H., Ackerman, M., Tubis, M., and Blahd, W. H.,** ^{111}In labeled antibody heavy metal chelate conjugates: a potential alternative to radioiodination, *Proc. Soc. Exp. Biol. Med.*, 151, 297, 1976.
51. **Ternynck, T., and Aurameas, S.,** A new method using p-benzoquinone for coupling antigens and antibodies to marker substances, *Ann. Immunol. (Poznan)*, 127, 197, 1976.
52. **Ohmomo, Y., Yokoyama, A., Yamauchi, Y., Horiuchi, K., Saji, H., Tanaka, C., and Torizuka, K.,** In vivo kinetics and thrombus accumulation of ^{67}Ga-labeled urokinose, *J. Nucl. Biol. Med.*, 12, 47, 1985.
53. **Peters, K. and Richards, F. M.,** Chemical cross-linking: reagents and problems in studies of membrane structure, *Annu. Rev. Biochem.*, 46, 523, 1977.
54. **Pilch, P. F. and Czech, M. P.,** Interaction of cross-linking agents with the insulin effector system of isolated fat cells, *J. Biol. Chem.*, 254, 3375, 1979.
55. **Eckelman, W. C., Gibson, R. E., Vieras, F., Rzeszotarski, W. J., Francis, B. F., and Reba, R. C.,** Receptor binding radiotracers: a class of potential radiopharmaceuticals, *J. Nucl. Med.*, 20, 350, 1979.
56. **Selikson, M., Gibson, R. E., Eckelman, W. C., and Reba, R. C.,** Calculation of binding isotherms when ligand and receptor are in different volumes of distribution, *Anal. Biochem.*, 108, 64, 1980.
57. **Larson, S. M., Carrasquillo, J. A., Krohn, K. A., Brown, J. P., McGuffin, R. W., Ferrens, J. M., Graham, M. M., Hill, L. D., Beaumier, P. L., Hellstrom, K. E., and Hellstrom, I.,** Localization of ^{131}I labeled p97-specific Fab fragments in human melanonas as a basis for radiotherapy, *J. Clin. Invest.*, 72, 2101, 1983.
58. **Humm, J. L.,** Dosimetric aspects of radiolabeled antibodies for tumor therapy, *J. Nucl. Med.*, 27, 1490, 1986.
59. **Eckelman, W. C., Tweedle, M., and Welch, M. J.,** NMR enhancement with Gd labeled antibodies, in *Radiolabeled Monoclonal Antibodies for Imaging and Therapy — Potential, Problems and Prospects*, Srivastava, S. C., Ed., Plenum Publishing, New York, 1988.
60. **Hnatowich, D. J., Childs, R. L., and Lanteigne, D.,** The preparation of DTPA-coupled antibodies radiolabeled with metallic radionuclides: an improved method, *J. Immunol. Methods*, 65, 147, 1983.
61. **Wang, T. S. T., Ng, A. K., Alsedairy, S., Fawwaz, R. A., Hardy, M. A., and Alderson, P. O.,** A method for direct quantification of the amount of DTPA In-111 monoclonal antibody preparations, *Appl. Radiat. Isot.*, 38, 315, 1987.
62. **Meares, C. F., Goodwin, D. A., Leung, C. S. H., Girgis, A. Y., Silvester, D. J., Nunn, A. D., and Lavender, P. L.,** Covalent attachment of metal chelates to proteins: the stability in vivo and in vitro of the conjugate of albumin with a chelate of ^{111}In, *Proc. Natl. Acad. Sci. U.S.A.*, 73, 3803, 1976.
63. **Pettit, W. A., DeLand, F. H., Bennett, S. J., and Goldenberg, D. M.,** Improved protein labeling with stannous tartrate reduction of pertechnetate, *J. Nucl. Med.*, 21, 59, 1980.

64. **Huang, J. T., Kaiszadeh, M., and Sakimura, I.,** Detection of bacterial endocarditis with ^{99m}Tc labeled antistaphylococcal antibody, *J. Nucl. Med.*, 21, 783, 1980.
65. **Rhodes, B. A., Torvestad, D. A., Breslow, K., Burchiel, S. W., Reed, K. A., and Austin, R. K.,** ^{99m}Tc labeling and acceptance testing of radiolabeled antibodies, in *Tumor Imaging*, Burchiel, S. W. and Rhodes, B. A., Eds., Masson, New York, 1982, 111.
66. **Sundrehage, E.,** Formation of ^{99m}Tc immunoglobulin G complexes free from radionuclides, quality controlled by radioimmunoelectrophoresis, *Eur. J. Nucl. Med.*, 7, 549, 1982.
67. **Eckelman, W. C., Meinken, G., and Richards, P.,** ^{99m}Tc-human serum albumin, *J. Nucl. Med.*, 12, 707, 1971.
68. **Steigman, J., Williams, H. P., and Solomon, N. A.,** The importance of the protein sulfhydryl group in HSA labeling with ^{99m}Tc, *J. Nucl. Med.*, 16, 573, 1975.
69. **Lanteigne, D. and Hnatowich, D. J.,** The labeling of DTPA-coupled proteins with ^{99m}Tc, *Int. J. Appl. Radiat. Isot.*, 35, 617, 1984.
70. **Paik, C. H., Phan, L. N. B., Hong, J. J., Sahami, M. S., Heald, S. C., Reba, R. C., Steigman, J., and Eckelman, W. C.,** The labeling of high affinity sites of antibodies with ^{99m}Tc, *Int. J. Nucl. Med. Biol.*, 12, 3, 1985.
71. **Khaw, B. A., Strauss, H. W., Carvalho, A., Locke, E., Gold, H. K., and Haber, E.,** ^{99m}Tc labeling of antibodies to cardiac myosin Fab and to human fibrinogen, *J. Nucl. Med.*, 23, 1011, 1982.
72. **Kasina, S., Vanderheyden, J. L., and Fritzberg, A. R.,** Application of diamide dimercaptide N_2S_2 bifunctional chelating agents for ^{99m}Tc labeling of proteins, Proc. 6th Int. Symp. on Radiopharmaceutical Chemistry, Boston, June 29—July 3, 1986, 269.
73. **Arano, Y., Yokoyama, A., Magata, Y., Saji, H., Horiuchi, K., and Torizuka, K.,** Synthesis and evaluation of a new bifunctional chelating agent for ^{99m}Tc labeling proteins: p-carboxyethylphenyl-glyoxal-di (N-methylthiosemicarbazone), *Int. J. Nucl. Med. Biol.*, 12, 425, 1985.
74. **Tolman, G. L., Hadjian, R. A., Morelock, M. M., Drozynski, C. A., and Cormier, T. A.,** The use of metalloproteins as bifunctional chelators, *J. Nucl. Med.*, 26, 438, 1985.
75. **Powe, J., Pak, K. Y., Paik, C. H., Steplewski, Z., Ebbert, M. A., Herlyn, D., Ernst, C., Alavi, A., Eckelman, W. C., Reba, R. C., and Koprowski, H.,** Labeling monoclonal antibodies and $F(ab')_2$ fragments with ^{111}In using cyclic DTPA anhydride and their in vivo behavior in mice bearing human tumor xenografts, *Cancer Drug Delivery*, 1, 125, 1984.
76. **Juarez-Salinas, H., Engelhorn, F., Bigbee, W. L., Lowry, M. A., and Stanket, L. H.,** Ultrapurification of monoclonal antibodies by high-performance hydroxyapatite (HPHT) chromatography, *Bio Techniques*, (Bio-Rad Laboratories, Richmond, Calif.), May/June 1984.
77. **Khaw, B. A., Fallon, J. T., Strauss, H. W., and Haber, E.,** Myocardial infarct imaging of antibodies to canine cardiac myosin with ^{111}In diethylenetriamine pentaacetic acid, *Science*, 209, 295, 1980.
78. **Meares, C. F., McCall, M. J., Reardan, D. T., Goodwin, D. A., Diamanti, C. I., and McTigue, M.,** Conjugation of antibodies with bifunctional chelating agents: isothiocyanate and bromoacetamide reagents, methods of analysis and subsequent addition of metal ions, *Anal. Biochem.*, 142, 68, 1984.
79. **Yokoyama, A., Omono, Y., Horiuchi, K., Saji, H., Yamamoto, K., Ishii, Y., Tanaka, H., and Torizuka, K.,** Deferoxamine, an excellent bifunctional chelating agent for labeling proteins with gallium: ^{67}Ga-HSA, *J. Nucl. Med.*, 22, 32, 1981.
80. **Anderson, W. T. and Strand, M.,** Stability, targeting and biodistribution of ^{46}Sc and ^{67}Ga-labeled monoclonal antibody in erythroleukemic mice, *Cancer Res.*, 45, 2154, 1985.
81. **Fairweather, B. A., Bradwell, A. R., Dykes, P. W., Vaughan, A. T., Watson-James, S. F., and Chandler, S.,** Improved tumor localization using indium-111 labeled antibodies, *Br. Med. J.*, 287, 167, 1983.
82. **Rainsbury, R. M., Westwood, J. H., Coombes, R. C., Neville, A. M., Ott, R. J., Kalirai, T. S., McCready, V. R., and Gazet, J. C.,** Localization of metastatic breast carcinoma by a monoclonal antibody chelate labeled with ^{111}In, *Lancet*, 22, 934, 1983.
83. **Wensel, T. G., and Meares, C. F.,** Binfunctional chelating agents for binding metal ions to protein, in *Radioimmunoimaging and Radioimmunotherapy*, Burchiel, S. W. and Rhodes, B. A., Eds., Elsevier, Amsterdam, 1983, 185.
84. **Fawwaz, R. A., Wang, T. S. T., Srivastava, S. C., Rosen, J. M., Ferrone, S., Hardy, M. A., and Alderson, P. O.,** Potential of palladium-109-labeled antimelanoma antibody for tumor therapy, *J. Nucl. Med.*, 25, 796, 1984.
85. **Millipore,** *Technical Bulletin*, L26/82528, Millipore, Bedford, Mass., January, 1985.

Chapter 7

PHYSIOLOGICAL, PHARMACOLOGICAL, AND IMMUNOLOGICAL ASPECTS OF ANTIBODY TARGETING

Howard Sands and Brian M. Gallagher

TABLE OF CONTENTS

I. INTRODUCTION

The development of monoclonal antibodies for the delivery in vivo of drugs, toxins, and radioisotopes for the detection and treatment of disease is currently an extremely active field of research. Exquisite specificity can be designed into these molecules, permitting the recognition of, and differentiation between, cell surface molecules and various other biological molecules in vitro, for example, fibrin vs. fibrinogen. It has frequently been assumed that this in vitro specificity could also be readily achieved in vivo. In practice, however, the various in vitro specificities and affinities for target vs. nontarget sites have not been reflected by the extent of in vivo localization. Much of the earlier work demonstrated poor in vivo localization, results which can be attributed to the methods employed to either produce, purify, or radiolabel the antibody. Current labeling and purification technology represents a significant improvement in the quality of these methods.[2-4] However, despite great improvements in the chemistry for generating immunoreactive and stable radiolabeled antibodies, the specificity of localization, particularly in tumors, remains significantly lower than predicted by in vitro assays.[5] This is due, at least in part, to a series of physiological, pharmacological, and immunological factors which have received very little attention. The vast majority of in vivo studies has employed various IgG isotypes which have evolved over millions of years to remain in the circulating plasma for relatively long periods of time in order to provide a protection against infections. It is not surprising that the intrinsic ability of these molecules to rapidly exist from the blood toward extravascular sites would be at least affected by the same physiological factors which limit the delivery of virtually any compound to tumor sites. These include such nonimmunological factors as capillary surface area, capillary permeability, regional perfusion within the tumor, and the percent of the cardiac output supplying the tumor. These must be considered in addition to the immunological factors relating to both the antibody specificity and affinity and antigen shedding, availability, and turnover.[5] In addition, pharmacological factors such as the dose of antibody injected, route of administration, and dose regimen can profoundly influence tumor localization.[6-8] This chapter presents a few examples of the above physiological, pharmacological, and immunological factors and their influence on antibody localization in human xenografts grown in mice. It is designed to give an overview of the state-of-the-art, rather than an exhaustive review of the literature.

II. PHYSIOLOGICAL FACTORS

A. Blood Flow

The relative vascular perfusion to various tissues can be measured using the diffusable tracer ^{86}Rb.[9-11] Following i.v. injection, this tracer equilibrates into tissues within 2 min in accord with regional vascular perfusion[11] (Figure 1). It is possible, therefore, to measure the relative blood flow to a tissue by sampling tissues 2 min after injection of ^{86}Rb and determining the activity within the tissue as percent injected ^{86}Rb dose per gram of tissue.

By employing this technique, the effect of tumor mass on blood perfusion was measured for the SL1/SL2 murine lymphoma over a tumor weight range from 20 to 1000 mg for tumors grown either subcutaneously or under the capsule of the kidney (subrenal capsule, see Figure 2).[10,12] Animals bearing tumors of various weights growing in either of these two sites were injected with ^{86}Rb. The results indicated that the murine lymphomas growing at the subrenal site had a considerably greater perfusion than the same tumors grown subcutaneously (Figure 3). In addition, subcutaneous tumors showed no weight dependent change in perfusion, whereas a significant decrease in the relative perfusion was observed with increased tumor mass in the subrenal site.

The relationship between these observations and the relative uptake of a monoclonal

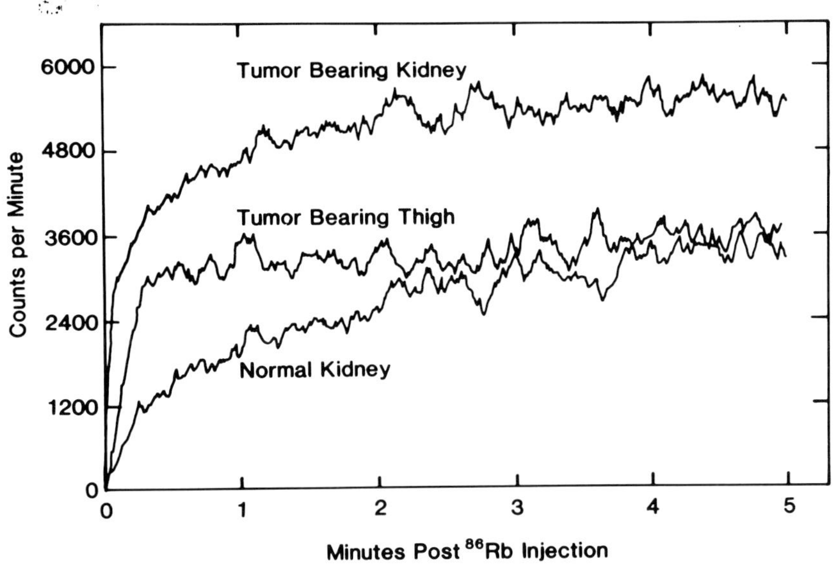

FIGURE 1. Time course of ^{86}Rb uptake by mouse tissues. (From Sands, H., Jones, P. L., Neacy, W. P., Shah, S. A., and Gallagher, B. M., *Cancer Immunol. Immunotherap.*, 22, 169, 1986. With permission.)

antibody OX7 directed against the THY 1.1 antigen expressed by SL1/SL2 cells[10] is shown in Table 1. Tumors growing at the subrenal site had approximately a fivefold greater blood perfusion than the same tumors growing subcutaneously. This difference appeared to correlate with the four- to fivefold difference in uptake for the specific OX7 antibody. Anti-horseradish peroxidase (anti-HRP) was also used as an isotype-matched nonspecific immunoglobulin which has no specificity for either the SL1 or SL2 tumor type. This nonspecific antibody showed a significantly lower accumulation in tumors than the OX7 antibody and further demonstrated no difference in accumulation between tumors growing at either site (Table 1). The amount of anti-HRP found associated with these tumors apparently reflects the nonspecific permeability of these tumors to macromolecules. The 2 to 3% I.D. per gram observed for these murine lymphomas is quite low compared with values seen with various tumor xenograft models.

In contrast to the excellent correlation between blood flow and antibody uptake observed in the homograft system employing the murine lymphoma growing in the mouse, interpretation of the data obtained for a human xenograft growing in the athymic mouse is more complicated. The Clouser human breast carcinoma was grown at three sites in the athymic mouse and blood flow and antibody (B6.2) uptake were determined in a manner similar to that described above. In addition to the subcutaneous and subrenal sites, tumors were also grown in the spleen of the animals (intrasplenic).[13] Despite large differences in blood flow, over a factor of approximately eight for subcutaneous vs. subrenal tumors as determined by ^{86}Rb, antibody uptake at all tumor sites was identical (Table 2). As in the homograft system described above, blood flow to the subrenal tumors decreased as tumor size increased, whereas no such relationship was seen for the subcutaneous tumors (Figure 4). It was observed, however, that the accumulation of anti-HRP, the nonspecific immunoglobulin, was significantly greater in the xenograft models than in the murine homograft model described above (4 to 8% I.D./g versus 2 to 3% I.D./g, respectively). This finding prompted further investigation to determine if other factors besides tumor perfusion could be affecting antibody targeting.

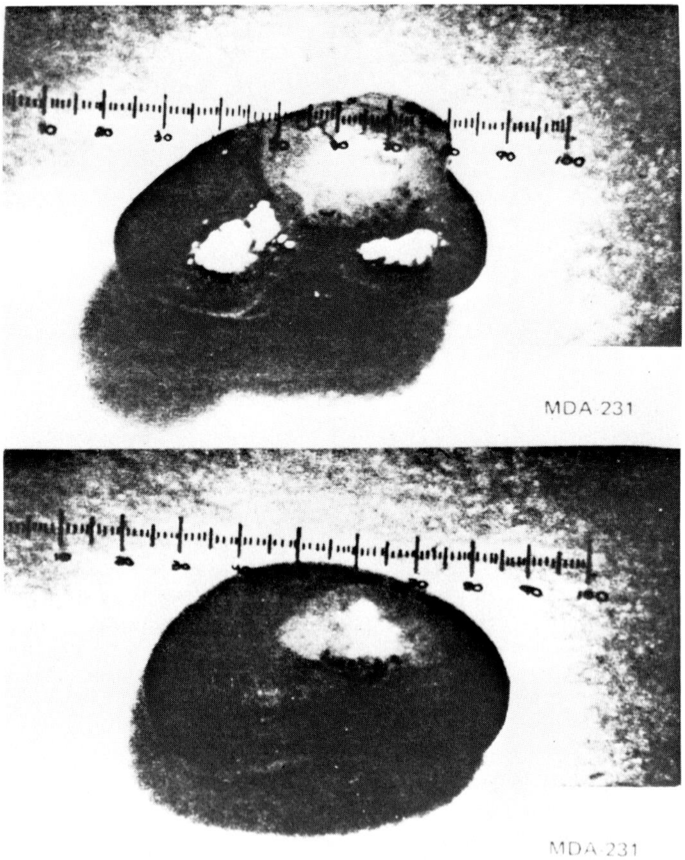

FIGURE 2. Visualization of the MDA-MB-231 human breast tumor implanted for 11 days under the renal capsule showing the ocular micrometer scale superimposed in control (top) and L-phenylalanine mustard treated (bottom) animals. (From Bodgen, A. F., Kelton, D. E., Cobb, W. R., and Esber, H. J., *Proc. Symp. on the Use of Athymic (Nude) Mice in Cancer Research*, Houchens, D. P. and Ovejera, A. A., Eds., Gustav Fisher, Stuttgart, 1978, 231. With permission.)

B. Vascular Volume and Vascular Permeability

In addition to blood flow, the vascular volume and vascular permeability of tumors may be major determinants of antibody uptake. The vascular permeability of tumors has been reported to be higher than that of nonmalignant tissues.[14-16] Localization studies of monoclonal antibodies in murine and human tumor xenografts have shown that the accumulation of nonspecific IgG was significantly greater in a human breast carcinoma than in a murine lymphoma.[17] These results could be explained by an increased vascular permeability of the human xenograft. Employing *in situ* ^{99m}Tc labeling of red blood cells and coinjection of ^{125}I-labeled bovine serum albumin and ^{131}I-labeled nonspecific IgG, the vascular volume and permeability to these two different proteins can be rapidly and simultaneously determined.[18] Results of such a study are presented in Figure 5 and show that the vascular permeability of the xenograft (Clouser) was significantly greater than that of the murine lymphoma (SL2). These results may explain the differences observed in the accumulation of monoclonal

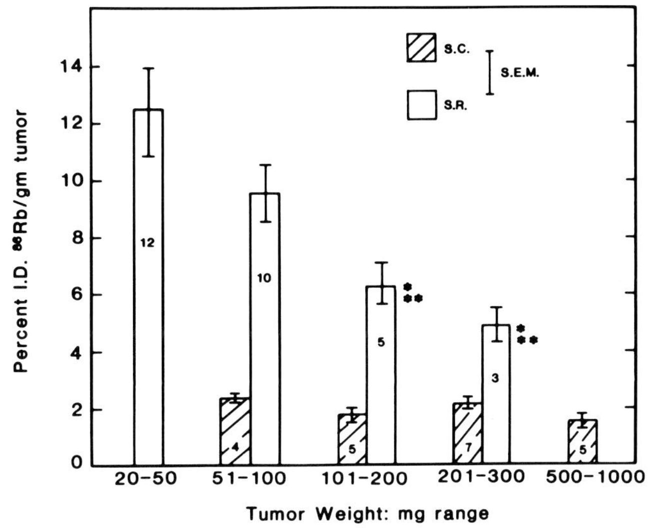

FIGURE 3. Effect of tumor size on relative blood flow of SL1 and SL2 tumors. Data from SL1 and SL2 tumors were pooled. The number in the bars indicate the number of tumors used to generate the mean. S.C. indicates subcutaneous tumors. S.R. indicates subrenal tumors. *, $p < 0.05$ compared with 20 to 50 mg and **, $p > 0.05$ compared with 51 to 100 mg. (From Sands, H., Jones, P. L., Neacy, W. P., Shah, S. A., and Gallagher, B. M., *Cancer Immunol. Immunotherap.*, 22, 169, 1986. With permission.)

Table 1
IN VIVO ACCUMULATION IN SUBRENAL AND SUBCUTANEOUS SL2 TUMORS 48 HR AFTER ANTIBODY INJECTION[9,10]

	Subcutaneous (% injected dose per gram)	Subrenal (% injected dose per gram)
^{86}Rb	2.20 ± 0.35	11.12 ± 2.85
OX7 (specific)	6.24 ± 3.59	27.44 ± 7.64
Anti-HRP (nonspecific)	2.26 ± 1.14	2.96 ± 0.18

Note: ±, Standard deviation

Table 2
ANTIBODY UPTAKE AND BLOOD FLOW TO CLOUSER TUMORS[5]

	Subcutaneous (% injected dose per gram)	Subrenal (% injected dose per gram)	Intrasplenic (% injected dose per gram)
^{125}I-B6.2	23.70 ± 7.3	18.7 ± 5.5	19.7 ± 3.4
^{86}Rb	1.10 ± 0.4	7.8 ± 3.5	3.3 ± 2.2
^{131}I-Anti-HRP	7.81 ± 1.1	6.1 ± 1.1	6.0 ± 2.4

Note: ±, standard deviation.

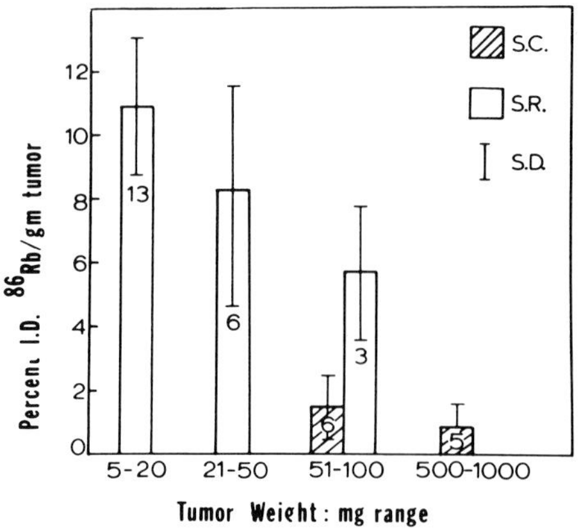

FIGURE 4. Effect of tumor size on relative blood flow of human xenografts (Clouser) growing in athymic mice. The number in the bars indicate the number of tumors used to generate the mean. S.C. indicates subcutaneous tumors. S.R. indicates subrenal tumors.

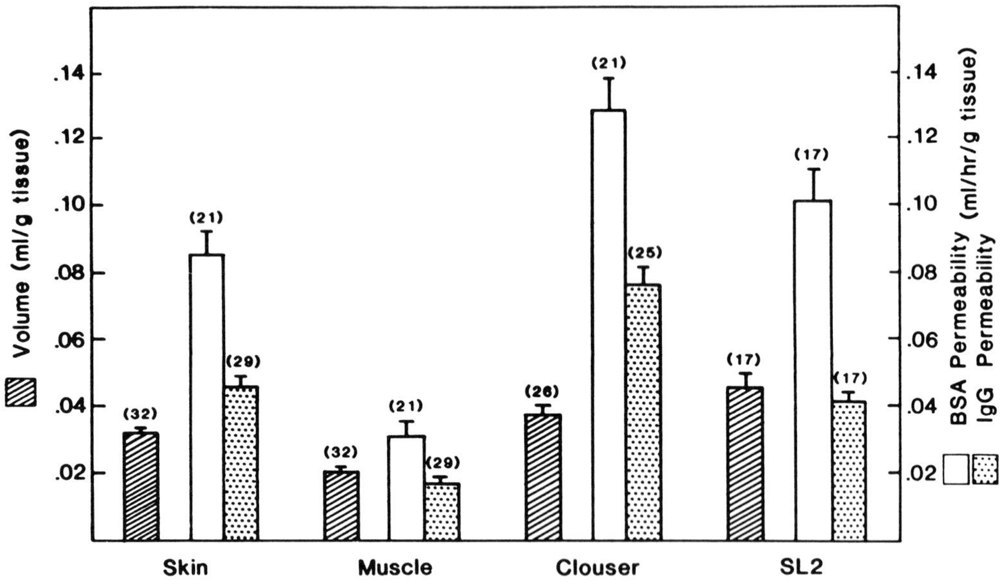

FIGURE 5. Vascular volume and permeability to IgG and BSA of various tissues. Data are presented as the mean ± S.E.M. Numbers in parentheses represent the number of individual observations. Range of tumor sizes: SL2, 35 to 1050 mg; Clouser, 35 to 835 mg. (From Sands, H., Shah, S. A., and Gallagher, B. M., *Cancer Lett.*, 27, 15, 1985. With permission.)

antibodies in human and murine tumors grown in the athymic mouse described earlier. In addition, the vascular permeabilities for both tumor types are significantly higher than those observed for normal skin and muscle (Figure 5). Again, these findings may explain the nonspecific accumulation of macromolecules by tumor model systems. If the tumor mass is sufficiently great, the extent of localization by nonspecific immunoglobulins may be sufficient to produce images by external scanning.[19]

Another example of the possible importance of vascular permeability was observed in the accumulation of a "tumor-associated antibody" (A6H) by a renal cell carcinoma (TK177G)

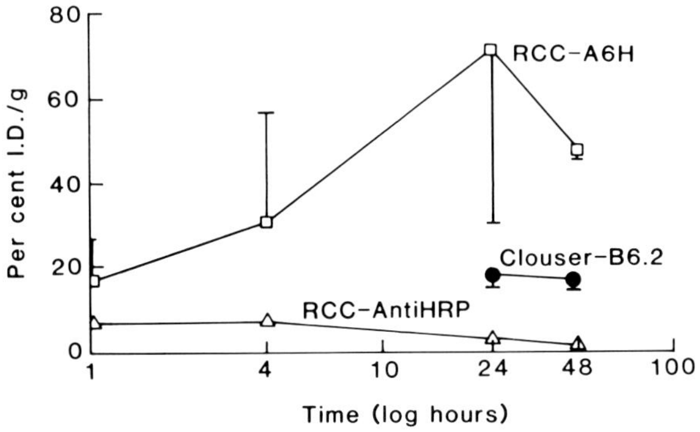

FIGURE 6. Percent of the injected dose per gram of tumor for two tumor-specific antibodies (A6H and B6.2) compared with the uptake of a nonspecific control antibody (anti-HRP). Data are the mean of 4 to 5 determinations ± S.D. RCC is the renal cell carcinoma, TK177G.

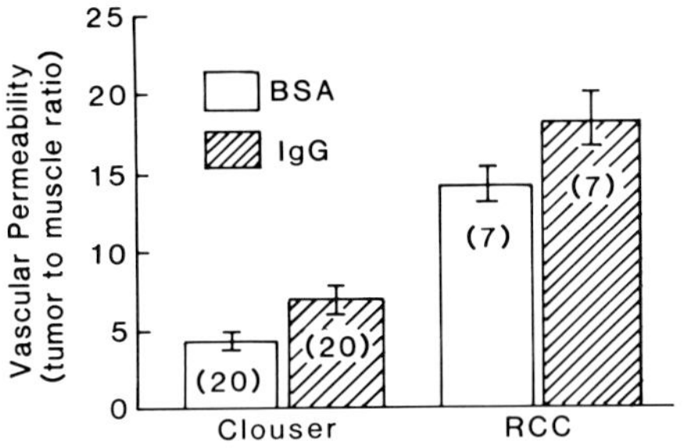

FIGURE 7. Relative vascular permeability of two tumor types, Clouser and renal cell carcinoma (RCC). The data are presented as the mean of the ratio of permeability of tumor to permeability of muscle in the same animal. Bar indicates S.E.M.; (), number of observations.

grown as a xenograft in mice. The specific uptake of antibody A6H by TK177g xenografts of the human renal cell carcinoma in the athymic mouse is three- to fourfold greater than that reported for most other human tumor xenografts and their associated antibodies such as the uptake of ^{125}I-B6.2 by the Clouser human breast carcinoma (Figure 6).[20,21]

Since vascular volume was similar in both tumor types and the differences in the relative blood flow were quite small, the data suggest that differences in vascular permeability may play an important role in determining the extent of specific antibody localization within different tumor types. Direct measure of the vascular permeability demonstrated significant differences between breast and renal cell tumor xenografts. These differences in vascular permeability were especially dramatic when the data were normalized to the vascular permeability of muscle (Figure 7). Although it s not yet clear if these differences are of clinical significance, these findings dramatically demonstrate the influence that vascular permeability can have on antibody localization in these xenograft systems.

The importance of tumor permeability is also illustrated in two additional studies. The first demonstrated the potential for radioimmunotherapy using an ^{131}I-labeled antibody[5] (Figure 8). In these experiments, xenografts of the human colorectal carcinoma LS174T were implanted under the capsules of the kidneys of athymic mice. One day after implantation, approximately 160 μCi of either the specific antibody ^{131}I-B72.3 or the nonspecific

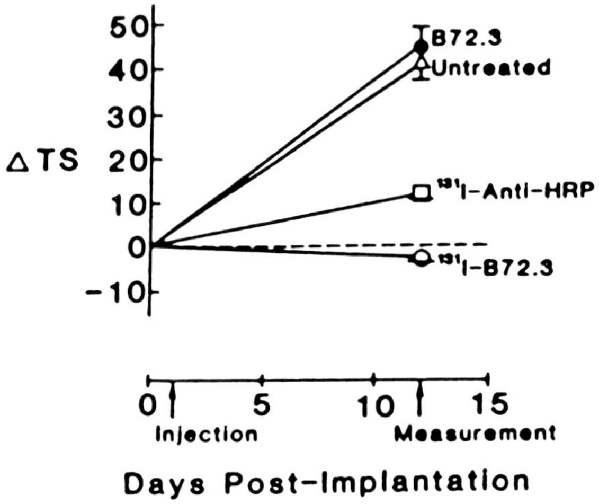

FIGURE 8. The therapeutic effect of ^{131}I-labeled antibodies on human colorectal tumors (LS174T) growing as a xenograft under the subrenal capsule of athymic mice. See text for details. ΔTS, change in tumor size. (From Sands, H., Shah, S. A., Jones, P. L., Neacy, W., and Gallagher, B. M., *Monoclonal Antibodies and Breast Cancer*, Ceriani, R. L., Ed., Martinus Nijhoff Publishing, Boston, Mass., 1985, 303. With permission.)

antibody ^{131}I-anti-HRP was injected intravenously. The tumors were measured 12 days after implantation and the changes in tumor size (ΔTS) were determined. LS174T tumors grew equally well in either untreated mice or in mice given equivalent quantities of unlabeled B72.3. A single dose of ^{131}I-B72.3 resulted in a marked inhibition of tumor growth. Of considerable surprise was the finding that an equivalent injected dose of the subclass-matched nonspecific antibody, ^{131}I-anti-HRP, also produced a significant therapeutic response. Since the nonspecific uptake of anti-HRP is approximately one third that of B72.3 due to the relatively high capillary permeability of these xenografts, these data suggest that at the dose of labeled antibody used, nonspecific uptake of an ^{131}I-IgG$_1$ resulted in a sufficient radiation dose to produce a therapeutic response. These results demonstrate the possible influence that increased capillary permeability may have on nonspecific antibody uptake in experimental animal studies.

In a second study, the uptake of antibody into tumor xenografts was increased using two procedures, external radiation and hyperthermia, both of which are thought to increase vascular permeability.[22] It may, therefore, be possible to increase specific tumor uptake of monoclonal antibodies through the use of either pharmacological or physiological manipulations which result in increased vascular permeability.

III. PHARMACOLOGICAL FACTORS

A. Dose Response

The relationship between the amount of antibody injected and the degree of tumor uptake has been studied both in human xenograft models and in patients. Using xenografts of the human colorectal carcinoma LS174T and radioiodinated B6.2, the percent of the injected radioactive dose taken up by the tumor remained constant over a large range of injected protein (1.0 to 25 μg). A reduction in the percent uptake was not observed until 100 μg of antibody was injected (Figure 9). Similar results have been reported in studies using anti-THY 1.1 antibody and the SL2 murine lymphoma in AKR/J mice.[23] These data suggest that at the protein doses normally used in athymic mouse-human xenograft systems, the available

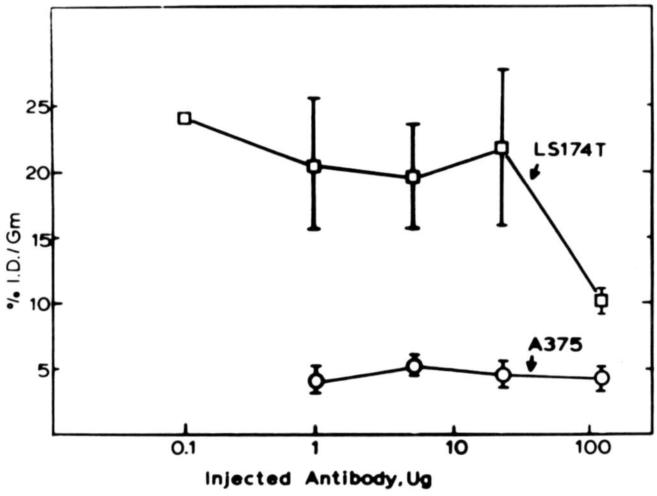

FIGURE 9. Dose response curve for the percent I.D. per gram of B6.2 uptake into a human colorectal xenograft (LS174T) growing in athymic mice. A375 is a control human melanoma xenograft which does not react with B6.2 antibody.

antigen is in great excess. When evaluating experiments of this type, it is important to consider that much of the antigen in tumors may not be accessible to bind antibody and, in addition, much of the radioactive antibody associated with the tumor may be present unbound in the extracellular fluid.

Several clinical trials have been reported in which a range of antibody doses was used. ^{131}I-B72.3 antibody has been used at doses of 0.27, 1.19, and 3.8 mg and no significant differences in blood clearances or in tumor uptake were reported.[24] In addition, no dose-dependent tumor uptake for ^{111}In-T101 was seen in a cutaneous T cell lymphoma using doses of 1 to 50 mg.[25] In contrast, an increased number of sites of metastases of malignant melanoma were detected when the dose of ^{111}In-ZME-018 was increased from 2.5 to 10 mg.[26] Therefore, a general statement on the dose response relationship for all antibody-tumor combinations cannot be made. Each antibody and tumor combination must be looked at separately. It is likely that higher doses of antibody may be required when levels of circulating antigen are significant, although conflicting reports exist in the literature.[27]

For therapeutic applications of radiolabeled antibodies, the dose response relationship with regard to the specific activity (μCi/μg) may be important although very few relevant studies have been published. Using ^{131}I-anti-THY 1.1 as a therapeutic agent for SL2 lymphomas in AKR/J mice, doses of 500 and 1000 μCi were found to be effective in prolonging survival. However, at doses of 1500 μCi, survival rates resembled those of untreated controls, possibly due to bone marrow toxicity.[23]

A study was done in athymic mice bearing large established human neuroblastomas using the antibody ^{131}I-3F8 at doses of 125 to 1000 μCi. Tumor *shrinkage* occurred only with the specific ^{131}I-labeled antibody. Both the degree of reduction in tumor size and the duration of the response were dependent on the dose of ^{131}I used. At higher doses, complete ablation of the neuroblastoma was seen.[28]

A similar study was done using ^{131}I-labeled B72.3 and employed small human colorectal xenografts of LS174T. Marked inhibition of tumor growth was seen at antibody doses of 430 and 320 μCi (Figure 10). Doses of 80 and 160 μCi also produced significant therapeutic effects in a dose dependent manner. There exists little published information on the relationship between the amounts of antibody and associated radioactivity and the effect on

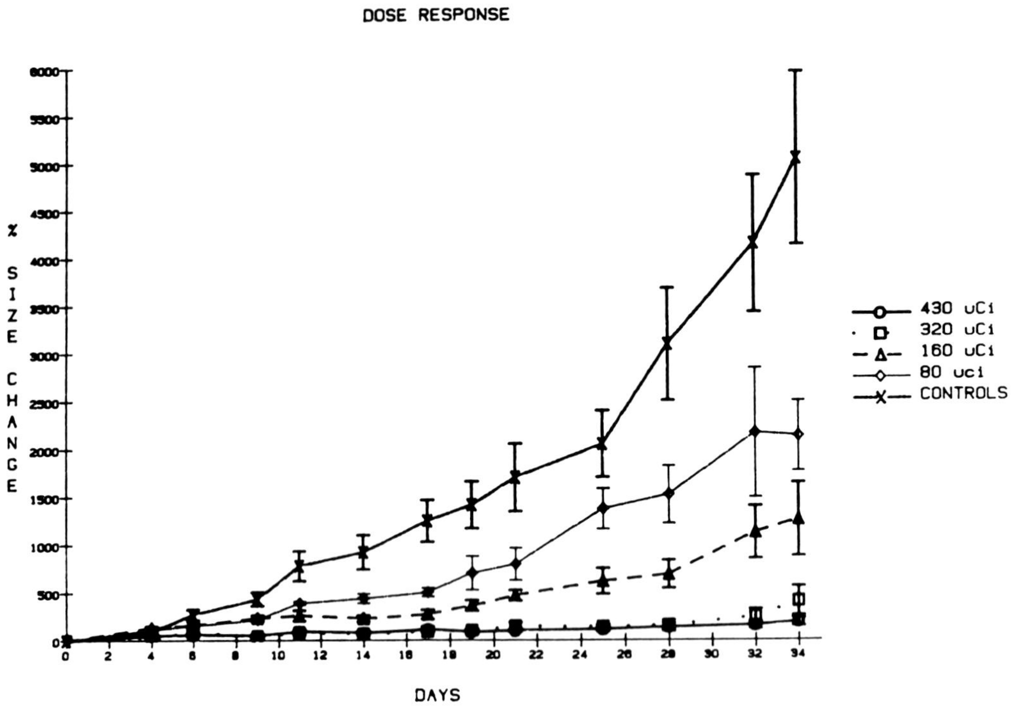

FIGURE 10. Therapeutic response to increasing concentrations of ^{131}I-labeled B72.3 on the growth of subcutaneous LS174T human colorectal xenografts after i.v. injection of radiolabeled antibody.

Table 3
PERCENT INJECTED DOSE PER GRAM OF B72.3 (MEAN ± SD) IN MICE WITH LS174T TUMORS

	6 hr		24 hr	
	i.p.	i.v.	i.p.	i.v.
Blood	13.18 ± 1.62	25.83 ± 5.15	11.87 ± 1.37	14.28 ± 2.61
Liver	4.56 ± 1.14	8.34 ± 2.18	6.66 ± 5.59	3.69 ± 0.76
Kidney	4.01 ± 1.02	5.94 ± 1.71	3.05 ± 0.45	3.39 ± 0.57
Muscle	0.92 ± 0.22	1.45 ± 0.33	1.09 ± 0.34	1.40 ± 0.59
Tumor	9.45 ± 0.39	7.58 ± 2.23	10.31 ± 8.99	11.61 ± 1.16

Note: n = 3 — 5; i.p., intraperitoneal; i.v., intravenous.

either the targeting or the therapeutic response. More research efforts are clearly needed to optimize this relationship both in animal models and in humans.

B. Route of Antibody Administration

Antibodies may be administered via different routes to target tumors in different locations. Intravenous (i.v.) administration has been by far the most commonly employed injection route and may be used for the detection of disseminated disease, whereas intraperitoneal (i.p.) injections have been used for the detection and treatment of colorectal and ovarian metastases of the peritoneal cavity.[6] The subcutaneous (s.c.) route may be of value for detection of metastatic lymph nodes using lymphoscintigraphy.[7,8,29,30]

The results presented in Table 3 compare the pharmacokinetics of ^{125}I-and ^{131}I-labeled

B72.3 after i.v. and i.p. injections into athymic mice bearing xenografts of a colorectal carcinoma. Despite differences in blood levels, tumor uptakes of antibody were similar at 24 hr. The i.p. route can be useful in the laboratory, particularly in experimental protocols requiring repetitive dosing in animals without tails. Furthermore, the intraperitoneal dissemination of tumor, particularly in ovarian carcinoma, remains a major clinical problem. It may be possible to enhance the delivery of therapeutic agents using the i.p. route.[6]

While s.c. injection has allowed the detection of tumors in a guinea pig model, clinical utility of this route of administration has yet to be demonstrated.[7,8,29,30] In one clinical trail, s.c. injection of an anti-melanoma IgG was compared with i.v. injection. Following the i.v. injection, six of six lesions greater than 3 cm and six of eight lesions 1.5 to 3 cm were detected, while after s.c. injection tumor negative and tumor positive lymph nodes could not be distinguished.[31] This may have resulted from aberrations in lymphatic flow and/or the presence of shed antigen in normal lymph nodes, which could appear as "tumor" positive upon scanning. More encouraging results have been reported using the IgM 3E-1.2 for thc detection of breast metastases in lymph nodes. Lymphoscintigraphy detected involved nodes that did not present as a palpable mass, whereas i.v. injection of 3E-1.2 did not produce useful images.[29] The clinical utility of monoclonal antibodies for lymphoscintigraphy is still an area that needs to be resolved.

C. Form of the Antibody

Most laboratory and clinical trials of monoclonal antibodies have used either intact IgG or its proteolytic $F(ab')_2$ or Fab fragments.[27,32,35] The molecular weight of intact IgG is 150,000 daltons. Maximum tumor uptake typically requires 24 to 48 hr in animals. Since the blood clearance of intact IgG is relatively slow, optimal clinical images are obtained at least 48 hr after injection of radiolabeled antibody.[35] Efforts to enhance the rate of blood clearance and improve the imaging sensitivity have focused on the use of IgG fragments. Blood clearance of $F(ab')_2$ is faster than that of intact IgG[32,36] and improved tumor imaging in animal and clinical studies using $F(ab')_2$ has been reported.[37-40] Blood clearance of Fab is even faster[32] than that of $F(ab')_2$. Depending upon the antibody, this may result in clearance rates and loss of avidity which markedly reduces absolute tumor uptake.[32,33,41] Clinical studies using the anti-melanoma antibody 96.5 have shown the Fab fragment to be the form of the antibody which gave the best tumor resolution and detection.[33,41-43] The affinity of the divalent IgG parent may play a significant role in influencing the utility of monovalent Fab since the avidity is greatly diminished by the loss of one of the combining sites.

In contrast to the wealth of data available for IgG and its fragments, there is relatively little information available on the experimental and clinical use of anti-tumor IgM (900,000 daltons). In animal studies, one radiolabeled IgM injected i.v. has been shown to target murine tumors and to localize in a human tumor grown in the Sprague-Daley rat,[44] while others have failed to localize in human xenografts in mice.[45,46] As mentioned previously, clinical results with labeled IgM have been mixed. An antibody to breast cancer successfully detected lymph nodal involvement after s.c. but not after i.v. injection.[29] Again, this suggests that employment of the optimal injection site may be necessary to maximize antibody targeting.

Novel fragments of antibodies can be made by methods other than proteolytic fragmentation. Several mutant antibodies deficient in either the heavy chain C_H2 or C_H3 domain (Figure 11) have been produced.[47,48] The blood clearances of these mutants are distinctly different from that of intact IgG (Figure 12).[48] These studies were carried out with antibodies directed at the non-tumor hapten p-azophenylarsonate (ARS). A micropore chamber filled with ARS conjugated to Sepharose® beads was used as a synthetic "tumor".[49] The ability of these antibodies to localize in and bind to this target was compared with their blood clearance (Table 4).[50] Biodistribution and imaging studies suggest that the blood clearance

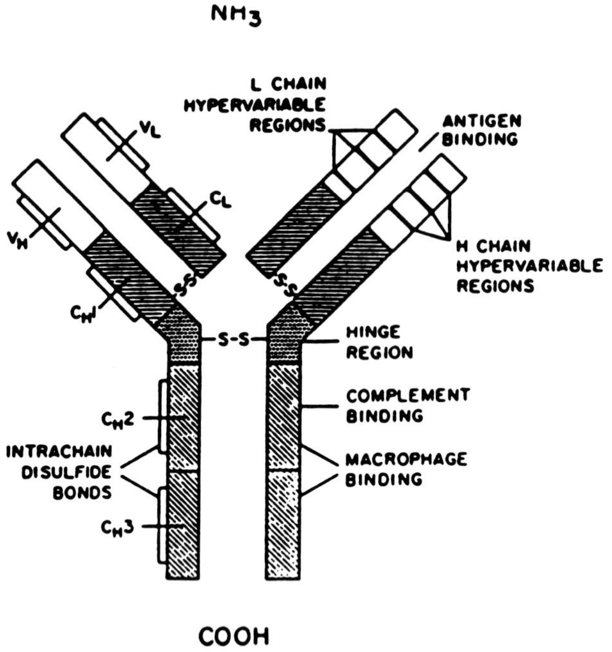

FIGURE 11. Structure of immunoglobulin molecules (IgG). (Reprinted with permission from Morrison, S. L. and Scharff, M. D., *Crit. Rev. Immunol.*, 3, 1, 1981. Copyright CRC Press, Inc., Boca Raton, Fla.)

and target accumulation of the C_H3 deficient antibody may make this mutant useful for tumor localization. By employing suitable genetic engineering, it is possible to generate a wide range of unique molecules which combine the desired antigen specificity with altered biological properties. The potential for exploiting these mutant molecules for targeting has received little attention.

D. Radionuclides

The whole body distribution of radiolabeled antibodies differs with the radionuclide as well as with the form of the antibody. Radioiodinated IgG clears from the blood rather slowly and clears from the liver and kidneys quickly with radioactivity accumulating in the thyroid. When antibodies are labeled with diethylenetriaminepentaacetic acid (DTPA) - ^{111}In, a large percentage of the ^{111}In localizes in the liver and remains there for an extended period of time.[34,35,51-53] Although this was originally thought to reflect antibody damage caused by the radiolabeling procedure, there are other possible explanations. The persistence of ^{111}In in the liver may result from antibody being accumulated as part of normal metabolic turnover. Within the liver, transchelation of ^{111}In from DTPA to indium-avid ferroproteins such as ferritin or transferrin may occur.[54] This could result in ^{111}In being bound in the liver to proteins which turn over very slowly. A similar process may occur within tumors which are known to have a high concentration of such ferroproteins and/or their receptors. Radioiodinated $F(ab')_2$ and Fab demonstrate little liver uptake but are rapidly cleared from the blood. ^{111}In-labeled DTPA-Fab and $F(ab')_2$ accumulate in the kidney and activity persists for days.[32] In general, following injection of labeled antibodies, tumor accumulation of ^{111}In is 25 to 400% greater than that of radioiodine.[35,51-53] The lower levels of radioiodine observed may be due to the lack of iodine-sequestering mechanism in these tissues. The different patterns of distribution which have been observed for the various forms of antibodies labeled with

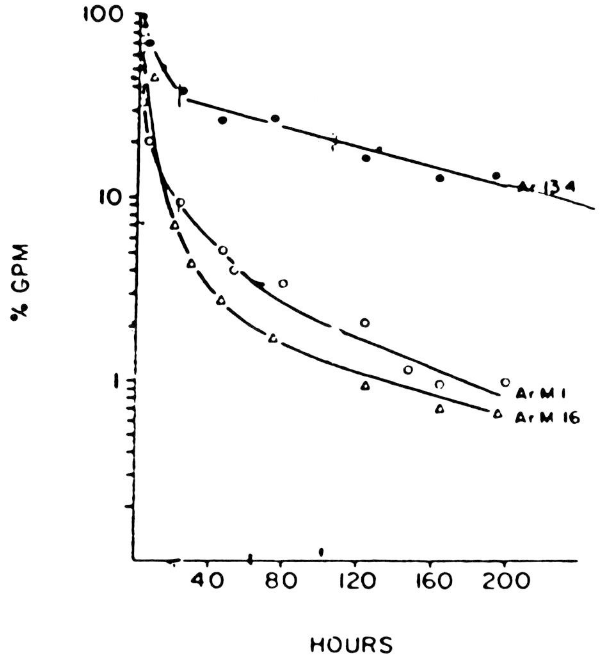

FIGURE 12. The intravascular disappearance of parental (Ar13.4) and mutant immunoglobulins (ArM1 and ArM16). The intravascular radioactivity present at 2 min was taken as 100%. Each point represents the average of samples taken from 2 to 3 animals. (From Pollock, R. R., Metlou, J., Thammana, P., Haseltine, B., Giusti, A., Zack, D., Fischberg, E., Yelton, D. E., and Scharff, M., *Radioimmunoimaging and Radioimmunotherapy,* Burchiel, S. W. and Rhodes, B. A., Eds., Elsevier, Amsterdam, 1983, 93. With permission.)

Table 4
ARS BEADS UPTAKE AND BLOOD VALUES FOR MUTANT ANTIBODIES

	5 days (injected dose per gram)			13 Days (injected dose per gram)		
	Chamber	**Blood**	**C/B**	**Chamber**	**Blood**	**C/B**
Parent IgG	43.7 ± 4.0	4.1 ± 0.5	10.6	39.4 ± 3.4	0.60 ± 0.1	65.7
C_H2 Deletion	9.0 ± 3.8	0.5 ± 0.0	18.0	8.0 ± 1.0	0.10 ± 0.0	80.0
C_H3 Deletion	11.8 ± 1.7	0.1 ± 0.3	118.0	16.8 ± 2.3	0.01 ± 0.0	1680

Note: C/B, The ratio of antibody in the chamber divided by the antibody in the blood.

different isotopes suggest that the most desirable combination of antibody form and radionuclide will depend on the intended use.

IV. IMMUNOLOGICAL FACTORS

A. Membrane Bound Antibody

In most animal and clinical studies in which the uptake of both a specific and a nonspecific antibody was determined, the specific antibody is found to localize in tumor to only a three-

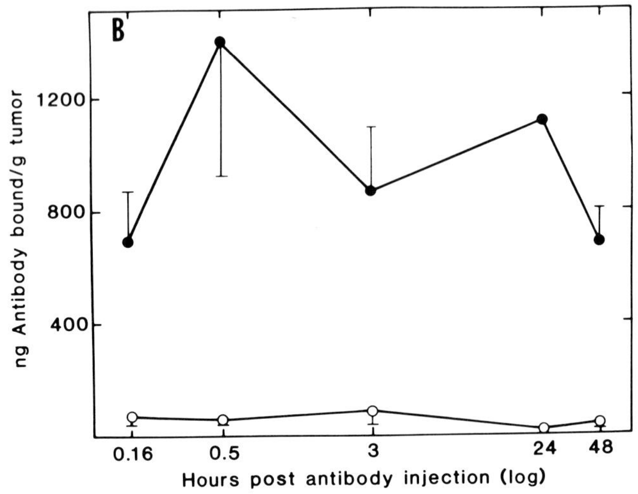

FIGURE 13. Membrane binding of tumor "specific" antibody 0X7 (●) and control antibody (anti-HRP) (0) by SL2 lymphomas. Antibody was injected intravenously and at the indicated times; mice were sacrificed and the amount of radiolabeled antibody binding to a crude membrane preparation was determined. Data are mean ± S.D. of 3 to 5 observations.

to fivefold greater extent than the nonspecific antibody. Several of the physiological and pharmacological factors already discussed appear to play a major role in governing this in vivo targeting ratio. In experiments in which tumors were removed from the animal, homogenized, and a membrane preparation made, a significantly greater amount of antibody was found specifically bound to tumor.[9,10] This result is illustrated in Figure 13 in which the amount of OX7 bound to the subrenal murine lymphoma (SL2) is compared with the membrane of a nonspecific antibody. Similar results have been observed in human breast, colorectal, and renal cell carcinomas using appropriate specific and nonspecific antibodies.[55] This suggests that although the specificity for targeting solid tumors may represent only a factor of three- to fivefold, within the tumor a much higher specificity similar to that obtained in vitro can be achieved. This specificity becomes masked, however, by nonspecific localization due to permeability and possibly by limitations on the antigen available for binding in vivo. This latter point will be discussed subsequently.

B. Shed Antigen

The effect of antigen shed into the circulation on antibody targeting is not clear. Clinical studies in patients having high circulating concentrations of CEA, AFP, and HCG using ^{131}I-antibody have found radionuclide distribution and imaging quality to be uneffected by the amount of antigen present.[27] In contrast, studies using athymic mice bearing xenografts which produce varying amounts of shed CEA have shown that liver uptake of ^{111}In increased and ^{125}I decreased as the CEA secretory rate of the tumor rose. The ratio of ^{111}In/^{125}I found in the tumor also varied with the degree of antigen shedding.[53] Perhaps the effects of circulating antigen were not noted in the clinical studies because only radioiodinated antibodies were studied.

C. Heterogeneity of Antibody Binding In Vivo

The cellular distribution of antibody may be more important for therapy than for diagnosis. Knowledge of antibody binding patterns may help in the design of antibody cocktails for imaging, while the three-dimensional distribution within tumors is important in choosing radionuclides for therapy. Using in vivo autoradiography, the binding patterns of several antibodies have been studied. Athymic mice bearing human tumor xenografts were injected with the appropriate antibody labeled with ^{125}I and, at the appropriate time, usually 24 hr, the tumors were removed, fixed, sectioned, covered with photographic emulsion, exposed, developed, and stained with hemotoxylin-eosin.[56,57] These in vivo results can be compared with binding patterns observed in vitro when tumors were removed from untreated mice, fixed, sectioned, and the sections incubated with radioiodinated antibody. After the appropriate incubation time, the slices were washed, coated with emulsion, exposed, developed, and stained as described above.

In one study, the targeting of monoclonal anibodies to human tumor xenografts in athymic mice was investigated by the analysis of the cellular distribution of two radioiodinated monoclonal antibodies, B6.2 and B72.3, which recognize different tumor-associated antigens.[56] The distribution of each antibody within Clouser human mammary carcinoma (B6.2 positive, B72.3 negative) and LS174T human colorectal carcinoma (B6.2 positive, B72.3 positive) were compared using the above autoradiographic techniques. Autoradiography was also used to determine the pattern of binding after in vitro incubation with radiolabeled antibody. Both in vivo and in vitro localization of ^{125}I-labeled B72.3 in LS174T tumors were characterized by the binding of antibody to antigen-rich, mucin-containing globules shed from the tumor cells (Figure 14A). In contrast, the in vivo localization of B6.2 was restricted to groups of cells at the tumor periphery and to well-vascularized regions of the tumor (Figure 14B). Thus, B6.2 and B72.3, with quantitatively similar tumor uptake in vivo (approximately 20% injected dose per gram), show very different spatial distributions within LS174T tumors. The in vivo binding of B6.2 in Clouser tumors was restricted to small clusters of cells scattered fairly evenly throughout the tumor. No evidence was found for the presence of such antigen-rich foci after in vitro incubation of tumor sections with B6.2; rather, a uniform binding of antibodies was observed. This suggests that the heterogeneity of regional uptake may be due to differences in antibody delivery rather than in antigenic expression (Figure 14C). Staining patterns similar to the B72.3 mucin localization have been reported using anti-CEA and CEA-secreting xenografts.[56]

An entirely different pattern was observed when the human lymphoma xenograft KG1-A was studied using the anti-human leukocyte antibody (Figure 14D). In this case, a wide zone of activity was found at the tumor periphery. Superimposed on a relatively high background staining, zones of high activity (one to ten cells in diameter) were distributed throughout the tumor.

Other studies employed an antibody directed against a human renal cell carcinoma. Athymic mice bearing subcutaneous TK177G renal cell carcinomas were injected with ^{125}I-labeled A6H and sacrificed at 24 hr. The distribution of activity in tumor sections was heterogeneous and concentrated at the tumor periphery and in structures characteristic of TK177G which histologically appears as highly differentiated (Figure 14E). Data of this type strongly suggest the importance of the availability of the target antigens within tumors growing in vivo.

Clearly, the discrepancies observed between in vitro staining, which reflects antigen expression, and the in vivo pattern, which reflects available antigen, suggest that the common practice of screening tumor sections with antibody in vitro may not be predictive of the true pattern of antibody distribution in vivo. This factor, in addition to those discussed earlier, can significantly effect the success of antibody delivered therapy. An increased understanding of antigen distribution patterns in vivo may provide a rational basis for the selection of appropriate therapeutic radioisotopes for radioimmunotherapy studies.

D. Antibody Cocktails

The combination of nonsaturating antibody binding and antigen heterogeneity reviewed above suggests that the use of cocktails containing two or more antibodies may be of value,

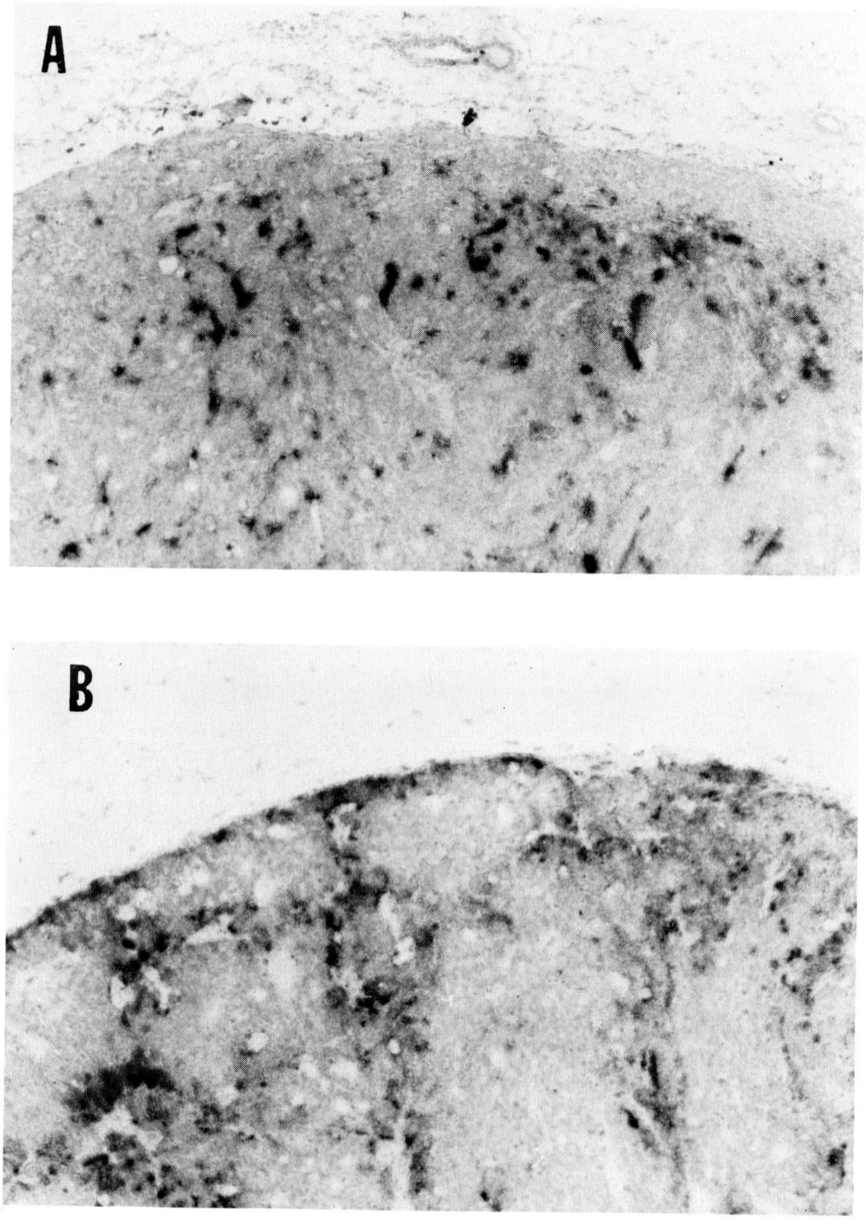

FIGURE 14. Autoradiographic analysis of the in vivo binding of antibodies. Antibodies were injected intravenously 24 hr before removal of the xenograft (Magnification × 80.) A, B72.3 binding to LS174T colorectal xenografts; B, B6.2 binding to LS174T colorectal xenografts; C, B6.2 binding to Clouser breast tumor xenografts; D, Anti-human leukocyte antibody binding to KG1-A lymphoma xenografts; and E, A6H binding to TK 177G renal cell carcinoma xenografts.

especially in antibody directed therapy using radioisotopes, toxins, or drugs. Data from well-controlled studies are not yet available. It is imperative that any study compare a twofold dose of antibody A and a twofold dose of antibody B with that of the combined dose of antibody A and antibody B in order to rule out the dose dependency discussed above. At present there is little published information available supporting the concept of antibody mixtures to overcome problems of heterogeneity.

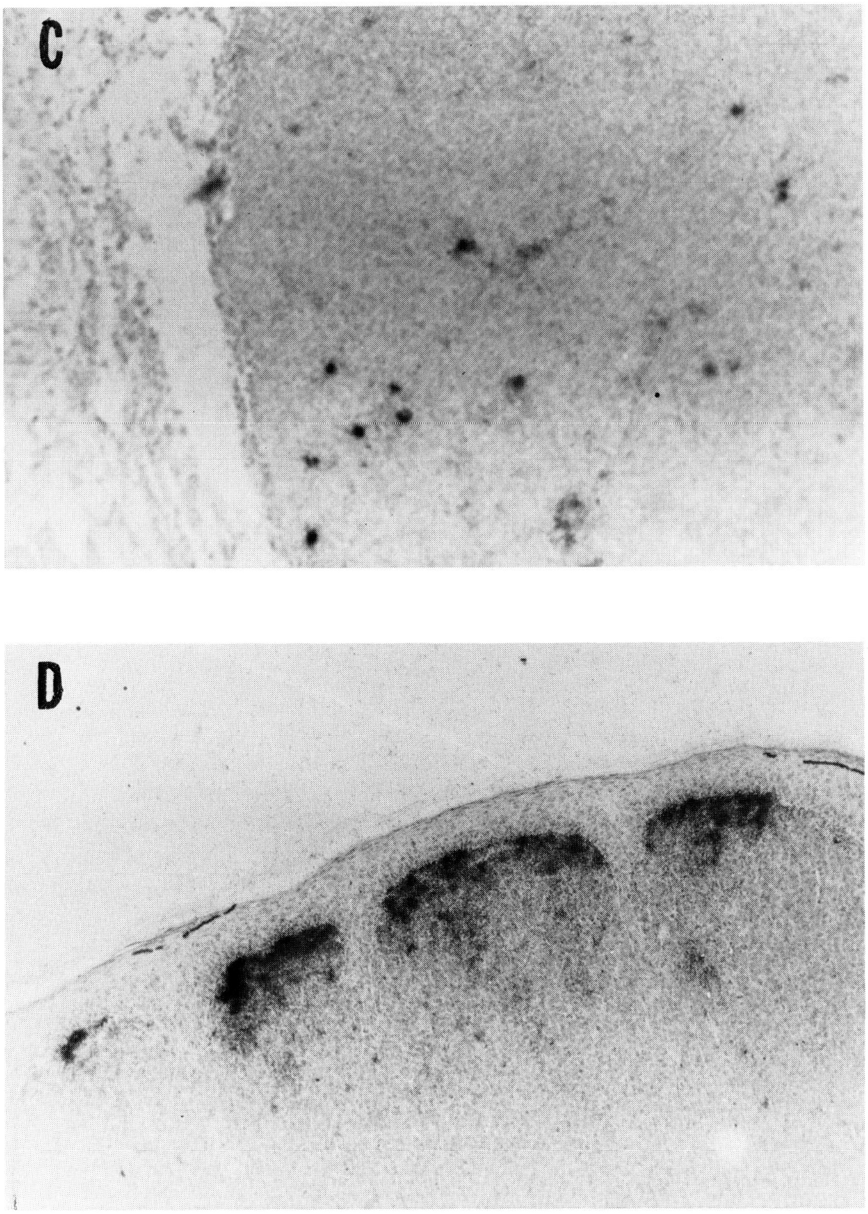

FIGURE 14 (continued).

E. Anti-Murine Responses

The i.v. injection of murine antibodies can produce an anti-murine response in patients. In most diagnostic protocols, a single injection of mouse antibodies has not produced toxic effects and a strong anti-murine response has generally not been observed. If, however, murine antibodies are to be useful for either repeated diagnosis or for repeated therapy, the degree and type of anti-murine response must be known. Few studies have routinely determined the anti-murine response of patients after either single or repeated injections. Anti-murine responses to intact IgG have been reported.[59-60] No comparisons of the immunogenicity of the IgG with that of $F(ab')_2$ or Fab have appeared.

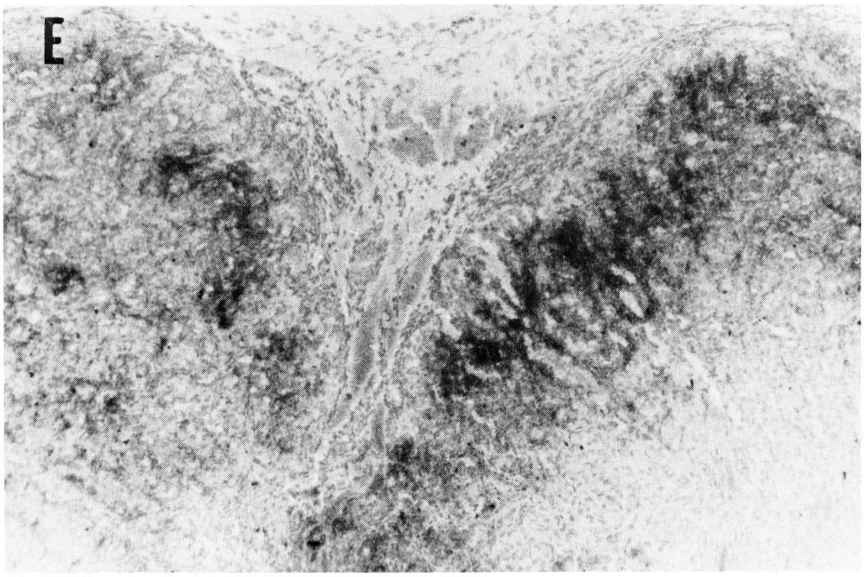

FIGURE 14 (continued).

Three recent studies have addressed the nature of the anti-murine response, i.e., whether it is against the framework (Fc) portion of the molecule or against the antigen binding sites. The response of patients given a single injection of the anti-colorectal antibody 17-1A was studied.[61] Of 21 patients, 18 produced anti-murine IgG, and this response was observed when the murine antibody was still present in the circulation. Of the 41 patients, 35 produced antibodies following single or multiple injections of 17-1A raised an anti-idiotypic response with the majority directed against the antigen combining site of 17-1A. Anti-idiotypic antibodies persisted in the circulation for up to 475 days following a single dose of 15 to 800 mg of 17-1A.[61]

In another study, the anti-murine response following injection of 200 μg of the anti-osteosarcoma antibody 791T/36 was studied in 11 patients. Plasma from all 11 patients inhibited the binding of fluorescein-labeled 791T/36 in vitro indicating the presence of anti-idiotypic antibodies which could be detected as early as 2 to 3 days after injection.[62]

A third study detected anti-idiotypic antibodies in five of ten cutaneous T cell lymphoma patients who had received multiple injections of the murine antibody T101. No anti-murine response was found in six chronic lymphocytic leukemia patients given the same antibody. Total doses ranged from 40 to 1000 mg.[63]

If the antigen to which the antibody is directed is truly a "tumor associated" protein, the patient may have mounted an immunological response against the antigen earlier in the natural history of the disease. A natural outcome would be the production of anti-idiotypic antibodies as part of the network control of specific immunoglobulin production.[64] The injection of a murine antibody with similar binding sites might later trigger the immunologic memory response. Thus, the rapid production of anti-idiotypic antibodies in cancer patients may not be surprising and anti-idiotype production may not be a characteristic of patients injected with antibodies directed at noncancer targets such as platelets or fibrin.

The finding that a major portion of the anti-murine response to antibodies is anti-idiotypic implies that the use of antibody fragments, human antibodies, or chimeric antibodies (antibodies composed of human constant and murine variable regions) will not totally overcome the anti-murine response problem. The production of anti-idiotypic antibodies clearly needs to be better understood and solutions to this problem will not be straightforward.

V. CONCLUSION AND SUMMARY

The application of monoclonal antibodies for specific tumor cell targeting in vivo continues to be an area of active research. Too often, however, the in vitro characteristics of these molecules have not been predictive of their behavior in animal models or in clinical studies. This is due, at least in part, to the various nonimmunological factors described in this chapter. The limitations imposed by tumor perfusion and capillary permeability appear to represent significant barriers to the delivery of macromolecules such as antibodies. Attempts to circumvent these problems have employed antibody fragments and deletion mutant immunolobulins which display altered pharmacokinetic distributions. The more rapid blood clearance of these molecules results in improved tumor to background ratios but with a decreased absolute delivery of antibody to the tumor. Other attempts to circumvent the difficulties in delivery have employed increased dose of antibody and alternative routes of administration. In the former case, the relationship between the dose administered and the extent of targeting specificity and sensitivity is still unresolved. In the latter case, antibody administration by nonintravenous routes appears to be promising, however only limited reports using this approach have appeared. The immunological factors of antigen expression and accessibility under physiological conditions present further complications for future consideration. The striking examples of the discordant results obtained in vitro vs. in vivo raise many additional questions about the ultimate success of either drugs or toxins linked to antibodies for therapeutic purposes. In this regard, radioimmunotherapy appears to have a significant advantage. The ability of particulate radiation to traverse several cell diameters and thereby to impact distant cells expressing little or no target antigen, may permit the delivery of an adequate radiation dose for decreasing the rate of tumor growth. If the encouraging results obtained in animal model systems can be reproduced in the clinic, a significant improvement in the management of cancer patients could be achieved. Finally, the immune response to foreign protein needs to be more completely understood to maximize the delivery of an effective therapeutic dose.

It should be emphasized that although much work has been carried out exploring the potential application of antibody directed diagnosis and therapy, our understanding of many of the fundamental factors influencing the delivery of antibodies and their conjugates remains limited. If the promise of antibody-mediated diagnosis and therapy is to be realized in the clinical setting, the questions highlighted in this brief overview need to be addressed.

NOTE ADDED IN PROOF

Since completion of this review there has been considerable progress and additional information made available in many of the topics covered. Several examples are the production and evaluation of chimeric antibodies,[65,66] a more detailed report on the role of vascular volume and permeability,[67] and critical comparisons in clinical trials of intravenous vs. intraperitoneal injection.[68,69] While more data is now available, the basic conclusion, i.e., the need for an increased understanding of the role of nonimmunological factors which influence tumor accretion of radiolabeled monoclonal antibodies, is still valid.

REFERENCES

1. **Hui, K-Y., Haber, E., and Matsueda, G. R.,** Monoclonal antibodies to a synthetic fibrin-like peptide bind to human fibrin but not fibrinogen, *Science*, 222, 1129, 1983.
2. **Brown, B. A., Comeau, R. D., Jones, P. L., Liberatore, F. A., Neacy, W. P., Sands, H., and Gallagher, B. M.,** Pharmacokinetics of monoclonal antibody B72.3 and its fragments labeled with either ^{125}I or ^{111}In, *Cancer Res.*, 47, 1149, 1987.
3. **Eckelman, W. C., Paik, C. H., and Reba, R. C.,** Radiolabeling of antibodies, *Cancer Res.*, 40, 3036, 1980.
4. **Hnatowich, D. J., Layne, W. W., Childs, R. L., Lanteigne, D., Davis, M. A., Griffin, T. W., and Doherty, P. W.,** Radioactive labeling of antibody: a simple and efficient method, *Science*, 220, 613, 1983.
5. **Sands, H., Shah, S. A., Jones, P. L., Neacy, W., and Gallagher, B. M.,** Non-immunological factors affecting the localization of monoclonal antibodies in xenografts of human breast and colon tumors, in *Monoclonal Antibodies and Breast Cancer*, Ceriani, R. L., Ed., Martinus Nijhoff Publishing, Boston, 1985, 303.
6. Hammersmith Oncology Group and Imperial Cancer Research Fund, Antibody guided irradiation of malignant lesion: three cases illustrating a new method of treatment, *Lancet*, 1, 1441, 1984.
7. **Weinstein, J. N., Steller, M. A., Keenan, A. M., Covell, D. G., Key, M. E., Sieber, S. M., Oldham, R. K., Hwang, K. M., and Parker, R. J.,** Monoclonal antibodies in the lymphatics: selective delivery to lymph node metastases of a solid tumor, *Science*, 222, 423, 1983.
8. **Weinstein, J. N., Parker, R. J., Kennan, A. M., Dower, S. K., Morse, H. C., III, and Sieber, S. M.,** Monoclonal antibodies in the lymphatics: toward the diagnosis and therapy of tumor metastases, *Science*, 218, 1334, 1982.
9. **Sands, H., Jones, P. L., Neacy, W., Shah, S. A., and Gallagher, B. M.,** The imaging of small experimental murine tumors grown in the subrenal capsule using monoclonal antibodies, *Cancer Lett.*, 24, 65, 1984.
10. **Sands, H., Jones, P. L., Neacy, W. P., Shah, S. A., and Gallagher, B. M.,** Site-related differences in the localization of the monoclonal antibody OX7 in the SL2 and SL1 lymphomas, *Cancer Immunol. Immunotherap.*, 22, 169, 1986.
11. **Gullino, P. M. and Grantham, F. H.,** Studies on the exchange of fluids between host and tumor. II. The blood flow of hepatomas and other tumors in rats and mice, *J. Natl. Cancer Inst.*, 27, 1465, 1961.
12. **Bodgen, A. F., Kelton, D. E., Cobb, W. R., and Esber, H. J.,** A rapid screening method for testing chemotherapeutic agents against human tumor xenografts, in *Proc. Symp. on the Use of Athymic (Nude) Mice in Cancer Research*, Houchens, D. P. and Ovejera, A. A., Eds., Gustav Fischer, Stuttgart, 1978, 231.
13. **Shah, S. A., Gallagher, B. M., and Sands, H.,** Radioimmunodetection of small human tumor xenografts of athymic mice by monoclonal antibodies, *Cancer Res.*, 45, 5824, 1985.
14. **Bauer, F. K., Tubis, M., and Thomas, H. B.,** Accumulation of homologous radioiodinated albumin in experimental tumors, *Proc. Soc. Exp. Biol. Med.*, 90, 140, 1955.
15. **Song, C. W. and Levitt, S. H.,** Effects of X-irradiation on vascularity of normal tissue and experimental tumor, *Radiology*, 94, 445, 1970.
16. **Ackerman, N. B. and Hechmer, P. A.,** Comparison of vascular permeability of tumors and liver host tissue, *Bibl. Anat.*, 15, 304, 1977.
17. **Sands, H., Jones, P. L., Neacy, W. P., Shah, S. A., and Gallagher, B. M.,** unpublished observation.
18. **Sands, H., Shah, S. A., and Gallagher, B. M.,** Vascular volume and permeability of human and murine tumors grown in athymic mice, *Cancer Lett.*, 27, 15, 1985.
19. **Mann, B. D., Cohen, M. B., Saxton, R. E., Morton, D. L., Benedict, W. F., Korn, E. L., Spolten, L., Grahman, L. S., Chang, C. C., and Burk, M. W.,** Imaging of human tumor xenografts in nude mice with radiolabeled monoclonal antibody: limitations of specificity due to nonspecific uptake of antibody, *Cancer (Philadelphia)*, 54, 1318, 1984.
20. **Sands, H., Jones, P. L., Shah, S. A., Palme, D., Chiou, R., Vessella, A., Lange, P., and Gallagher, B. M.,** Physiological factors affecting the uptake of antibody by renal cell carcinoma (RCC) xenografts grown in athymic mice, *Cancer Drug Delivery*, 2, 225, 1985.
21. **Zalutsky, M. R., Colcher, D., Kaplan, W. D., and Kufe, D. W.,** Radioiodinated B6.2 monoclonal antibody: further characterization of a potential radiopharmaceutical for the identification of breast tumor, *Int. J. Nucl. Med. Biol.*, 12, 227, 1985.
22. **Stickney, D. R., Gridley, D. S., Kirk, G. A., and Slater, J. M.,** Enhancement of monoclonal antibody (MAb) binding to melanoma with single dose radiation or hyperthermia, *Cancer Drug Delivery*, 2, 225, 1985.
23. **Badger, C. C., Krohn, K. A., Peterson, A. V., Shulman, H., and Bernstein, I. D.,** Experimental radiotherapy of murine lymphoma with ^{131}I-labeled anti-THY 1.1 monoclonal antibody, *Cancer Res.*, 45, 1536, 1985.

24. **Carrasquillo, J. A., Colcher, D., Sugarbaker, P., Reynolds, J. R., Keenan, A. M., Simpson, D., Bryants, G., Thor, A., Perentesis, P., Esteban, J., Horowitz, M., Schlom, J., and Larson, S. M.,** Radiolocalization of colon cancer with I-131 B72.3, *J. Nucl. Med.*, 26, 15, 1985.
25. **Carrasquillo, J. A., Bunn, J. A., Keenan, A. M., Reynolds, J. C., Schroff, R. W., Foon, K. A., Ming-Hsu, S., Gazdar, A. F., Mulshine, J. M., Perenteis, P., Horowitz, M., and Larson, S. M.,** Imaging of cutaneous T cell lymphoma (CTCL) with T101 monoclonal antibody, *J. Nucl. Med.*, 26, 16, 1985.
26. **Murray, J. L., Rosenblum, M., Lamki, L., Haynie, T. P., Glenn, H., Jahns, M., Plager, C., Hersh, E. M., Unger, M., and Carlo, D. L.,** Imaging findings and pharmacokinetics of 111-Indium ZME-018 monoclonal antibody (MOAB) in malignant melanoma, *J. Nucl. Med.*, 26, 16, 1985.
27. **Goldenberg, D. M. and Deland, F. H.,** History and status of tumor imaging with radiolabeled antibodies, *J. Biol. Response Modif.*, 1, 121, 1982.
28. **Cheung, N-K., V., Landmeier, B., Kallick, S., Nelson, D., Ellery, S., Adams, R., Neely, J., Coccia, P., and Miraldi, F.,** Complete tumor ablation with Iodine 131 radiolabeled monoclonal antibody (MAb) against human neuroblastoma (NB) xenografted in nude mice, *Proc. Am. Assoc. Cancer Res.*, 26, 270, 1985.
29. **Stacken, S., Lowe, M. G., McKatee, K., Thompson, C. H., Lichenstein, M., Leyden, M., Salehi, N., Andrews, J., and McKenzie, I. F. C.,** Detection of breast cancer using the monoclonal antibody 3E-1.2, in *Monoclonal Antibodies and Breast Cancer,* Ceriani, R. L., Ed., Martinus Nijhoff Publishing, Boston, 1985, 233.
30. **Keenan, D. M., Weinstein, J. N., Carrasquillo, J. A., Reynolds, J. C., Perentesis, P., Foon, K. A., Mulshine, J. L., Bunn, P. A., and Larson, S. M.,** Immunolymphoscintigraphy with Indium 111 labeled T101 monoclonal antibody, *J. Nucl. Med.*, 26, 54, 1985.
31. **Engelstad, B., Khentigan, A., Del Rio, M., Rosendorf, F. L., Ramos, E., Reinhold, C., Hattner, R., Okerlano, M., Spitler, L., and Scannon, P.,** Clinical trials with intravenous (IV) and subcutaneous (SQ) In-111 antimelanoma monoclonal radioimmunoimaging, *Clin. Nucl. Med.*, 10, 22, 1985.
32. **Brown, B. A., Comeau, R. D., Jones, P. L., Liberatore, F. A., Neacy, W. P., Sands, H., and Gallagher, B. M.,** Comparison of the pharmacokinetics of ^{125}I and ^{111}In labeled intact and proteolytic fragments of a monoclonal antibody, *Cancer Drug Delivery*, 2, 219, 1985.
33. **Carrasquillo, J. A., Krohn, K. A., Beaumier, P., McGuffin, R. W., Brown, J. P., Hellstrom, K. E., Hellstrom, I., and Larson, S. M.,** Diagnosis of and therapy for solid tumors with antibodies and immune fragments, *Cancer Treat. Rep.*, 68, 317, 1984.
34. **Halpern, S. E., Hagan, P. S., Witztum, K. F., and Dillman, R. O.,** Radioimmunoscintigraphy using ^{111}In-labeled monoclonal antibodies and the case for immunotherapeutics, *J. Med. Technol.*, 2, 301, 1985.
35. **Perkins, A. C. and Pimm, M. V.,** Differences in tumor and normal tissue concentrations of iodine- and indium-labelled monoclonal antibodies. I. The effect on image contrast in clinical studies, *Eur. J. Nucl. Med.*, 11, 295, 1985.
36. **Burchiel, S. W., Khaw, B. A., Rhodes, B. A., Smith, T. W., and Haber, E.,** Immunopharmacokinetics of radiolabeled antibodies and their fragments, in *Tumor Imaging: The Radioimmunochemical Detection of Cancer,* Burchiel, S. W., Rhodes, B. A., and Friedman, B. E., Eds., Masson Publishing, New York, 1982, 125.
37. **Moldofsky, P. J., Powe, J., Mulhern, C. B., Jr., Hammond, N., Sears, H. F., Gatenby, R. A., Steplewski, Z., and Koprowski, H.,** Metastatic colon carcinoma detected with radiolabeled $F(ab')_2$ monoclonal antibody fragments, *Radiology*, 149, 549, 1983.
38. **Wahl, R. L., Parker, C. W., and Philpott, G. W.,** Improved radioimaging and tumor localization with monoclonal $F(ab')_2$, *J. Nucl. Med.*, 24, 316, 1983.
39. **Powe, J., Pak, K. Y., Paik, C. H., Steplewski, Z., Ebbert, M. A., Herlyn, D., Ernst, C., Alavi, A., Eckelman, W. C., Reba, R. C., and Koprowski, H.,** Labeling monoclonal antibodies and $F(ab')_2$ fragments with (^{111}In) indium using cyclic DTPA anhydride and their in vivo behavior in mice bearing human tumor xenografts, *Cancer Drug Delivery*, 1, 125, 1984.
40. **Buchegger, F., Haskell, C. M., Schreyer, M., Scazziga, B. R., Randin, S., Carrel, S., and Mach, J-P.,** Radiolabeled fragments of monoclonal antibodies against carcinoembryonic antigen for localizaton of human colon carcinoma grafted into nude mice, *J. Exp. Med.*, 158, 413, 1983.
41. **Larson, S. M., Carrasquillo, J. A., Krohn, K. A., Brown, J. P., McGuffin, R. W., Ferens, J. M., Graham, M. M., Hill, L. D., Beaumier, P. L., Hellstrom, K. E., and Hellstrom, I.,** Localization of ^{131}I-labeled p97 specific Fab fragments in human melanoma as a basis for radiotherapy, *J. Clin. Invest.*, 72, 2101, 1983.
42. **Larson, S. M., Brown, J. P., Wright, P. W., Carrasquillo, J. A., Hellstrom, I., and Hellstrom, K. E.,** Imaging of melanoma with I-131-labeled monoclonal antibodies, *J. Nucl. Med.*, 24, 123, 1983.

43. **Larson, S. M., Carrasquillo, J. A., McGuffin, R. W., Krohn, K. A., Ferens, J. M., Hill, L. D., Beaumier, P. L., Reynolds, J. C., Hellstrom, K. E., and Hellstrom, I.,** Using I-131 labeled, murine Fab against a high molecular weight antigen of human melanoma: preliminary experience, *Radiology,* 155, 487, 1985.
44. **Zimmer, A. M., Rosen, S. T., Spies, S. M., Polovina, M. R., Minna, J. D., Spies, W. C., and Silverstein, E. A.,** Radioimmunoimaging of human small cell lung carcinoma with I-131 tumor specific monoclonal antibody, *Hybridoma,* 4, 1, 1985.
45. **Menard, S., Miotti, S., Tagliabue, E., Parmi, L., Buraggi, G. L., and Colnaghi, M. I.,** Tumor radioimmunolocalization in murine systems using monoclonal antibodies, *Tumori,* 69, 185, 1983.
46. **Pimm, M. V. and Baldwin, R. W.,** Distribution of IgM monoclonal antibody in mice with human tumor xenografts: lack of tumor localization, *Eur. J. Cancer Clin. Oncol.,* 21, 765, 1985.
47. **Morrison, S. L. and Scharff, M. D.,** Mutational events in mouse myeloma cells, *Crit. Rev. Immunol.,* 3, 1, 1981.
48. **Pollock, R. R., Metlay, J., Thammana, P., Haseltine, B., Giusti, A., Zack, D., Fischberg, E., Yelton, D. E., and Scharff, M.,** Generation of mutant monoclonal antibodies with changes in biological function, in *Radioimmunoimaging and Radioimmunotherapy,* Burchiel, S. W. and Rhodes, B. A., Eds., Elsevier, Amsterdam, 1983, 93.
49. **Jain, R. K., Shah, S. A., and Finney, P. L.,** Continuous noninvasive monitoring of pH and temperature in rat Walker 256 carcinoma during normoglycemia and hyperglycemia, *J. Natl. Cancer Inst.,* 73, 429, 1984.
50. **Shah, S. A., Pollock, R. R., Brown, B. A., Gallagher, B. M., Scharff, M. D., and Sands, H.,** Pharmacokinetics and imaging using mutant anti-ARS antibodies, *J. Nucl. Med.,* 27, 1023, 1986.
51. **Pimm, M. V., Perkins, A. C., and Baldwin, R. W.,** Differences in tumour and normal tissue concentration of iodine- and indium-labeled monoclonal antibodies. II. Biodistribution studies in mice with human xenografts, *Eur. J. Nucl. Med.,* 11, 300, 1985.
52. **Halpern, S. E., Hagan, P. L., Garver, P. R., Koziol, J. A., Chen, A. W. N., Frincke, J. M., Bartholomew, R. M., David, G. S., and Adams, T. H.,** Stability, characterization, and kinetics of ^{111}In-labeled monoclonal anti-tumor antibodies in normal animals and nude mouse-human tumor models, *Cancer Res.,* 43, 5347, 1983.
53. **Hagan, P. L., Halpern, S. E., Chen, A., Krishnan, L., Frincke, J., Bartholomew, R. M., David, G. S., and Carlo, D.,** In vivo kinetics of radiolabeled monoclonal antiCEA antibodies in animal models, *J. Nucl. Med.,* 26, 1418, 1985.
54. **Hnatowich, D. J., Griffin, T. W., Koscinczyk, C., Rusckowiski, M., Childs, R. L., Mattis, J. A., Shealy, D., Doherty, P. W.,** Pharmacokinetics of an Indium-111 labeled monoclonal antibody in cancer patients, *J. Nucl. Med.,* 26, 849, 1985.
55. **Sands, H., Jones, P. L., Shah, S., Palme, D., and Vessella, R.,** Unpublished observation.
56. **Jones, P. L., Gallagher, B. M., and Sands, H.,** Autoradiographic analysis of monoclonal antibody distribution in human colon and breast tumor xenografts, *Cancer Immunol. Immunotherap.,* 22, 139, 1986.
57. **Pimm, M. V., Armitage, N. C., Perkins, A. C., Smith, W., and Baldwin, R. W.,** Localization of an antiCEA monoclonal antibody in colorectal carcinoma xenografts, *Cancer Immunol. Immunotherap.,* 19, 8, 1985.
58. **Dillman, R. O., Shawler, D. L., Dillman, J. B., and Royston, I.,** Therapy of chronic lymphocytic leukemia and cutaneous T cell lymphoma with T101 monoclonal antibody, *J. Clin. Oncol.,* 2, 881, 1984.
59. **Sears, H. F., Alkison, B., Mattis, J., Ernst, C., Herlyn, D., Steplewski, Z., Hayry, P., and Koprowski, H.,** Phase I. Clinical trials of monoclonal antibody treatment of gastrointestinal tumors, *Lancet,* 1, 762, 1982.
60. **Sears, H. F., Herlyn, D., Steplewski, Z., and Koprowski, H.,** Effects of monoclonal antibody immunotherapy on patients with gastrointestinal adenocarcinoma, *J. Biol. Response Mod.,* 3, 138, 1984.
61. **Herlyn, D., Lubeck, M., Sears, H., and Koprowski, H.,** Specific detection of anti-idiotypic immune responses in cancer patients treated with murine monoclonal antibodies, *J. Immunol. Methods,* 85, 27, 1985.
62. **Rowe, R. W., Pimm, M. V., and Baldwin, R. W.,** Anti-idiotype antibody responses in cancer patients receiving a murine monoclonal antibody, *IRCS Med. Sci.,* 13, 936, 1985.
63. **Shawler, D. L., Bartholomew, R. M., Smith, L. A., and Dillman, R. O.,** Human immune response to multiple injections of murine monoclonal IgG, *J. Immunol.,* 135, 1530, 1985.
64. **Jerne, N. K.,** Towards a network theory of the immune system, *Ann. Immunol.* (Inst. Pasteur), 125C, 373, 1971.
65. **Sahagan, B. G., Dorai, H., Saltzbaber-Muller, J., Toneguzzo, F., Guindon, C. A., Lilly, S. P., McDonald, K. W., Morrissey, D. V., Stone, B. A., Davis, G. L., McIntosh, P. K., and Moore, G. P.,** A genetically engineered murine/human chimeric antibody retains specificity for human tumor-associated antigen, *J. Immunol.,* 137, 1066, 1986.

66. **Brown, B. A., Davis, G. L., Saltzbaber-Muller, J., Simon, P., Ho, M.-K., Shaw, P. S., Stone, B. A., Sands, H., and Moore, G. P.,** Tumor-specific genetically engineered murine/human chimeric monoclonal antibody, *Cancer Res.*, 47, 3577, 1987.
67. **Sands, H., Jones, P. L., Shah, S. A., Palme, D., Vessella, R. L., and Gallagher, B. M.,** Correlation of vascular permeability and blood flow with monoclonal antibody uptake by a human Clouser and renal cell xenografts, *Cancer Res.*, 48, 188, 1988.
68. **Colcher, D., Esteban, J., Carrasquillo, J. A., Sugarbaker, P., Reynolds, J. C., Bryant, G., Larson, S. M., and Schlom, J.,** Complementation of intracavitary and intravenous administration of a monoclonal antibody (B72.3) in patients with carcinoma, *Cancer Res.*, 47, 4218, 1987.
69. **Ward, B. D., Mather, S. J., Hawkins, L. A., Crowther, M. E., Shepherd, J. H., Granowska, M., Britton, K. E., and Slevin, M. L.,** Localization of radioiodine conjugated to the monoclonal antibody $HMFG_2$ in human ovarian-carcinoma-assessment of intravenous and intraperitoneal routes of administration, *Cancer Res.*, 47, 4719, 1987.

Chapter 8

IMMUNOLYMPHOSCINTIGRAPHY AND OTHER NONINTRAVENOUS APPLICATIONS OF MONOCLONAL ANTIBODIES

John N. Weinstein

TABLE OF CONTENTS

I. INTRODUCTION

Monoclonal antibodies have generally been administered intravenously, for scintigraphic imaging and for other in vivo applications. The rationale is clear: intravenous (i.v.) injection gives access to almost all tissues, with the exception of those in the central nervous system. However, regional routes of delivery should be considered when the location of the target antigen is anatomically restricted.

A small calculation will serve to illustrate the rationale for regional administration of antibodies: consider the proverbial 1 g solid tumor is a 70 kg human. If the blood flow per gram of tumor were, on average, equal to that in other parts of the body, then a molecule injected intravenously would pass through the tumor capillaries only once every 49 days (if it happened to remain in the circulation that long). Even then, the molecule would be statistically unlikely to leave the circulation and encounter antigen on the cells of a solid tumor. A similar inefficiency of delivery applies, of course, to low molecular weight diagnostic agents and drugs (except that everything happens faster), and the edifice of classical pharmacology has been built on functional selectivities obtained in the face of very low-efficiency delivery. With macromolecules such as the immunoglobulins, however, regional delivery provides a feasible alternative; macromolecules can be confined to anatomically defined compartments and tissues more easily than can small molecules. Most of the work to date on regional delivery of antibodies has been done in the lymphatic system, the target being either normal lymphoid or malignant cells in lymph nodes. Hence, lymphatic delivery will occupy the bulk of this chapter. Other possibilities that have been considered include intraperitoneal administration (principally for ovarian carcinoma), intraarterial infusion, and injection into the cerebrospinal fluid. The major emphasis, again because of the weight of experience thus far, will be on oncological and immunological applications.

II. LYMPHATIC DELIVERY OF ANTIBODIES: THE CLINICAL RATIONALE

Diagnostic assessment of lymph node status is important in the staging of most malignancies, including Hodgkin's disease, non-Hodgkin's lymphoma, melanoma, and carcinomas of breast, testis, prostate, colon, cervix, and lung. Current techniques for noninvasive detection of metastases are limited in sensitivity. Physical examination, X-ray, computerized tomography, gallium scanning, and magnetic resonance imaging are all unreliable for detecting tumors much less than about 1 cm in diameter (i.e., 1 g or roughly 1 billion tumor cells). Lymphangiography with radiologic contrast material is a cumbersome procedure requiring cannulation of lymph vessels, and the only site of injection in routine clinical practice is the foot.

Lymphoscintigraphy with ^{99m}technetium colloid has been considered, primarily for detection of internal mammary metastases of breast cancer.[1-3] Colloid is injected under the costal margin, and its uptake by macrophages in the lymph nodes monitored using a gamma camera. A positive reading is obtained only if the lymph node chain or architecture of individual nodes is grossly disrupted.

The problem is that this approach is essentially nonspecific. In principle, imaging with antibodies directed against tumor cells could be thousands of times more sensitive.[4] Regional delivery via the lymphatics represents an attempt to overcome some of the pharmacologic problems associated with i.v. administration of antibodies. The price is that this approach will not detect tumor in other common sites such as the lungs, liver, and bone (except in so far as antibody passes from the lymphatics to the systemic circulation, as described in the next section).

The term "lymphatic delivery" is intended to include both direct injection into cannulated

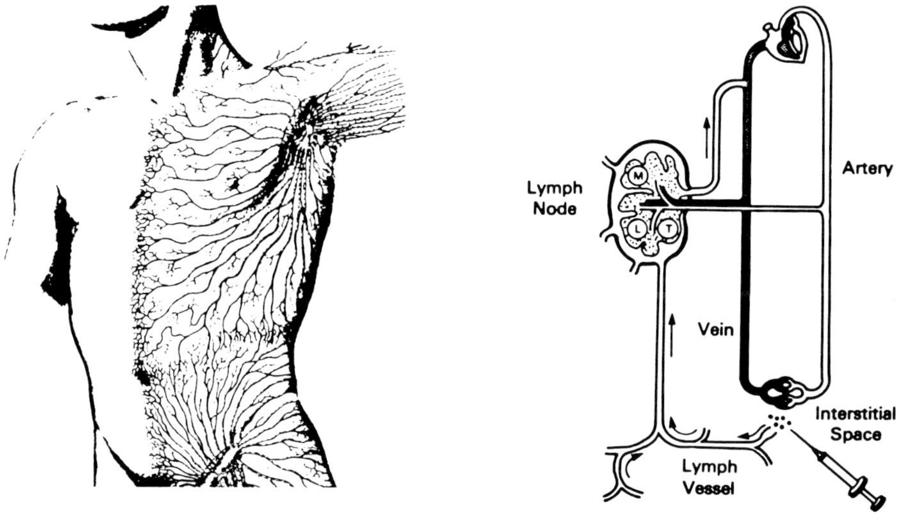

FIGURE 1. Passage of monoclonal antibodies through the lymphatics. Left: lymphatics of the torso (due to Sappey). Right: schematic view of the passage of an antibody molecule from a s.c. injection site into the lymphatics through clefts in the endothelium of the terminal lymphatic capillary. In the first node encountered, or in more distant nodes of the chain, antibody may bind to normal cells such as the (M) macrophages and (L) lymphocytes, or to (T) tumor cells. Antibody not removed from the lymph flow finally passes into the bloodstream, largely via the thoracic duct. (Modified from Weinstein, J. N., Parker, R. J., Keenan, A.M., Dower, S. K., Morse, H. C., III, and Sieber, S. M., *Science*, 218, 1334, 1982.)

lymphatic vessels (analogous to standard contrast lymphangiography) and injection into an interstitial space for uptake by the lymphatic capillaries. Most of the experience to date has involved the latter.

III. LYMPHATIC DELIVERY OF ANTIBODIES: THE PHYSIOLOGICAL BACKGROUND

The lymphatic system is most familiar in the immunological context, but it is also responsible for scavenging proteins (including immunoglobulins) that have leaked out of the circulation, filtering them through lymph nodes, and returning them to the bloodstream. This is an absolutely essential function, and death would result within a day or two if it ceased. This specialization of lymphatic capillaries for protein uptake provides the basis for lymphatic delivery of antibodies. The following description of lymphatic physiology draws on information from the classical literature[5] supplemented by findings from studies in our laboratory.

When small, water-soluble drugs are injected subcutaneously, the vast majority of them are cleared via the blood capillaries. However, molecules the size of immunoglobulins do not pass readily into the local blood capillaries. They are prevented from doing so by the continuous endothelial lining of the vessels and perhaps also by the presence of an intact basement membrane. Instead, as shown in Figure 1, a considerable percentage of the macromolecules pass into lymphatic capillary endings, which lack a basement membrane[6] and possess specialized clefts between their endothelial cells.[7] The clefts are thought to open and close in response to hydrostatic pressure differences and local muscle activity. They have been hypothesized to remain open in the face of external pressure (such as that of a local injection) because of fibers which pass like guy wires from collagen fibers in the interstitium to endothelial flaps bordering the clefts.

Whatever the details may be, once lymph has formed in the lymphatic capillaries, it flows into larger and larger tributary vessels, propelled by the contraction of smooth muscle in the vessel walls, by the activity of extrinsic skeletal muscles, and by hydrostatic pressure differences (generated, for example, by the volume of an injectate). Retrograde flow is prevented by a system of unidirectional valves. Upon reaching a lymph node, lymph flows into the marginal sinus located beneath the external capsule, then through a set of sinusoids in the medulla, and out of the node via an efferent vessel. In passing through the node, immunoglobulin molecules carried in the lymph may bind to target cells or be removed from the flow nonspecifically. Molecules remaining in the lymph pass to more distant nodes in the chain. If still not removed from the flow, they then pass into the bloodstream, by way of the thoracic duct and other lymphatico-venous connections. Thereafter, the immunoglobulin would be expected to distribute to the organs of the body as though injected i.v. in the first place. The lymphatic system is not a true ''circulation''. Rather, it is single-pass — like a great river system of merging tributaries which, collectively, drain the various watershed regions of the body.

IV. LYMPHATIC DELIVERY OF ANTIBODIES: MONOCLONAL ANTIBODIES DIRECTED AGAINST NORMAL CELLS IN ANIMALS

Initial studies of lymphatic delivery using monoclonal antibodies were done with monoclonals directed against normal lymph node cells, rather than against tumor.[8,9] Those studies were intended to delineate the pharmacology in a quantitatively reproducible system before introducing the complexities of a metastatic model. They also pointed the way to later clinical studies of patients with lymphoma and to possible attempts at modifying immune function.

The experiments[10] were done with a murine IgG_{2a} (36-7-5) that reacts with a private specificity of the mouse class I major histocompatibility antigen H-K^k. The antigen is expressed on over 90% of the lymphocytes of K^k positive mouse strains and (usually at lower levels) on almost all other cell types in those animals.

Iodine-125-labeled anti-H-2K^k was injected subcutaneously in the hind footpads of K^k positive mice. Two hours later, 10 to 20% of the injected radioactivity was found in the ipsilateral popliteal node, 50-fold more than in the popliteal nodes of K^k negative mice. High selectivity ratios were also observed for the lumbar and renal nodes, which are further along in the drainage pathway from the hind foot. Little radioactivity was found in the axillary and cervical nodes, or in contralateral popliteal and lumbar nodes, thus indicating that accumulation in the ipsilateral regional nodes had taken place regionally, via the lymphatics, not through the bloodstream. The popliteal nodes contained approximately 16,000% of dose per gram, whereas the figure for liver was 2000-fold less. Hence, the lymphatic route was clearly very efficient for reaching target antigens on the lymphoid cells. Figure 2 shows a pair of animals imaged 2 hr after injection in the hind footpads with ^{125}I-labeled anti-K^k. Popliteal and lumbar nodes were easily visualized in the K^k-positive mouse within 5 min after injection.

Further experiments showed the importance of antibody dose.[11,12] Above a dose of about 0.5 μg, k^k binding sites in the popliteal nodes became saturated, and antibody overflowed to the lumbar and renal nodes. At about 1 μg, those nodes also saturated. Antibody overflowed into the bloodstream and distributed to the liver, spleen, lungs, and other organs. Doses of about 0.3 μg optimized the ratio of node image to body background, as indicated by Figure 3.

Quantitative kinetic models[13,14] developed to describe and predict the pharmacology of lymphatic delivery in such systems indicated a pattern of ''sequential overflow'' from one node to the next, and finally to the systemic organs. However, the data also indicated a component of functional bypass such that the nodes could not be considered simply as being

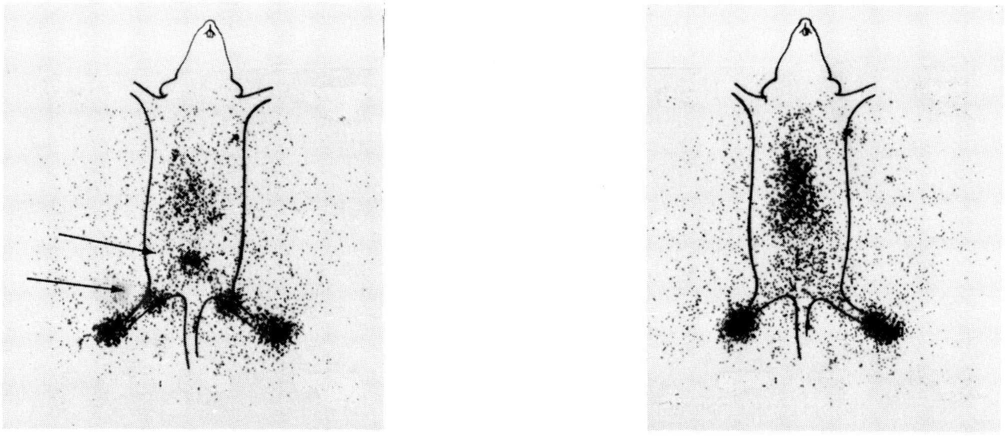

FIGURE 2. Gamma camera images of H-2K^k-positive (left) and H-2K^k-negative (right) mice 2 hr after injection in both hind footpads with ^{125}I-labeled anti-H-2K^k IgG (0.25 μCi/foot). The most prominent spots are the injection sites. Popliteal nodes (behind the knees) and lumbar nodes (in the lower abdomen) are also prominent in the K^k-positive mouse, but not the K^k-negative animal. Body background radioactivity is much more pronounced in the negative animal, largely because less antibody has bound in the feet and nodes, whereas more has overflowed into the systemic circulation. (Modified from Weinstein, J. N., Parker, R. J., Holton, O. D., III, Keenan, A. M., Covell, D. G., Black, C. D. V., and Sieber, S. M., *Cancer Investigation,* 3, 85, 1985.)

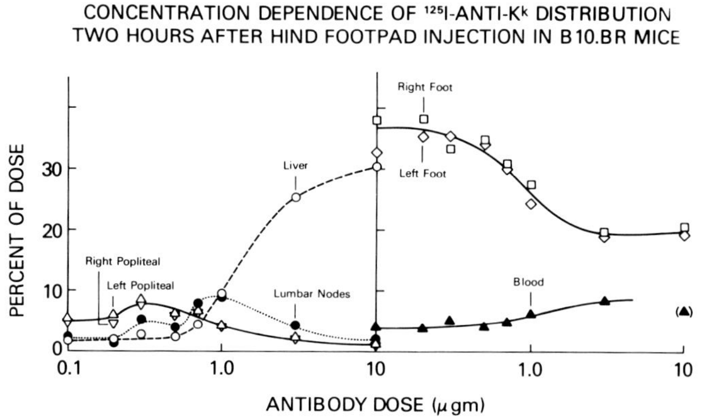

FIGURE 3. Dose dependence of ^{125}I-labeled anti-K^k distribution 2 hr after injection in the hind footpads of K^k-positive mice. The injection volume was 50 μl, and there were four animals per group. The liver (and other body organs) increase dramatically in uptake at doses above about 0.8 μgm, thus reflecting the sequential overflow along the lymphatics and into the bloodstream. (From Weinstein, J. N., Steller, M. A., Covell, D. G., Holton, O. D., III, Keenan, A. M., Sieber, S. M., and Parker, R. J., *Cancer Treat. Rep.,* 68, 257, 1984.)

in series with one another. A preliminary report[15] indicates that IgM is cleared from the injection site much more slowly than is IgG.

Those initial animal experiments provided data on two extreme cases: an antibody which bound to nothing (i.e., in the antigen-negative mouse strain) and one which bound to virtually all cells (in the positive strain). Other studies of antibodies against lymphoid cells have dealt with antigens of more restricted distribution. In one such instance, fluorescein-labeled IgG anti-Lyt 2 was injected in the hind footpads of mice. It reached and labeled all of the Lyt

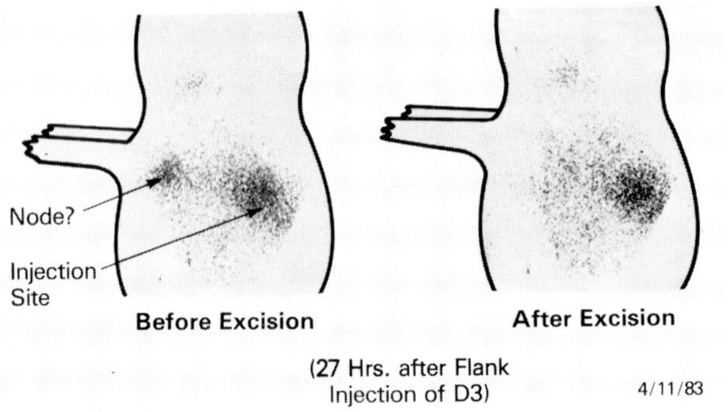

FIGURE 4. Gamma camera image of a lymph node metastasis of line 10 hepatocarcinoma implanted intradermally in the flank of a guinea pig. The animal was imaged 27 hr after s.c. injection of ^{125}I-labeled D3 (anti-tumor) antibody in the flank. The left hand panel shows the injection site and an image thought to be a cancerous draining lymph node. Upon excision of the node under anesthesia, a corresponding area of increased accumulation in the image disappeared. (From Weinstein, J. N., Keenan, A. M., Holton, O. D., III, Covell, D. G., Sieber, S. M., Black, C. D. V., Barbet, J. and Parker, R. J., in *Monoclonal Antibodies and Breast Cancer*, Ceriani, R. L., Ed., Martinus Nijhof, Boston, 1985, 218.)

2-positive subpopulation in the popliteal node, as assessed by fluorescence microscopy and flow cytometry. However, some nodes appeared to be segmented functionally and to label unevenly with dye injected at one site in the watershed region.[40] Experiments with antibody directed against lymphoid cells have provided a preclinical basis for imaging of lymphoma and also of normal human lymphoid cells, as a possible alternative to lymphoscintigraphy with nonspecific ^{99m}Tc-labeled colloids.

V. LYMPHATIC DELIVERY: MONOCLONAL ANTITUMOR ANTIBODIES IN ANIMALS

Only one set of animal studies on lymphatic delivery has been reported using monoclonal antibodies directed against tumor cells. With respect to solid tumors, the reason may be the difficulty of finding an immunogenic animal model which metastasizes with regularity to the lymph nodes. Few, if any, human tumor xenografts in nude mice metastasize in a suitable way.

In the one study reported, an antitumor antibody (D3) was used to detect lymph node metastases of line 10 hepatocarcinoma in guinea pigs.[16,17] Line 10 is a chemically-induced, transplantable tumor. When inoculated intradermally in the flank of a guinea pig, it metastasized within a week to the ipsilateral superficial distal axillary (SDA) node. D3, a monoclonal IgG_1 directed against a 290,000 dalton dimer on line 10 cells, had previously been found to localize selectively in line 10 tumor after i.v. administration.[18,19] To test the feasiblity of lymphatic delivery, the antibody was injected subcutaneously either in the front paw or in the flank near the tumor. Figure 4 shows a gamma camera image which suggested accumulation of D3 in a cancerous SDA node after injection in the flank. Without moving the anesthetized animal from its position under the gamma camera, the SDA node was dissected out. The area of increased accumulation in question disappeared, thus substantiating its identification as the lymph node.

Such images did not suffice to prove specificity of binding. Antibody might, for example, have been taken up nonspecifically in hyperplastic nodes. Specificity was demonstrated by double-label experiments with ^{125}I-labeled D3 and an isotype-matched nonbinding antibody labeled with ^{131}I. Figure 5 shows the radioactivity that was measured in SDA nodes and other organs after co-injection of the two immunoglobulins. Nodes ipsilateral to the primary

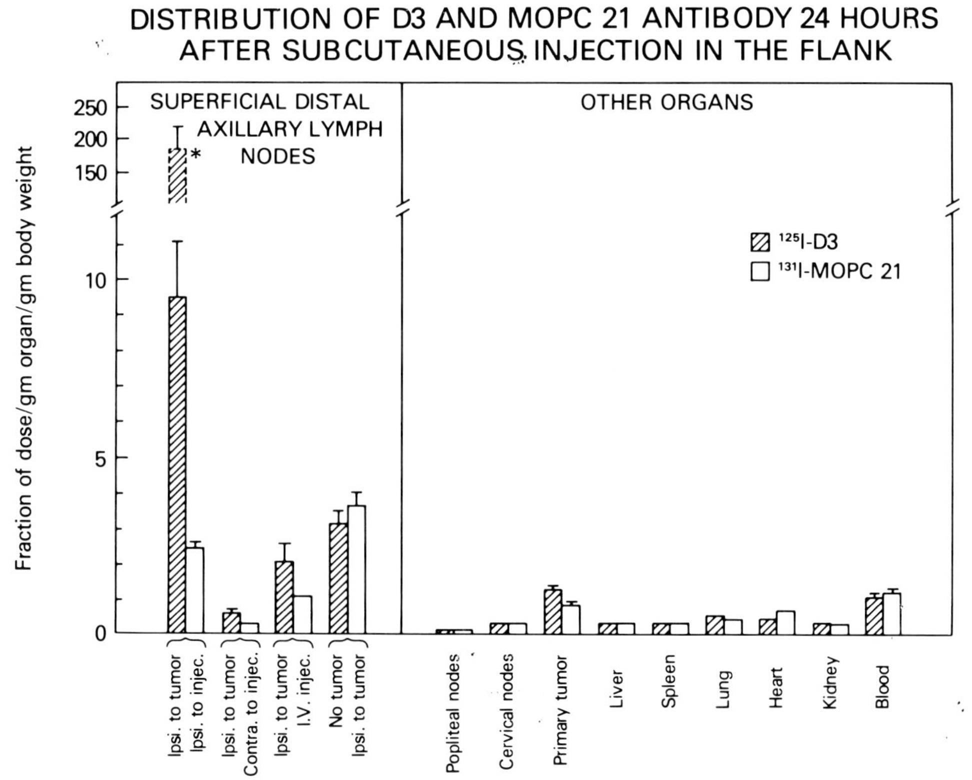

FIGURE 5. Distribution of ^{125}I-labeled D3 and ^{131}I-labeled control antibody (MOPC 21) 24 hr after coinjection in guinea pigs with line 10 tumors. Injections were subcutaneous in the flank, except where indicated as i.v. Studies were done 17 to 20 days after implanting 10^6 line 10 cells intradermally in the flank. On average, 4% of the node weight was tumor. The dashed bar (with asterisk) indicates radioactive uptake normalized by tumor weight rather than by node weight. The selectivity ratio within tumor substance was approximately 100 to 1. Injections contained 0.3 μg of ^{125}I-labeled D3 (1.9 μCi) and 0.3 μg of ^{131}I-labeled MOPC 21 (0.6 μCi). The data are geometric means (+/− standard error where large enough to be visible). (Modified from Weinstein, J. N., Steller, M. A., Keenan, A. M., Covell, D. G., Key, M. E., Sieber, S. M., Oldham, R. K., Hwang, K. M., and Parker, R. J., *Science*, 222, 423, 1983.)

tumor and to the injection site showed, on average, a 3.9 to 1 ratio of specific (D3) to nonspecific (MOPC 21) binding. However, this figure did not reflect the full extent of selectivity obtained. Only 4% of the weight of the nodes was tumor at the time of the injection, hence the specific-to-nonspecific ratio within the tumor itself was much higher, approximately 100 to 1. The lack of radioactivity in nodes ipsilateral to the tumor but contralateral to the site of injection indicated that delivery to ipsilateral nodes was principally regional, through lymphatic drainage, not via the bloodstream. Normal nodes and other organs showed no selectivity.

It remained possible that antibody delivered via the lymphatics was not bound to metastatic cells, but rather to antigen shed from the primary tumor into lymphatic vessels and filtered out by the lymph nodes. This may have been the case in clinical studies,[20,21] to be discussed later, with polyclonal antibody to human carcinoembryonic antigen. In the case of D3, however, localization in early metastatic tumor was demonstrated directly by autoradiography,[16] as shown in Figure 6. However, when a lymph node metastasis grew larger, to several hundred milligrams in the guinea pig node, antibody reached only part of the mass. This last finding indicated a possible major limitation of lymphatic delivery, an inability to permeate,[22] or even reach, large metastases.

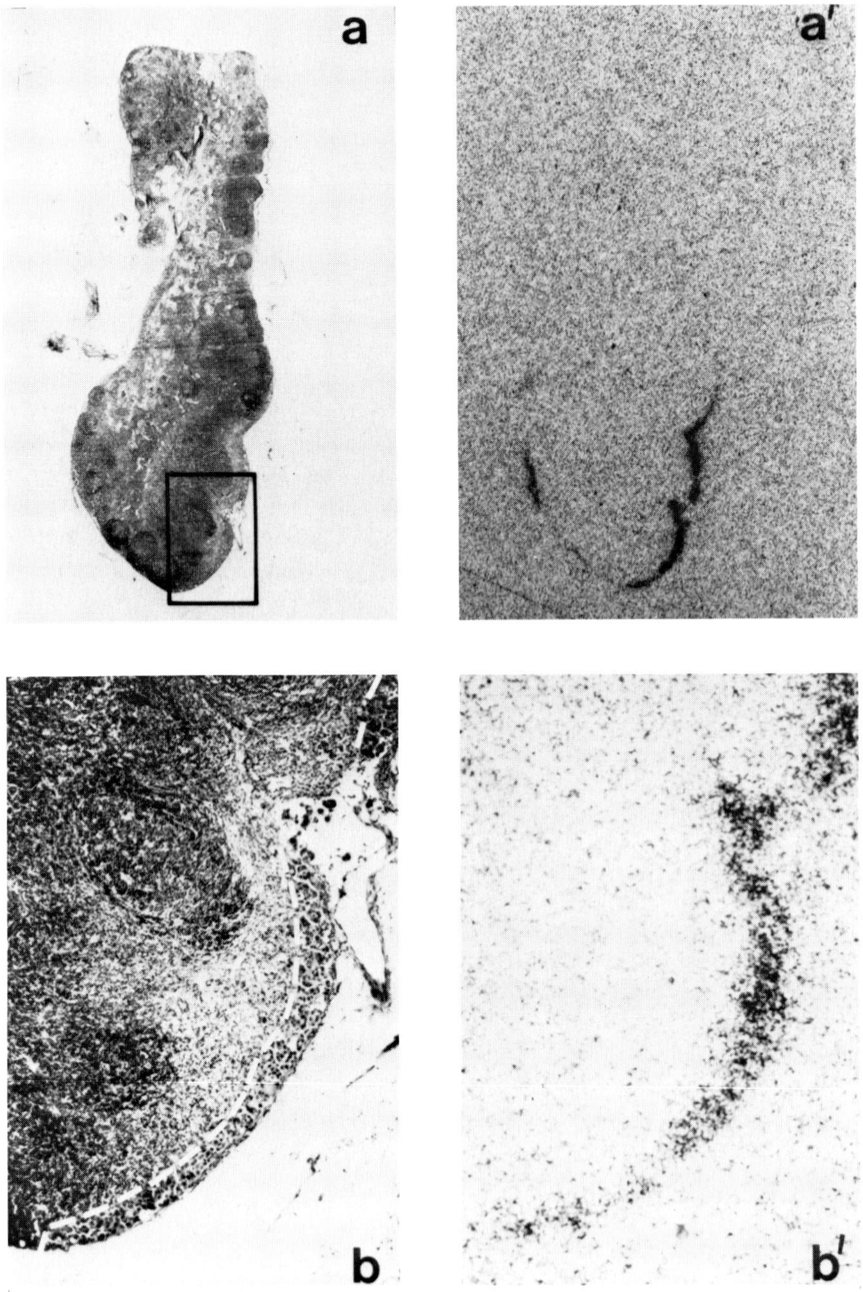

FIGURE 6. Autoradiographic study of a cancerous superficial distal axillary node 24 hr after ipsilateral s.c. injection of ^{125}I-labeled D3 IgG. The guinea pig was injected with 34 μgm D3 (3.4 μCi) on day 21 after implantation of 10^6 L10 cells. (a) Paraffin-embedded section stained with hematoxylin and eosin. Tumor occupied 2% of the node area. (a') Autoradiogram of 6 μm section cut adjacent to that in (a). Grains representing ^{125}I-labeled antibody are seen along the rim of the node at one end. (b) Higher magnification corresponding to the insert box in (a). Large, pleiomorphic tumor cells occupy the area demarcated by white dashed line. (b') Autoradiogram of section adjacent to that in (b). (Magnification of (a) and (a'), 14 ×; of (b) and (b'), 57 ×. From Weinstein, J. N., Steller, M. A., Keenan, A. M., Covell, D. G., Key, M. E., Sieber, S. M., Oldham, R. K., Hwang, K. M., and Parker, R. J., *Science,* 222, 423, 1983.)

Experiments were also done to test the feasibility of two-antibody techniques for visualizing both malignant and normal lymph node cells.[23] ^{125}I-labeled D3 was injected in the flank of the animal, and the superficial distal axillary node on that side was visualized 24 hr later. ^{125}I-labeled antibody (8BE6) directed against guinea pig T-cells was then injected in the forepaw, and the same node showed additional uptake (on the basis of its normal T-cell component). As long as the radioactivity in the second injection was kept sufficiently high, both images could thus be obtained and quantitated independently, even though only a single label was used. If labeled with different isotopes, the two antibodies could instead be coinjected and imaged separatedly, provided appropriate energy windows could be set for the gamma camera.

VI. ENDOSCOPIC ADMINISTRATION FOR LYMPHATIC UPTAKE

Subcutaneous (s.c.) injection suffices to reach many lymph node groups. It was clear, however, that another approach would be required for access to the nodes draining visceral organs. To reach the hilar and mediastinal nodes in which lung cancers can seed, antibody might be injected through the bronchial wall in the area of the primary tumor using a cytology needle and fiberoptic bronchoscope.[24] The antibody would then be expected to follow the same drainage path as do metastatic tumor cells, toward nodes of the carina and mediastinum. A feasibility study of this strategy has been conducted using an I-131-labeled murine IgG_{2b} reactive with mouse I-E^k. The anti-I-E^k was known to cross react with determinants on antigen-presenting cells in a number of species, including the dog.[25] Initial experiments in dogs by Mulshine et al.[24] showed uptake in hilar and carinal nodes that was antigen specific and approximately 100-fold greater than in distant lymph nodes. Analogous endoscopic techniques may be applicable to colorectal carcinoma. In particular, the status of regional nodes can determine whether the anal sphincter is saved at surgery or whether a patient with low rectal carcinoma will require a permanent colostomy.

VII. THERAPY VIA THE LYMPHATICS

Studies thus far have focused on the basic pharmacology or else on diagnostic applications. The potential for therapy via the lymphatics is more limited. In the case of breast carcinoma, for example, regional lymph node status is considered an indicator of metastatic spread, not a site at which the spread can be prevented. Surgical removal of the axillary nodes is not thought to influence survival,[26] but it is possible that lymphatic delivery of antitumor antibodies would provide advantages over external beam radiotherapy for local control of the disease. Current conventional therapy does indicate some settings in which more definitive benefit might be realized from the lymphatic approach; irradiation of regional nodes appears to improve the prognosis for selected patients with tumors which disseminate early via the lymphatics — malignancies such as Hodgkin's disease, some non-Hodgkin's lymphomas, and seminomatous testicular carcinoma.

In deciding on an isotope for therapeutic use in the lymphatics, the characteristics required may differ from those for i.v. administration. It may, for example, be possible to use short-lived species if accumulation in the target nodes is sufficiently quick. Because of rapid accumulation, Black et al.[41] have been able to use conjugates of ^{212}bismuth, which has a half-life of 61 min, to obtain selective killing of B-cells in the lymph nodes of mice. This represented the first antigen-selective use of alpha-emitter/antibody conjugates in vivo. The antibody used was a murine IgG_1 anti-Lyb 8.2 designated CY-34. The antibody was labeled with ^{212}Bi by chelation and injected into the footpads of mice. There was approximately a one order of magnitude selectivity (with respect to T-cells in the target lymph nodes of Lyb 8.2 positive mice and with respect to B-cells in the target nodes of Lyb 8.2 negative mice).

Although there was no direct proof, this selectivity probably required the short range of an alpha emitter (range about 70 μm for ^{212}Bi), given the size of follicles in mouse lymph nodes. When high spatial resolution is not required, beta emitters may be useful.

VIII. CLINICAL STUDIES OF LYMPHATIC DELIVERY: POLYCLONAL ANTIBODIES

In 1975 Order et al.[27] reported a case study using the polyclonal gamma globulin fraction of an antiserum raised against ferritin, a "tumor-associated" antigen. The preparation was injected directly into a cannulated lymphatic vessel for detection of lymph node metastases in a patient with Hodgkin's disease. Gamma camera images showed accretions of radioactivity in a region of known lymph node tumor. The study was not designed to give evidence of antigenic specificity or to demonstrate histological localization in tumor substance. A second patient[28] did not show similar deposition of radioactivity and, correspondingly, had no axial disease demonstrable by Ethiodol contrast lymphangiography.

In 1980 DeLand et al.[20,21] reported a series of patients injected subcutaneously with ^{131}I-labeled goat IgG directed against carcinoembryonic antigen. Cancerous nodes were imaged, but anomalous findings complicated the issue of antigenic specificity. To explain cases in which the histology revealed no metastatic tumor in highly radioactive nodes, the investigators made the compelling suggestion that antibody might be binding to antigen shed from the primary tumor and sequestered in the regional lymph nodes.

IX. CLINICAL STUDIES OF LYMPHATIC DELIVERY: MONOCLONAL ANTIBODIES

Thompson et al.[29] have injected ^{131}I-labeled monoclonal 3E1.2 in the finger webs of patients with breast cancer in an attempt to image axillary nodes. The antibody is a murine IgM reactive with membrane and cytoplasm of breast carcinoma cells, as well as with the luminal membranes of normal breast. The study (nine patients) suggested a generally positive correlation between accumulation of label at 16 to 24 hr and the presence of disease. Nonspecific uptake was approximated in some patients by injection of ^{125}I-labeled control antibody. The attenuation factor for ^{125}I in nodes of the axilla was estimated by placing a bottle source containing ^{125}I in that location. Ratios of 2:1 were obtained for specificity, and one patient with non-Hodgkin's lymphoma injected similarly with 3E1.2 showed less accumulation in the nodes. These findings suggested an element of specificity to the localization, but surgical specimens were not available for verification.

Other studies have been directed against metastases of malignant melanoma. At our own institution, several different preparations have been used in patients with stage II melanoma: ^{131}I-labeled Fab fragments of 96.5 (anti-P97) and 48.7 (anti-GP240), as well as whole IgG 9.2.27 (anti-GP240). Some patients were injected subcutaneously near the site from which the primary tumor had been removed surgically. Others were injected in the web spaces between the fingers to reach axillary nodes or between the toes to reach lymph node groups in the groin. The pharmacological, histochemical, and clinical data are currently being analyzed in detail, but a preliminary report[30] indicates no reliable localization in cancerous nodes. It is not clear at this point whether optimal choice of reagent, label, and method of administration will change that picture. It may be that lymph node metastases of melanoma preclude effective access to the involved nodes, even at an early stage of growth. Alternatively, there may be nonspecific uptake due to reactive cells within cancerous nodes. Despite the reported success with breast cancer,[29] these may be rather general problems with respect to metastases of solid tumors.

The situation appears quite different for T-cell lymphoma, as reported by Keenan et al.[31]

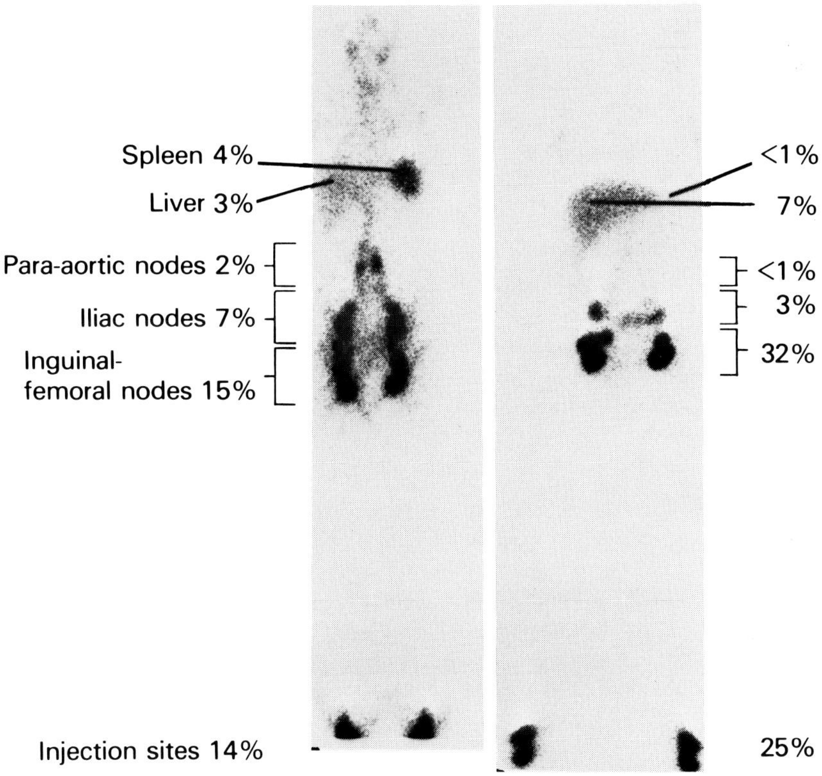

FIGURE 7. Anterior whole body gamma camera scans 2 to 3 days after administration of ^{111}In-labeled T101 in the toe webs of both feet. Numbers indicate percentages of injected activity in organs, nodes, and injection sites. Values for iliac and inguinal-femoral nodes represent the means of those obtained separately for left and right sides. The patient on the left had only minimal disease in the nodes. (The feet were partly out of the camera view, but percentages were calculated from region of interest scans taken at about the same time.) The patient on the right had large, bulky disease. Double foci in the feet of the right hand patient resulted from dorsiflexion and plantar flexion during imaging. The efficiencies of lymph node imaging were orders of magnitude higher than after i.v. injection. (From Keenan, A. M., Weinstein, J. N., Mulshine, J. L., Carrasquillo, J. A., Bunn, P. A., Jr., Reynolds, J. C., Foon, K. A., Perentesis, P., Ghosh, B., and Larson, S. M., *J. Nucl. Med.*, in press.)

T101 is a murine IgG_{2a} directed against the T65 antigen[32] on cells of chronic lymphocytic leukemia and cutaneous T-cell lymphoma (CTCL). The antigen is also expressed on normal T cells. In-111-labeled T101 was injected in the toe webs of patients with CTCL. Serial gamma camera imaging showed large concentrations of activity in the inguinal-femoral lymph nodes within 3 hr of injection. The node chains reached peak activity within 24 hr, and the indium levels then declined slowly. The first patient imaged had only minimal involvement of the lymph nodes (LN 2); the second had bulky disease in the nodes. Images of those two patients are shown in Figure 7. The 24 and 36% of dose imaged in nodes of those patients constituted by far the most efficient targeting of antibody achieved clinically by any noninvasive means. Additional patients have shown similar efficient uptake. The imaging appeared to be largely antigen specific,[31] but not tumor specific since T101 reacts also with normal T cells. Antibodies having greater selectivity for neoplastic cells would permit more sensitive and accurate assessment of lymph node status.

Table 1
COMPARISON OF SUBCUTANEOUS AND INTRAVENOUS INJECTION OF MONOCLONAL ANTIBODIES FOR DELIVERY TO TUMOR IN LYMPH NODES

Possible limitations of subcutaneous administration	Possible advantages of subcutaneous administration
Restriction to regional nodes	Lower dose
Requirement that lymph vessels be patent	Detection of smaller masses
	Can be faster
Possible toxicity at injection site	Less systemic toxicity
Possible sensitization to mouse immunoglobulin	Less competition by circulating antigen
Biological variability of lymphatics	Less cross reaction with antigen expressed on normal cells

Modified from Weinstein, J. N., Keenan, A. M., Holton, O. D., III, Covell, D. G., Sieber, S. M., Black, C. D. V., Barbet, J., and Parker, R. J., in *Monoclonal Antibodies and Breast Cancer,* Ceriani, R. L., Ed., Martinus Nijhof, Boston, 1985, 218.

X. OTHER REGIONAL ROUTES OF DELIVERY

Many, but not all, of the same advantages and disadvantages apply for other regional routes of delivery besides the lymphatics. The first studies[33-36] have now appeared on intraperitoneal administration, for detection or treatment of ovarian and colorectal carcinoma in the peritoneal cavity. Localization has also been attempted in the pericardial and pleural cavities[36] and intraarterially for irradiation of brain gliomas.[37]

XI. LIMITATIONS OF LYMPHATIC DELIVERY

Some of the possible advantages and limitations of lymphatic delivery with respect to i.v. administration are indicated in Table 1.

Lymphatic delivery is, of course, limited to tumor (or perhaps other disease) in the regional lymph nodes. Except for overflow of antibody into the bloodstream, metastases in such common sites as brain, lung, and liver will not be detected. A second limitation is that the lymphatic vessels must be patent if antibody is to reach its target. Large masses displace normal nodal tissue and can distort or block local lymph flow. The lymphatic approach was, therefore, expected to work best for small, early metastases. The lack of success with melanoma may reflect a problem of this sort. The much greater success with lymphoma may reflect easier penetration to and into the mass of cells. Lymphatic delivery will probably be used in tandem with i.v. injection, the former to detect small masses, the latter to detect large, well-vascularized ones. There may also be an advantage to using antitumor antibody in conjunction with an antibody directed against normal cells in the node, the latter to demonstrate gross distortion or blockage of the lymphatic chain. The feasibility of that approach has been demonstrated in guinea pigs,[23] as described earlier.

Since s.c. injection tends to be more effective for immunization than i.v. injection, it was thought that sensitization to mouse globulin might be an especially great problem. At this point it is clear that patients do develop anti-mouse antibodies after s.c. injection, but the author is not aware of any compilation of data on the dose dependence or on the relative frequencies of occurrence after i.v. and s.c. administration. Such information will be available from multiple sources very soon.

Radiotoxicity at the injection site appears not to be a major problem even with ^{131}I. No local damage has been reported in animals or in patients. For therapy with armed antibodies, however, local toxicity is likely to be a major problem. Cannulation of a lymphatic vessel and direct injection may be necessary.

XII. POSSIBLE ADVANTAGES OF LYMPHATIC DELIVERY

The most important possible advantage is sensitivity, as reflected in the ability to detect small numbers of cancer cells with low doses of radioactivity. Mouse popliteal nodes weighing less than 1 mg were imaged within a few minutes using less than a microCurie of ^{125}I-labeled anti-K^k antibody.[8] As little as 3 mg of early metastatic tumor in guinea pig nodes was also imaged, though not as soon after injection.[16] In studies of T-cell lymphoma, the efficiency of the imaging was sufficiently high that (by calculation) less than 10 mg of cells could have been identified.

The theoretical limit of sensitivity (the same for both i.v. and s.c. administration) is set by the number of antigenic determinants per cell, the specific activity of the labeled antibody, and the detection system. Assume, for example, a highly expressive tumor whose cells bind 500,000 antibody molecules at saturation. If the antibody was labeled to a specific activity of 10 mCi/mg with ^{131}I, then at saturation of binding there would be 1.25×10^{-9} mCi/cell, or 2.75 disintegrations per minute per cell. The practical lower limit of detection on one current clinical gamma camera (in the presence of spontaneous background only) is on the order of 100,000 disintegrations per minute. Therefore, approximately 40,000 antibody-labeled cells (0.04 mg) could, in principle, be detected.[38] That is about 25,000 times fewer cells than can be detected by other current noninvasive techniques. A more favorable isotope such as ^{111}indium of ^{99m}Tc would yield an even lower limit of detectability.

This calculation makes clear that diagnostic imaging with monoclonal antibodies will not be limited by intrinsic sensitivity. Rather, the limits will be set by pharmacologic factors, including the degree of saturation achievable and the background noise due to radionuclide not bound to tumor cells. The direct route via lymphatic vessels will be useful for diagnosis if it improves the signal-to-noise ratio.

Sequestering antibody in the lymphatics is expected to reduce cross-reactive binding. Studies[8] in mice with anti-K^k (these studies were described earlier) represented the logical extreme of "cross-reactive" binding. Nonetheless, localization in the nodes was profound. Antitumor antibodies inappropriate for i.v. use because of poor selectivity might be satisfactory for delivery via the lymphatics (except perhaps if the antigen were expressed on normal cell types in the lymphatics or shed in large amounts into lymph nodes from the primary tumor). It might be possible, for example, to use a monoclonal antibody equally reactive with normal and cancerous breast cells. In carefully selected cases, cross reaction could even be an *advantage* for diagnostic studies. For example, an antibody raised against malignant melanoma (designated 96.5) is removed from the circulation by the liver more quickly than are most antibodies,[39] probably because of cross-reactive binding. The liver is sufficiently large that there would presumably be no toxicity at diagnostic doses, and hepatic accumulation would tend to clear away background radioactivity due to antibody which overflowed the lymphatics into the bloodstream.

NOTE ADDED IN PROOF

Material for this chapter was compiled prior to July 1986.

REFERENCES

1. **Ege, G. N.,** Internal mammary lymphoscintigraphy, *Radiology,* 118, 101, 1976.
2. **Ege, G. N.,** Lymphoscintigraphy — techniques and applications in the management of breast cancer, *Semin. Nucl. Med.,* 13, 26, 1983.
3. **Kaplan, W. D.,** Iliopelvic lymphoscintigraphy, *Semin. Nucl. Med.,* 13, 42, 1983.
4. **Weinstein, J. N., Keenan, A.M., Holton, O. D., III, Covell, D. G., Sieber, S. M., Black, C. D. V., Barbet, J., and Parker, R. J.,** Use of monoclonal antibodies to detect metastases of solid tumors in lymph nodes, in *Monoclonal Antibodies and Breast Cancer,* Ceriani, R. L., Ed., Martinus Nijhoff, Boston, 1985, 218.
5. **Yoffey, J. M. and Courtice, F. C.,** *Lymphatics, Lymph and the Lymphomyeloid Complex,* Academic Press, Orlando, 1970, 1.
6. **Barsky, S. H., Baker, A., Siegal, G. P., Togo, S., and Liotta, L. A.,** Use of anti-basement membrane antibodies to distinguish blood vessel capillaries from lymphatic capillaries, *Am. J. Surg. Pathol.,* 7, 667, 1983.
7. **Leak, L. V.,** Studies on the permeability of lymphatic capillaries, *J. Cell Biol.,* 50, 300, 1971.
8. **Weinstein, J. N., Parker, R. J., Keenan, A. M., Dower, S. K., Morse, H. C., III, and Sieber, S. M.,** Monoclonal antibodies in the lymphatics: toward the diagnosis and therapy of tumor metastases, *Science,* 218, 1334, 1982.
9. **Parker, R. J., Weinstein, J. N., Keenan, A. M., Dower, S. K., Steller, M. A., Holton, O. D., and Sieber, S. M.,** Targeting of radiolabelled monoclonal antibodies in the lymphatics, *Cancer Res.,* in press.
10. **Sachs, D. H., Mayer, N., and Ozato, K.,** in *Monoclonal Antibodies and T-Cell Hybridomas,* Hammerling, U. and Kearney, J. F., Eds., Elsevier, Amsterdam, 1981, 95.
11. **Steller, M. A., Parker, R. J., Covell, D. G., Holton, O. D., III, Keenan, A. M., Sieber, S. M., and Weinstein, J. N.,** Optimization of monoclonal antibody delivery via the lymphatics: the dose-dependence, *Cancer Res.,* 46, 1830, 1986.
12. **Weinstein, J. N., Steller, M. A., Covell, D. G., Holton, O. D., III, Keenan, A. M., Sieber, S. M., and Parker, R. J.,** Monoclonal anti-tumor antibodies in the lymphatics, *Cancer Treat. Rep.,* 68, 257, 1984.
13. **Weinstein, J. N., Steller, M. A., Covell, D. G., Dower, S. K., Segal, D. M., Keenan, A. M., Sieber, S. M., and Parker, R. J.,** Use of monoclonal antibodies for diagnosis and therapy of tumor metastases in lymph nodes, in *Affinity Chromatography and Biological Recognition,* Chaiken, I. M., Wilchek, M., and Parikh, I., Eds., Academic Press, New York, 1983, 337.
14. **Covell, D. G., Steller, M. A., Parker, R. J., and Weinstein, J. N.,** Delivery of monoclonal antibodies through the lymphatics: characterization by compartmental modeling, *Comput. Appl. Med. Care,* 10, 884, 1985.
15. **Halpern, S. E., Hagan, P. L., Bartholomew, R. M., Frincke, J. M., Poggenburg, J. K., Merchant, E. B., and Carlo, D. J.,** Kinetics and distribution of subcutaneously administered 111-In IgG and IgM antibodies (A) in a mouse model, *J. Nucl. Med.,* 27 (Abstr.), 902, 1986.
16. **Weinstein, J. N., Steller, M. A., Keenan, A. M., Covell, D. G., Key, M. E., Sieber, S. M., Oldham, R. K., Hwang, K. M., and Parker, R. J.,** Monoclonal antibodies in the lymphatics: selective delivery to lymph node metastases of a solid tumor, *Science,* 222, 423, 1983.
17. **Weinstein, J. N., Holton, O. D., III, Black, C. D. V., Covell, D. G., Spaulding, G. F., Barbet, J., Steller, M. A., Sieber, S. M., Talley, M. J., and Parker, R. J.,** Regional delivery of monoclonal antitumor antibodies: detection and possible treatment of lymph node metastases, in *Cancer Metastasis: Experimental and Clinical Strategies,* Welch, D. R., Bhuyan, B. K., and Liotta, L. A., Eds., Alan R. Liss, New York, 1986, 169.
18. **Key, M. E., Bernhard, M. I., Hoyer, L. C., Foon, K. A., Oldham, R. K., and Hanna, M. G.,** Guinea pig line 10 hepatocarcinoma model for monoclonal antibody serotherapy. II. In vivo localization of a monoclonal antibody in normal and malignant tissues. *J. Immunol.,* 130, 1451, 1983.
19. **Bernhard, M. I., Hwang, K. M., Foon, K. A., Keenan, A. M., Kessler, R. M., Frincke, J. M., Tallam, D. J., Hanna, M. G., Peters, L., and Oldham, R. K.,** Localization of ^{111}Indium and ^{131}Iodine labeled monoclonal antibody in guinea pigs bearing line 10 hepatocarcinoma tumors, *Cancer Res.,* 43, 4429, 1983.
20. **DeLand, F. H., Kim, E. E., Corgan, R. L., Casper, S., Primus, F. J., Spremulli, E., Estes, N., and Goldenberg, D. M.,** Axillary lymphoscintigraphy by radioimmunodetection of carcinoembryonic antigen in breast cancer, *J. Nucl. Med.,* 20, 1243, 1979.
21. **DeLand, F. H., Kim, E. E., and Goldenberg, D. M.,** Lymphoscintigraphy with radionuclide-labeled antibodies to carcinoembryonic antigen, *Cancer Res.,* 40, 2997, 1980.
22. **Weinstein, N., Parker, R., Holton, O. D., III, Black, C. D. V., Sieber, S. M., and Covell, D. G.,** The pharmacology of monoclonal antibodies, in *Membrane-Mediated Cytotoxicity,* Reisfeld, R., Ed., Alan R. Liss, New York, in press.

23. **Weinstein, J. N., Black, C. D. V., Keenan, A. M., Holton, O. D., III, Larson, S. M., Sieber, S. M., Covell, D. G., Carrasquillo, J., Barbet, J., and Parker, R. J.**, Use of monoclonal antibodies for detection of lymph node metastases, in *Monoclonal Antibodies in Cancer Therapy*, Alan R. Liss, New York, 1986, 473.
24. **Mulshine, J. L., Keenan, A. M., Carrasquillo, J. A., Walsh, T., Linnoila, R. I., Holton, O. D., Harwell, J., Larson, S. M., Bunn, P. A., and Weinstein, J. N.**, Immunolymphoscintigraphy of pulmonary and mediastinal lymph nodes: a new approach to lung cancer imaging, *Cancer Res.*, submitted.
25. **Watanabe, M., Suzuki, T., Taniguchi, M., Shinohara, N.**, Monoclonal anti-Ia murine alloantibodies crossreactive with the Ia-homologues of other species including humans, *Transplantation*, 36, 712, 1983.
26. **Hellman, S., Harris, J. R., Canellos, G. P., and Fisher, B.**, Cancer of the breast, in *Cancer Principles and Practice of Oncology*, De Vita, V. T., Jr., Hellman, S., and Rosenberg, S. A., Eds., Lippincott, Philadelphia, 1982, 914.
27. **Order, S. E., Bloomer, W. D., Jones, A. G., Kaplan, W. D., Davis, M. A., Adelstein, S. J., and Hellman, S.**, Radionuclide immunoglobulin lymphangiography: A case report, *Cancer*, 35, 1487, 1975.
28. **Order, S. E.**, Immunospecific radionuclide immunoglobulin lymphography, in *Clinical Lymphography*, Vol. 7, Clouse, M. E., Ed., Williams & Wilkins, Baltimore, 1977, 316.
29. **Thompson, C. H., Stacker, S. A., Salehi, N., Lichtenstein, M., Leyden, M. J., Andrews, J. T., and McKenzie, I. F. C.**, Immunoscintigraphy for detection of lymph node metastases from breast cancer, *Lancet*, 2, 1245, 1984.
30. **Lotze, M. T., Carrasquillo, J. A., Weinstein, J. N., Bryant, G. J., Perentesis, P., Reynolds, J. C., Matis, L. A., Eger, R. R., Keenan, A. M., Hellstrom, I., Hellstrom, K. E., and Larson, S. M.**, Monoclonal antibody imaging of human melanoma: radioimmunodetection by subcutaneous or systemic injection, *Ann. Surg.*, in press.
31. **Keenan, A. M., Weinstein, J. N., Mulshine, J. L., Carrasquillo, J. A., Bunn, P. A., Jr., Reynolds, J. C., Foon, K. A., Perentesis, P., Ghosh, B., and Larson, S. M.**, Evaluation of lymphoma by immunolymphoscintigraphy: subcutaneous injection of indium-111-labeled T101 monoclonal antibody, *J. Nucl. Med.*, in press.
32. **Royston, I., Majda, J. A., Baird, S. M., Meserve, B. L., and Griffiths, J. C.**, Human T cell antigens defined by monoclonal antibodies: the 65,000-dalton antigen of T cells (T65) is also found on chronic lymphocytic leukemia cells bearing surface immunoglobulin, *J. Immunol.*, 125, 725, 1980.
33. **Epenetos, A. A.**, Antibody guided lymphangiography in the staging of cervical cancer, *Br. J. Cancer*, 51, 805, 1985.
34. **Wahl, R. L. and Fisher, S.**, Intraperitoneal delivery of radiolabeled monoclonal antibodies: enhanced regional delivery advantage using IV unlabeled anti-mouse antibody, *J. Nucl. Med.*, 27 (Abstr.), 921, 1986.
35. **Colcher, D., Esteban, J., Carrasquillo, J. A., Sugarbaker, P., Reynolds, J. C., Bryant, G., Larson, S. M., and Schlom, J.**, Comparison of route of administration of radiolabeled monoclonal antibodies in patients with colorectal cancer, *J. Nucl. Med.*, 27 (Abstr.), 902, 1986.
36. Hammersmith Oncology Group and the Imperial Cancer Research Fund, Antibody-guided irradiation of malignant lesions: three cases illustrating a new method of treatment, *Lancet*, 1, 1441, 1984.
37. **Epenetos, A. A., Courtenay-Luck, N., Pickering, D., Hooker, G., Durbin, H., Lavender, J. P., and McKenzie, C. G.**, Antibody guided irradiation of brain glioma by arterial infusion of radioactive monoclonal antibody against epidermal growth factor receptor and blood group A antigen, *Br. Med. J.*, 290, 1463, 1985.
38. **Weinstein, J. N., Parker, R. J., Holton, O. D., III, Keenan, A. M., Covell, D. G., Black, C. D. V., and Sieber, S. M.**, Lymphatic delivery of monoclonal antibodies: potential for detection and treatment of lymph node metastases, *Cancer Invest.*, 3, 85, 1985.
39. **Larson, S. M., Brown, J. P., Wright, P. W., Carrasquillo, J. A., Hellstrom, I., and Hellstrom, K. E.**, Localization of ^{131}I-labeled p97-specific Fab fragments in human melanoma as a basis for radiotherapy, *J. Nucl. Med.*, 24, 123, 1983.
40. **Weinstein, J. N.**, Unpublished data.
41. **Black**, In preparation.

Chapter 9

RADIOIMMUNOSCINTIGRAPHY WITH POLYCLONAL OR MONOCLONAL ANTIBODIES

Jorge A. Carrasquillo

TABLE OF CONTENTS

I. INTRODUCTION

Radioimmunoscintigraphy (RIS) of tumors is a technique in which radioactively labeled anti-tumor antibodies are administered to patients with malignant disease as diagnostic agents for tumor detection. This diagnostic modality has been possible due to advances in tumor immunology which have identified a multitude of "tumor associated antigens" present on human tumors and to the ability to produce antibodies which recognize these antigens. Since these antigens have a much higher expression in tumor than in normal tissue, the underlying principle is that when radiolabeled antibodies specific for the antigen are administered to a patient, they will be carried passively to all tissues; however, because the tumor has the antigen, the antibody will bind, progressively accumulate in the tumor, and be detected utilizing conventional nuclear medicine gamma cameras.[1] This specificity offers a distinct advantage over the majority of diagnostic methods available today which are indirect and dependent on differences in attenuation, mass effect, or ultrasound reflection.

Although on theoretical grounds, and based on results reported in animal tumor models, favorable targeting of radiolabeled antibodies should be easily obtained,[2-9] much of the work in humans with polyclonal and monoclonal antibodies has not shown the expected sensitivity for tumor imaging.[10-13] There are several factors which may be of importance in tumor targeting: stability of radiolabeled antibody, affinity, antigen concentration, cross-reacting antigens in normal tissue, antigen heterogeneity, circulating antigen, tumor blood flow, tumor capillary permeability, mass of antibody, choice of fragment or whole IgG, and gamma camera limitations. Human imaging trials addressing these issues are in progress. Some of the clinical trials that have been conducted with intravenous (i.v.) administration of radiolabeled antibody and some of the parameters that may be important in optimizing tumor uptake will be reviewed in this chapter. Review of RIS via lymphatic[14-16] or intracavitary delivery[17] can be found in Chapter 8.

II. HISTORICAL PERSPECTIVE

Pressman et al.[18,19] were among the first to explore the use of radiolabeled antibodies for tumor localization. They developed a simple and elegant technique which corrected for passive diffusion of radiolabeled protein in the extracellular space of tumors and demonstrated that tumor localization is secondary to antigen-specific binding. By injecting ^{131}I-labeled rabbit polyclonal anti-Wagners osteogenic sarcoma antibodies and a ^{125}I-labeled rabbit non-immune sera into rats bearing Wagners osteogenic sarcoma, preferential tumor uptake of the specific antibody was documented. Others soon corroborated these findings in animal models.[20,21]

As discussed in Chapter 7, efficient and specific delivery of radiolabeled antibody in tumor bearing animals models has been observed. The development of athymic strains of mice that will grow heterotransplants of human tumor has provided a particularly useful tumor model.[22] These results encouraged targeting tumors in humans, initially utilizing polyclonal antibodies, some of which were directed at normal body protein.[23] The monoclonal antibody (MoAb) technology[24] has had a great positive impact on the field in two general ways. First, using the technology as a tool, many tumor-associated antigens have been discovered which have been exploited for tumor targeting. Second, it has permitted production of unlimited amounts of well-characterized antibodies with little variation between lots.

III. IMAGING STUDIES

A. Carcinoembryonic Antigens

In 1965 Gold and Freeman described carcinoembryonic antigen (CEA) indicating that it was a tumor marker for gastrointestinal (GI) malignancies.[25] While subsequent studies have shown that CEA is not specific for cancer,[26,27] the clinical utility of serial serum CEA measurements for monitoring patients with gastrointestinal malignancies[28,29,30] has been documented. Because of the high incidence of expression and elevated concentration in most GI tumors, CEA has been one of the most frequently targeted antigens for radioimmunoscintigraphy.[10,31-44]

Goldenberg et al. were the first to successfully utilize ^{131}I affinity purified goat polyclonal antibodies against CEA to target a variety of tumors. Utilizing blood pool subtraction techniques, they reported 91% detection rate of CEA containing tumors which included ovarian, cervix, breast, lung, endometrium, and choledocus.[31] In a separate series of patients with colon cancer, they also reported 86 to 91% detection rates.[32] Although several series have been reported with ^{131}I anti-CEA, intercomparison is difficult because of the small number of patients in most series and the differences in antibody preparations utilized which could target one of several epitopes of the CEA antigen. Several other series have reported good tumor detection utilizing anti-CEA of polyclonal,[41] rat MoAb[37] or murine MoAb[33] origin. Unfortunately other investigators using polyclonal antibodies against CEA have not been able to duplicate these results. Mach et al. utilized ^{131}I anti-CEA antibodies in 25 patients with tumors of various origins including colon, breast, pancreas, ovarian, uterus, and stomach.[10] Utilizing blood pool subtracted scans, 11 of 27 patients had detectable disease while eight patients had questionable concentration in tumor which could not be recognized prospectively leading them to conclude that "this discrepancy, in results with Goldenberg's, could be due to difference in photoscanning technique or differences in interpretation of the results".

Other investigators using polyclonal anti-CEA of horse,[35] sheep[34] or baboon origin[44] observed limited tumor detection in patients with gastrointestinal and nongastrointestinal (CEA-containing) malignancies. Studies with ^{131}I murine MoAb anti-CEA demonstrated unequivocal uptake in less than 50% of patients studied with conventional gamma camera and blood pool subtraction techniques while the same MoAb resulted in 94% sensitivity for tumor detection when utilizing SPECT technology,[36] indicating the importance of technical factors unrelated to the MoAb.

The high levels of circulating antigen which intuitively, and based on animal studies,[45,46] were expected to have an adverse effect on tumor imaging do not appear to completely neutralize the injected antibody and its ability to localize in tumor sites.[31,32]

In summary, the sensitivity for tumor detection with ^{131}I labeled anti-CEA antibodies has been inconsistent. Even in those series with good lesion detection, the tumor-to-nontumor ratios have been suboptimal for routine clinical application although application of SPECT and more suitable isotopes warrant further investigation.

B. Colon Cancer

Much of the initial RIS of colon cancer (Table 2) was performed with radio-labeled anti-CEA antibodies. More recently several non-CEA tumor associated antigens expressed in colon cancer cells and other malignancies have been described and targeted with radiolabeled antibodies. The antibody 17-1A which recognizes a noncirculating cell surface antigen associated with human colon carcinoma has been studied extensively in vitro,[47] as part of a serotherapy trial[48] and in RIS trials.[13,49,50] Three different groups have studied over 130 patients with the IgG or $F(ab')_2$ with similar results. The sensitivity of lesion detection ranged from 51% to 69%. Mach et al. also studied 20 patients with noncolon carcinoma tumors (who did not express the antigen) with no localization by gamma scintigraphy indicating the specificity of targeting.[49] It was very encouraging that tumor detection was observed without the need for blood pool subtraction. In addition to imaging with ^{131}I-labeled 17-1A, Chatal et al.[50] utilized MoAb 19-9 which recognizes a monoganglioside that is shed into

Table 1
ANTI-CEA

Antibody	Dose (mg)	Isotope	Patients	Positive patients	Positive lesions	Ref.
Goat Anti-CEA IgG	<0.4	^{131}I 0.6—1.6 mCi	18 Various carcinomas	15 of 16	10 of 11 Primary 24 of 29 Metastases	31
Goat Anti-CEA IgG and $F(ab')_2$	1	^{131}I 1 mCi	27 Total 25 GI 2 Others	11 of 27	12 of 30	10
Goat Anti-CEA IgG	2—3 μg/kg	^{131}I 2 mCi	51 GI	41 of 43	49 of 53	32
Anti-CEA Goat and murine MoAb $F(ab')_2$	0.3	1—1.5 mCi	13 (Polyclonal) 26 Colon (MoAb) 2 Pancreas (MoAb)	5 of 13 (Poly) 14 of 28 (MoAb)	n/a	33
Sheep Anti-CEA IgG	0.1—02	^{131}I 0.3—1 mCi	13 GI	10 of 13	12 of 15	34
Horse Anti-CEA IgG	0.1	^{131}I 1 mCi	6 Colon and others	3 of 6	n/a	35
Murine MoAb Anti-CEA	0.3	^{131}I 1.5 mCi	5 Medullary thyroid 11GI	n/a	9 of 21 Rectilinear 16 of 17 SPECT	36
Rat MoAb YPC2/12.1	1	^{131}I 1 mCi	16 Colon 11 Others	13 of 16	n/a	37
Goat Anti-CEA	0.4—0.6	^{131}I < 2 mCi	3 Colon 2 Others	3 of 5	n/a	38
Goat Anti-CEA With liposome Entrapped horse Anti-goat	0.1	^{131}I 0.8—1.7 mCi	4 Colon 1 Appendix	4 of 5	n/a	39
Goat	0.3	^{131}I	5 Colon	5 of 7	7 of 9	40

Anti-CEA Sheep Anti-CEA	<1	0.5—1 mCi ^{131}I 0.5—1.8 mCi ^{111}In <1.8 mCi	2 Breast 8 Colon 3 Others 5 Dual studies (^{131}I and ^{111}In)	n/a	28 of 31 (^{131}I) Dual Studies 13 of 15 (^{111}In) 8 of 15 (^{131}I)	41
Sheep Anti-CEA	0.13	^{131}I 0.4—0.65 mCi	5 Head and neck	3 of 4	6 of 7	42
Murine MoAb Anti-CEA	3—6	^{111}In <5 mCi	5 Colon	0 of 5	none	43
Goat and Baboon anti-CEA	0.1—0.3	^{131}I 1—2 mCi	20 Breast 5 Medullary thyroid 2 Colon	3 of 20 0 of 5 1 of 2	n/a	44

Table 2
COLON CANCER

Antibody	Dose (mg)	Isotope	Number of patients	Positive patients	Positive lesions	Ref.
Murine MoAb 17-1A (IgG and F[ab']$_2$)	0.2—0.5	^{131}I <2 mCi	52 Colon	28 of 52 Overall 17 of 35 (IgG) 11 of 17 (F[ab']$_2$)	34 of 63 (overall) 51% (IgG) 61% (F[ab']$_2$)	49
Murine MoAb 17-1A	0.3—1.5	^{131}I 0.8—3 mCi	46 Colon 24 Others	n/a	27 of 46 (overall)	50
19-9			40 (17-1A, IgG) 12 (17-1A,F[ab']$_2$) 2 (19-9, IgG) 24 (19-9, F[ab']$_2$) 12 (19-9 Plus 17-1A or anti-CEA)		21 of 35 (17-1A, IgG) 6 of 11 (17-1A, F[ab']) 1 of 2 (19-9, IgG) 18 of 27 (19-9, F[ab']) 10 of 13 (Combination)	
Murine MoAb 17-1A (F[ab']$_2$)	0.15—0.4	^{131}I 0.7—1.4 mCi	8 Colon	7 of 8	22 of 32	13
Murine MoAb 791T/36 IgG	0.2	^{131}I 2 mCi	11 Colon	10 of 11	n/a	54
Murine MoAb 19-9 F(ab')$_2$	1	^{111}In 1—2 mCi	8 Colon 6 Others	n/a	8 of 12	62
Murine MoAb B72.3 IgG1	0.27—1.19	^{131}I 1.3—9 mCi	19 Colon	10 of 19	n/a	60

the circulation and present on colon carcinoma.[51] The sensitivity for tumor detection was slightly higher than that of 17-1A with 66% of the lesions detected. On immunohistochemical evaluation of tumor biopsies, they found significant antigen heterogeneity. This suggested the use of cocktails of 17-1A and 19-9, which permitted the localization of 10 of 13 tumor metastases. While the numbers are small and of questionable statistical significance, the use of cocktails is appealing on theoretical grounds and warrants further investigation.

Two other antibodies which have been used to target colon cancer, 791T/36[52] and B72.3,[53] were originally developed against osteogenic sarcoma and breast cancer, respectively. Further testing has shown that both antibodies recognize a variety of tumors including colon and ovarian cancer. The ability to target a host of different tumors is very helpful. Farrands et al. reported localization in 10 of 11 patients with colon cancer utilizing ^{131}I-labeled 791T/36.[54] In addition, they have reported successful imaging of osteosarcoma,[55] ovarian carcinoma,[56] and other tumors.[57] Blood pool subtraction was necessary and resulted in poor quality images. This antibody has the disadvantage that it cross reacts with normal peripheral blood elements.[58]

Utilizing ^{131}I-labeled B72.3 MoAb, we have targeted a novel high molecular weight antigen termed TAG-72 (tumor associated glycoprotein) with characteristics of a mucin.[53] Extensive studies by Colcher et al.[59] have shown that this is a carcinoma-associated antigen present in 85% of colon carcinoma, 50% of breast cancer, and 95% of ovarian carcinomas. We have studied 19 patients with colon cancer and have localized disease in 10 of these patients without blood pool subtraction techniques.[60] The antibody has no significant cross reactivity with normal tissues. Serial plasma measurements show 50% of the antibody clearing in the first 24 hr and a whole body half time of approximately 3.5 days. Because of the prolonged circulation and whole body retention, optimal images are obtained after 72 hr (Figure 1). The specificity of targeting has been documented by well counting of surgical specimens from patients receiving both ^{131}I-labeled B72.3 and ^{125}I-labeled nonspecific isotype-matched control. The limited sensitivity for detection is likely to be secondary to several factors including those related to delivery, accessibility of antigen, and dehalogenation (up to 20% days). Because of the very high tumor-to-nontumor ratios observed,[61] we plan further studies with more favorable isotopes and labeling methods as well as with fragments of B72.3.

C. Melanoma

We have had a large experience in RIS of melanoma (Table 3). Although several groups have utilized different MoAb for RIS, two melanoma-associated antigens have been the main targets. The best characterized antigen is p97, a 97,000 mol wt cell surface glycoprotein that is present in concentrations of up to 400,000 molecules per cell.[63,64] The second antigen that has been targeted is a high molecular weight melanoma-associated antigen (HMWA), which is a proteoglycan on the cell surface, with a molecular weight of 250,000 and 400,000.[65] Both antigens are expressed abundantly in the majority of melanoma tumors and do not modulate. Several MoAb have been developed against various of the epitopes on these antigens.

Utilizing 96.5 or 8.2 IgG (anti-p97) in patients with metastatic melanoma, Larson et al. demonstrated antigen specific uptake with 88% of metastatic lesions detected in patients with advanced disease.[66] The two major problems identified in this study were the prolonged MoAb circulation in the blood pool, with reduced target-to-non-target ratios (Figure 2), and the rapid development of human anti-mouse antibodies after a single injection.

In an attempt to improve the targeting and imaging as well as to minimize the immune response, we investigated the use of Fab fragments of anti-p97 antibodies.[11] We reported improved imaging using the Fab fragments with better contrast than seen previously with IgG (Figure 3) and without the need for blood pool subtraction. Nevertheless only 20 of 33 patients had positive scans. In a second series of ten patients, we were able to detect all

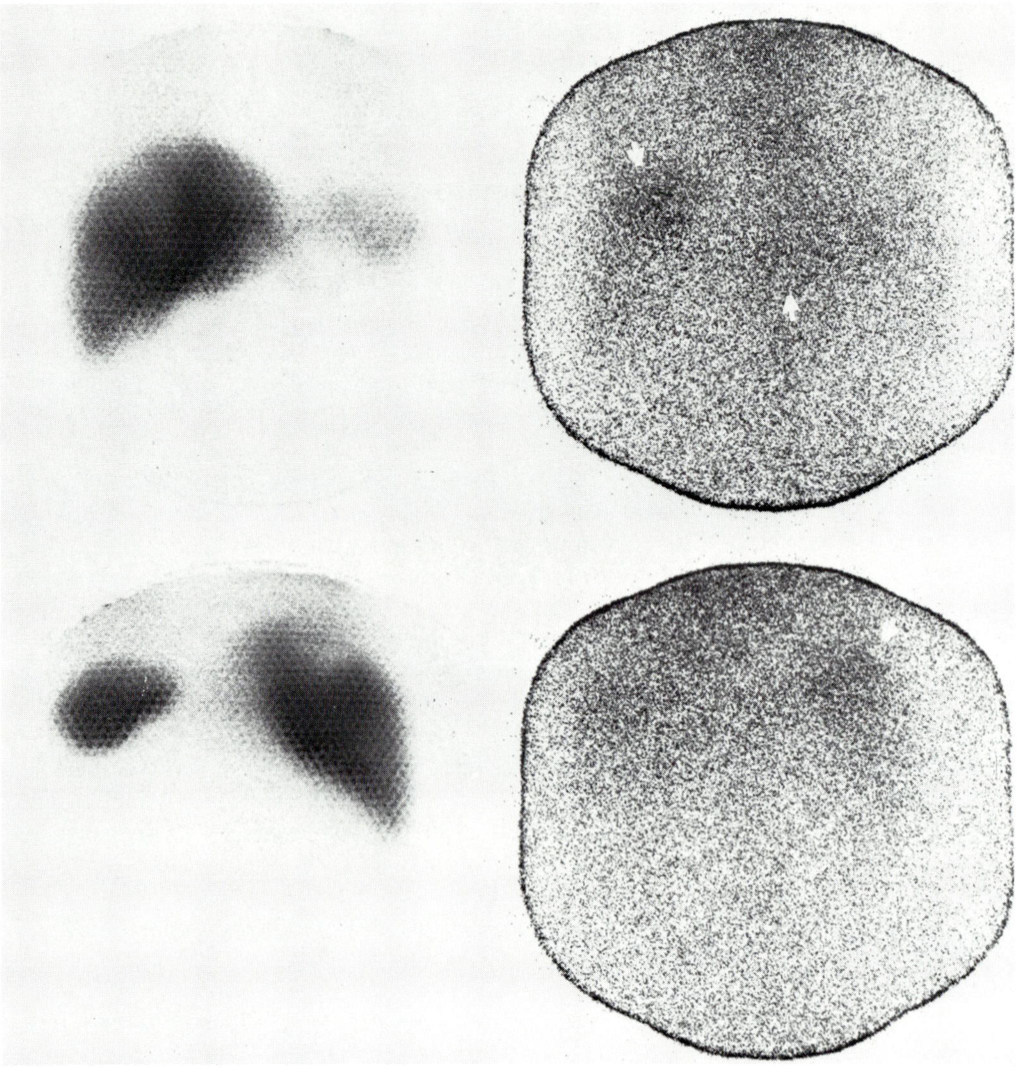

FIGURE 1. Imaging with ^{131}I B72.3. At 6 days postinjection, there is localization in upper portion of right lobe of liver, left lobe of liver (arrows) in anterior projection (right upper panel), and posterior projection (right lower panel). Left hand panel shows corresponding ^{99}mTc-sulfur colloid liver image, anterior (upper), and posterior (lower). Filling defect in right upper lobe is best seen in posterior view. Relatively thin and diffuse metastasis in left lobe of liver is not well seen in anterior ^{99m}Tc-sulfur colloid image. (From Larson, S. M., Radiolabeled monoclonal anti-tumor antibodies in diagnosis and therapy, *J. Nucl. Med.*, 26, 538-545, 1985. With permission from The Society of Nuclear Medicine.)

eight lesions present which were larger than 1.5 cm (Figure 4) utilizing Fab 48.7.[67] Targeting using Fab resulted in more favorable kinetics with earlier localization in tumor and faster whole body clearance; this was responsible for the improved contrast. The fast kinetics resulted in more favorable dosimetry[11] which is being exploited in a phase 1 therapy trial which is currently underway.[68] Fab 96.5 was labeled at high specific activities (up to 300 mCi per 100 mg) with good retention of immunoreactivity[69] and tumor targeting (Figure 5).

Other groups have targeted the p97 antigen with ^{111}In-labeled 96.5 IgG (anti-p97) antibody and were able to detect 50% of metastatic lesions overall and 81 to 83% at optimal dose levels.[70-72] These dose escalation studies documented dose dependent alterations in biodis-

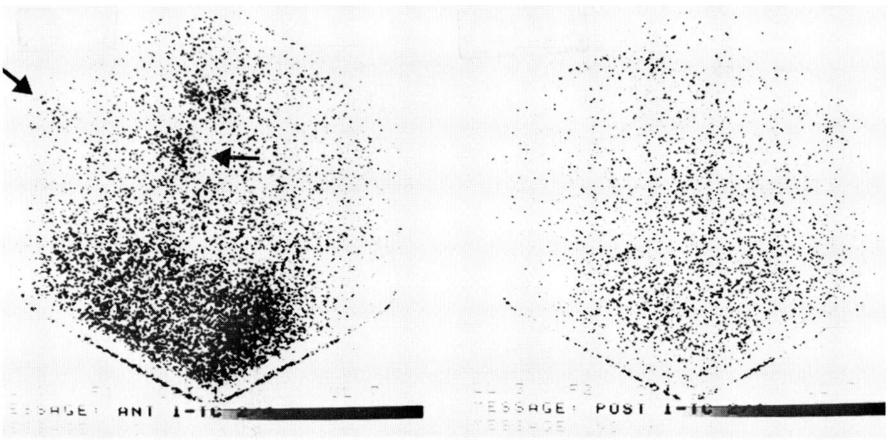

FIGURE 2. MM, patient with melanoma metastatic to right pulmonary hilum, s.c. tissue over back, and border of left heart. Blood pool subtraction images of the anterior (left) and posterior (right) chest are seen. There is focal uptake at right hilum, and some activity suggestive of metastases to right axilla are observed (arrows). (From Larson, S. M., Radiolabeled monoclonal anti-tumor antibodies in diagnosis and therapy, *J. Nucl. Med.*, 26, 538-545, 1985. With permission from The Society of Nuclear Medicine.)

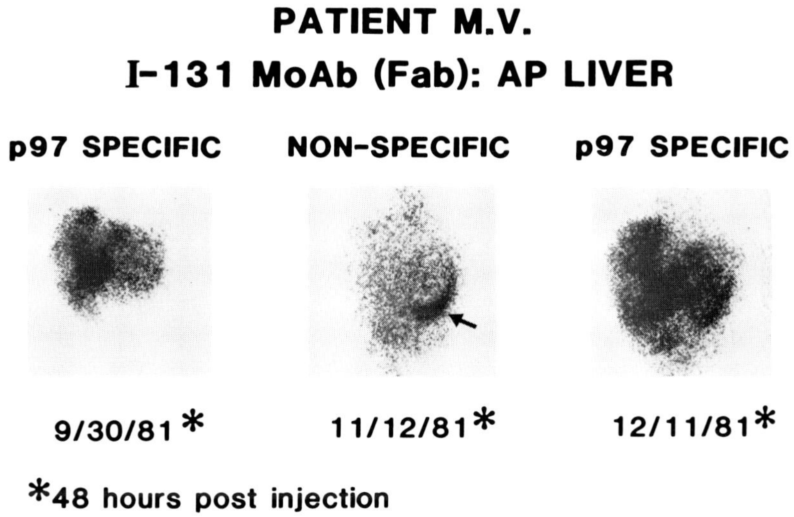

FIGURE 3. Gamma camera images from M. V., a patient with metastatic melanoma to liver. 4 mCi of ^{131}I-(anti-p97) Fab (monoclonal antibody) (8.2; 0.8 mg, cell binding assay (CBA) = 53%) was injected intravenously on September 30, 1981. Uptake in the periphery of a large intrahepatic tumor mass was observed. A control ^{131}I-Fab preparation (nonspecific, Fab 1.4; 1.32 mg, CBA = 1%) was injected 2 weeks later on November 12, 1981. No uptake was observed in tumor. A repeat ^{131}I-(anti-p97) Fab injection (8.2; 0.76 mg, CBA = 69%) was given 1 month after the nonspecific study (December 11, 1981). Tumor localization was again seen. Uptake in stomach and intestine (arrow) was seen on November 12, 1981, and December 11, 1981, and represents ^{131}I concentrating in these organs. (Reproduced from *The Journal of Clinical Investigation,* 1983, 72, 2101-2114, by copyright permission of the American Society for Clinical Investigation.)

Table 3
MELANOMA

Antibody	Dose (mg)	Isotope	Number of patients	Positive patients	Positive lesions	Ref.
Murine MoAb 96.5 or 8.2 (IgG)	1	^{131}I 1—2.5 mCi	6 Melanoma	6 of 6	22 of 25	66
Murine MoAb Fab 96.5 or 8.2	1—20	^{131}I <10 mCi	33 Melanoma	20 of 33	n/a	1
Murine MoAb Fab 48.7	1—10	^{131}I 2—10 mCi	10 Melanoma	8 of 10	17 of 23	67
Murine MoAb 9.2.27 IgG2a	1—50	^{111}In 5 mCi	9 Melanoma	2 of 5 (1 mg) 4 of 4 (50 mg)	2 of 8 (1 mg) 19 of 22 (50 mg)	73
Murine MoAb 96.5 (anti-p97) IgG2a	1—20	^{111}In 5 mCi	21 Melanoma	21 of 21	48 of 79 (Overall) 3 of 10 (1 mg) 19 of 32 (3 mg) 11 of 19 (5 mg) 5 of 16 (10 mg) 10 of 12 (20 mg)	70
Murine MoAb 96.5 (anti-p97) IgG2a	0.5—20	^{111}In 2.5—5 mCi	31 Melanoma	18 of 31	50 of 100 (Overall) 0 of 1 (.5 mg) 2 of 23 (1 mg) 5 of 10 (2 mg) 4 of 10 (5 mg) 9 of 12 (10 mg) 4 of 13 (20 mg, 2.5 mCi) 25 of 31 (20 mg, 5 mCi)	71
Murine MoAb 228.25S anti-HMWA IgG2a & F(ab′$_2$)	0.014—0.71	^{131}I 0.7—1.4 mCi	4 (IgG) Melanoma 4 (F[ab′]$_2$)	1 of 4 (IgG) 3 of 4 (F[ab]$_2$)	1 of 6 (IgG) 10 of 13 (F[ab′]$_2$)	74

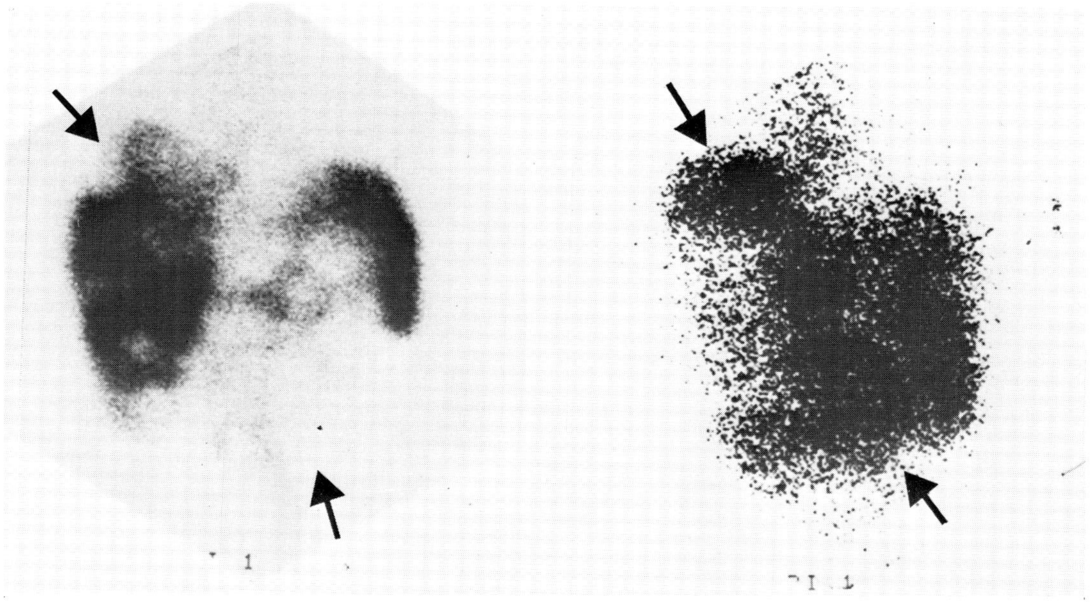

FIGURE 4. Localization of ^{131}I-(anti-chondroitin sulfate proteoglycan)-Fab in malignant melanoma metastatic to the liver. In left panel, a (^{99m}Tc) sulfur colloid liver spleen scan is shown (anterior projection). Dark area shows where functioning hepatic parenchyma is present. There are many space-occupying lesions throughout liver, and left lobe (arrow), is virtually replaced by tumor. In right panel, there is avid localization in invading tumor, in same location (arrow), after i.v. injection of ^{131}I-Fab (10 mCi, 10 mg). (From Larson, S. M., Carrasquillo, J. A., McGuffin, R. W., et al., Use of I-131 labeled, murine Fab against a high molecular weight antigen of human melanoma: preliminary experience, *Radiology*, 155, 487—492, 1985. With permission.)

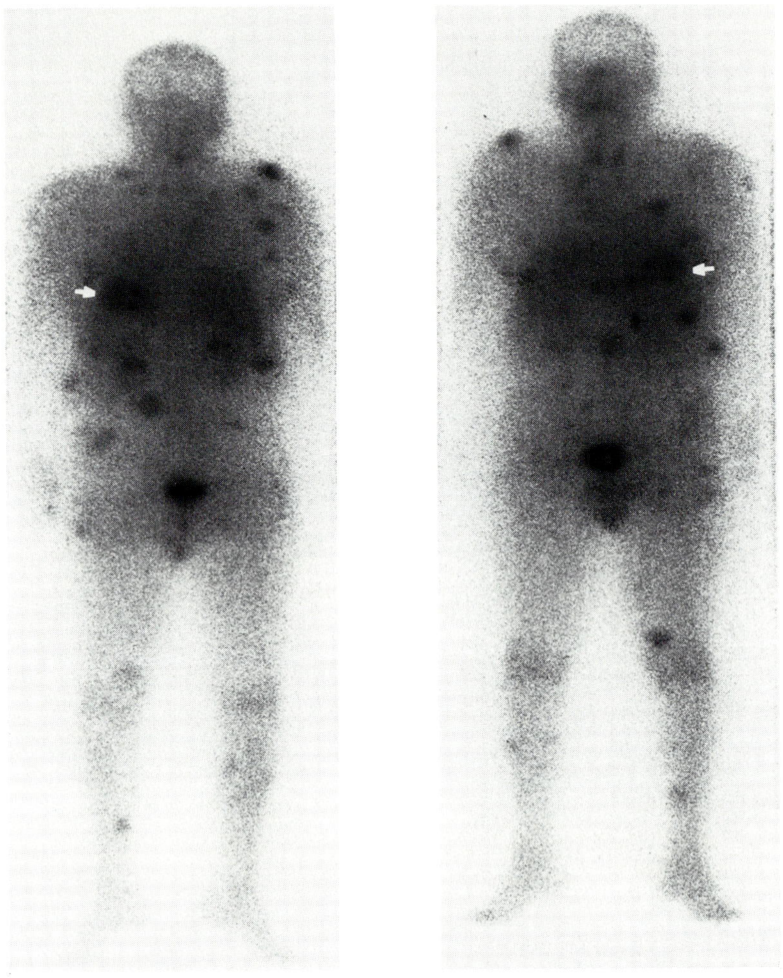

FIGURE 5. Localization of p97 specific Fab fragments (^{131}I MoAb), in multiple s.c. metastases from malignant melanoma, 48 hr after injection of 50 mg and 100 mCi of ^{131}I MoAb. In left panel, posterior projection, and right panel, anterior projection, of whole-body image, is shown. There is diffuse body background of radioactivity throughout extracellular space and also in liver. Some iodide is concentrated in thyroid, stomach (left upper quadrant, arrow), and bladder. Multiple subcutaneous (s.c.) deposits of radiolabeled antibody are seen throughout s.c. tissues, in masses that varied from 2 to 4 cm in diameter. Pattern of uptake was reproducibly seen on three other occasions, one with diagnostic and two other therapy doses. (From Larson, S. M., Radiolabeled monoclonal anti-tumor antibodies in diagnosis and therapy, *J. Nucl. Med.*, 26, 538-545, 1985. With permission from the Society of Nuclear Medicine.)

tribution and improved targeting at higher doses. A comparison of ^{111}In-labeled 96.5 images with images obtained with ^{131}I-labeled 96.5 IgG by our group shows superior contrast between tumor and nontumor with more easily evaluable images using ^{111}In as the label. Good targeting was also obtained utilizing ^{111}In-labeled 9.2.27 MoAb directed at the HMWA of melanoma. At the optimum dose, all four patients studied had positive images with 19 of 22 sites being localized on scan.[73] As with ^{111}In-labeled 96.5, dose-dependent alterations in biodistribution with improved images at higher doses (50 mg) were observed. Burraggi et al.,[74] targeting the same antigen with a different MoAb, ^{131}I-labeled 225.28S, were able to localize 10 of 18 lesions. This lower sensitivity was perhaps related to the relatively small dose of antibody utilized and to the use of ^{131}I as the radiolabel.

Immunohistologic studies with unlabeled antibody 9.2.27 using a modified PAP assay[75] showed that the localization of MoAb at lower doses was limited to the perimeter of the tumor but with doses above 250 mg, there was more uniform staining throughout the tumor.

Saturation of tumor antigen sites was not obtained at these dose levels. These studies with radiolabeled and unlabeled antibody show dose dependent alteration in the biodistribution with improved targeting at the higher doses. Many of these changes could be due to cross reactivity of the radiolabeled antibody with liver, spleen, and bone marrow, with saturation at higher doses. Whether this will hold true with other antibodies is not clear, but the effect dose escalation warrants further systematic investigation with other antibodies.

D. Human Chorionic Gonadotropin (HCG)

HCG (Table 4) is an extensively studied tumor marker[76] which has been associated most notably with trophoblastic or germ cell tumors, but can also be synthesized by other tumors without significant shedding into plasma.[77] Goldenberg et al. studied five patients with ^{131}I-labeled goat polyclonal anti-HCG and was able to detect disease in the majority of patients imaged and in all of those with high circulating levels of HCG.[78] As with other work by this group, blood pool subtraction was necessary for image interpretation. Morrison et al. utilized ^{99m}Tc labeled anti-HCG $F(ab')_2$ to localize disease in 13 of 14 patients studied, although only 54 to 64% of the lesions were visualized.[79] The short life of ^{99m}Tc (6 hr) did not appear to be a major problem when the $F(ab')_2$ fragment was utilized. The latter strategy lends itself to a kit labeling system, but the issue of stability of the label has not been exhaustively investigated.

As with CEA, this antigen is secreted into the plasma. Even though patients exhibited high circulating levels of antigen, tumor targeting was still observed.

E. Alpha-Fetoprotein

Alpha-fetoprotein (Table 5) is an oncofetal antigen frequently associated with hepatoma and other GI malignancies as well as germ cell tumors.[81] This antigen has been used successfully to monitor the serum of patients with a variety of malignancies. Goldenberg et al. utilized goat anti-AFP successfully in a variety of AFP producing tumors.[82] All sites of disease in patients with hepatocellular carcinoma and metastatic germ cell tumor of the testis were detected. As with other tumors with circulating antigen, high antigen levels of up to 15,000 ng/mℓ did not prevent tumor localization.

Hasall et al. were also successful in localizing the majority of AFP producing tumors.[83] In patients with low circulating levels of AFP, no tumor localization was observed after successful treatment indicating the specificity of targeting. As with many other antigen-antibody systems, variable targeting of the same antigen, in apparently similar patient populations, has been reported. For example, Ishii et al. localized disease in 47% of patients with no improvement with MoAb (22% positive images).[35]

F. Ovarian Carcinoma

Malignant ovarian tumors (Table 6) are among the most frequent problems in gynecological oncology, with 60% of epithelial cancer patients with advanced disease.[84] Several groups have targeted ovarian carcinoma of various histology.

Both Epenetos and Pateisky et al., utilizing ^{123}I-labeled antibodies against a component of the human milk fat globule membrane (HMFG1 and/or HMFG2),[85] were able to target 8 of 10 and 17 of 19 malignant ovarian carcinoma patients, respectively.[86-88] The negative studies were attributed to either technical difficulties or small disease (<1.5 cm). The tumors were seen as early as 3 min to 18 hr following antibody injection without the need for

Table 4
HUMAN CHORIONIC GONADOTROPIN (HCG)

Antibody	Dose (mg)	Isotope	Number of patients	Positive patients	Positive lesions	Ref.
Goat Anti-HCG	2—3 μg/kg	^{131}I 1—2.5 mCi	13 Testis 4 Hydatiform 8 Others	10 of 10 (Testis) Hydatiform mole 4 of 4	14 of 14 (Testis)	78
Murine MoAb Anti-HCG $F(ab')_2$	0.15	^{99m}Tc	14 Various carcinomas	13 of 14	18 of 28	79
Goat Anti-HCG IgG	1.0	^{131}I 1.2—1.8 mCi	5 Throphoblastic and germ cell	3 of 5	5 of 10	80

Table 5
ALPHA-FETOPROTEIN

Antibody	Dose (mg)	Isotope	Number of patients	Positive patients	Positive lesions	Ref.
Goat Anti-AFP IgG	0.1—0.6	^{131}I 1—4.4 mCi	12 Various tumors	9 of 12 (Overall) 4 of 4 (AFP)	11 of 11 (AFP producing)	82
Horse Anti-AFP IgG	0.1	^{131}I 1 mCi	15 Hepatoma (polyclonal) 9 Hepatoma (MoAb)	7 of 15		35
Murine MoAb Anti-AFP IgG				2 of 9		
Sheep Anti-AFP IgG	0.6	^{131}I 0.6 mCi	12 (Germ cell tumors)	10 of 12 8 of 8 (Increased AFP in serum)	12 of 15	83

Table 6
OVARIAN CARCINOMA

Antibody	Dose (mg)	Isotope	Number of patients	Positive patients	Positive lesions	Ref.
Murine MoAb	0.2	^{131}I	11 Ovarian	11 of 11	n/a	56
791T/36		<2 mCi	1 Benign cyst			
Murine MoAb	0.4	^{123}I	10 Ovarian	8 of 10	n/a	86
HMFG1 and HMFG2		0.5—2 mCi				
IgG1						
Murine MoAb	0.001—2	^{123}I	12 Ovarian	15 of 20 (All)	24 of 32 (Overall)	87
HMFG1 and HMFG2		<2 mCi	6 Breast			
IgG1			2 Colon	11 of 12 (Ovarian)		
Murine MoAb	0.4	^{123}I	19 Ovarian	18 of 20	17 of 19	88
HMFG2		0.5—2.2 mCi	4 Others			
IgG						
Murine MoAb	<1	^{111}In	6 Ovarians	10 of 11	13 of 14	89
H17E2(anti-PLAP)	IgG	1 mCi	8 Testis			
			1 Cervical			
Murine MoAb	<1	^{123}I	13 Ovarian	11 of 13	n/a	90
NDOG(anti-PLAP)		<2.2 mCi	2 Others			
IgG2b						

background subtraction. These improved images and detection rates are probably related to the quality of the MoAb as well as the excellent imaging characteristics of ^{123}I. Davies et al. targeted placental alkaline phosphatase (PLAP) with ^{123}I-labeled NDOG2 MoAb and were able to localize tumors in 10 of 13 patients with proven metastatic disease, in most cases, without the need for blood pool subtraction.[90] In many instances, the scan was the only test documenting metastases, leading the authors to suggest a clinical utility for the techinque.

G. Lymphoma

The majority of work performed to date has involved the targeting of solid tumors, both those described above and other solid tumors.[91-94] Most of the antigens on these tumors are on the cell surface or are secreted and do not modulate. Modulation is a phenomenon that can occur when an antibody comes in contact with the antigen on the cell surface; it causes a redistribution of the antigen on the cell surface and in the case of some antigens, the antigen-antibody complex is internalized.[95,96] This can have significant implications on tumor imaging since it can decrease the number of antigens available for targeting and, in addition, the processing of the labeled antibody once internalized can result in loss of the radiolabel from the tumor.

We have targeted cutaneous T-cell lymphoma and chronic lymphocytic leukemia (CLL) with ^{111}In-labeled T101. T101 is a murine IgG2a MoAb that recognizes a pan T-cell antigen (T65) present in normal T-lymphocytes and cutaneous T-cell lymphoma (CTCL) and also paradoxically expressed on CLL.[97,98] In contrast to other solid tumors, the targeting of CTCL and CLL is more favorable since the malignant cells are often found in the circulation and on the spleen and marrow which renders them readily accessible to circulating antibody. These malignant cells once targeted can modulate and internalize the radiolabeled MoAb[95] and the available evidence suggests that these cells will then carry the radioactivity to the involved sites. Utilizing ^{111}In-labeled T101, Bunn et al. have reported excellent targeting in CTCL.[99] Other studies reported by our group have shown excellent targeting of nodal as well as cutaneous sites (erythroderma and tumor) of CTCL involvement[100] (Figure 6). Many of the sites identified were previously not suspected to be involved. Biopsy specimens have documented lymphomatous involvement in positive sites with concentrations of ^{111}In in nodes consistently 10 to 100 times higher than those previously reported for solid tumor uptake following i.v. administration.

In contrast, ^{131}I-labeled T101 has given suboptimal images (submitted for publication).[121] Although it appears to be handled similarly to ^{111}In-labeled T101 initially, it is likely that once the MoAb is internalized, the ^{131}I is separated from the MoAb and then the ^{131}I is removed from the cell and excreted.[95] This appears to contrast with the ^{111}In label which probably binds to intracellular proteins after separation[101] from the T101.

IV. HUMAN ANTI-MURINE ANTIBODY RESPONSE (HAMA)

In utilizing MoAb for imaging as well as for serotherapy trials, the presence or the development of a host anti-murine antiglobulin response has been of great concern because of the potential for allergic reactions as well as alterations in biodistribtion.[66] Although several investigators have detected low levels of human IgG and IgM reactive with MoAb in healthy individuals as well as patients with malignancies who have not previously received murine MoAb, in this setting clinical side effects have rarely been seen.[102] The occurrence of HAMA after antibody administration is relatively high when utilizing whole immunoglobulin with 12 of 37 patients receiving single injections developing HAMA in one series[103] with similar experiences reported for smaller series by other investigators.[104,105] The administration of MoAb after development of HAMA has been associated with alterations in

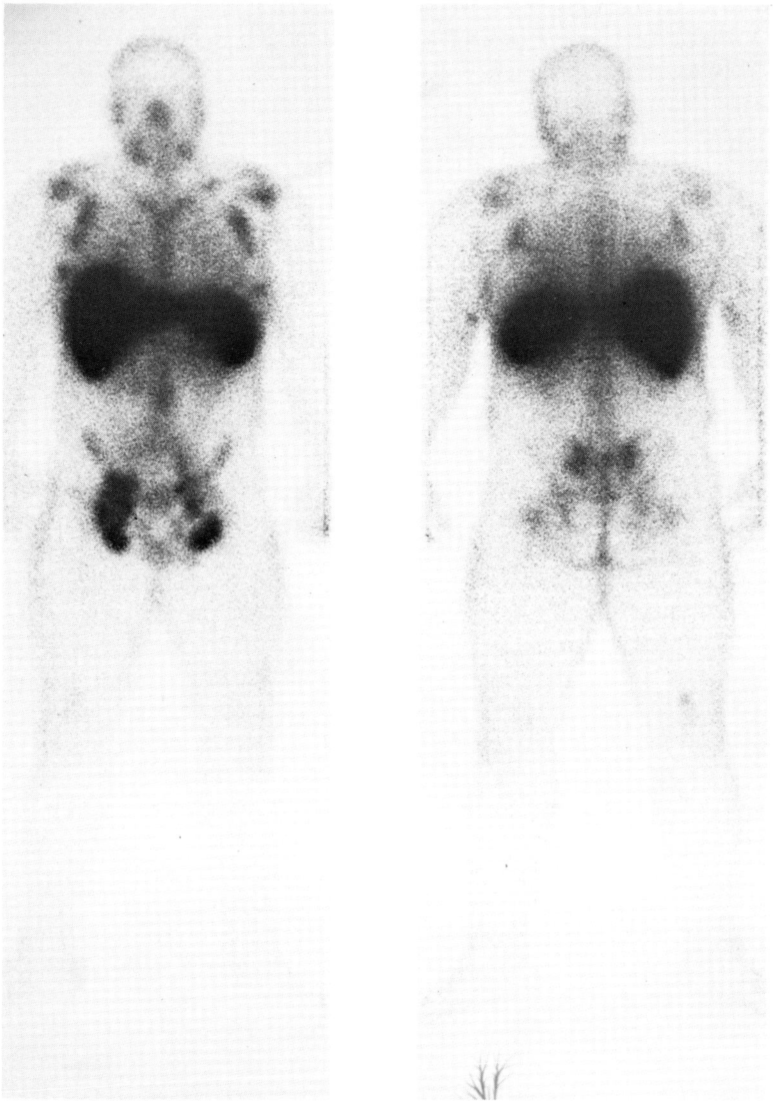

FIGURE 6. Whole body scans 72 hr after i.v. injection of 5 mCi (11 mg) of ^{111}In-T101 monoclonal antibody. The study shows uptake in cervical, axillary, inguinal-femoral, iliac, epitrochlear, and popliteal nodes. Uptake in skin (erythroderma) is also visualized. In addition liver, spleen, and bone marrow uptake is seen. (Reproduced with permission from *Nucl. Med. Biol.*, Vol. 13, Larson, S. M., Carrasquillo, J. A., Reynolds, J. C., Hellstrom, I., Hellstrom, K. E., Mulshine, J. C., and Mayptis, L. E., Therapeutic applications of radiolabelled antibodies; current situation and prospects, copyright 1986, Pergamon Journals Ltd.)

biodistribution and interference with tumor imaging[66,106] and with minor allergic side effects. The development of HAMA has been reduced significantly by utilizing Fab fragments. In contrast with intact IgG (incidence of HAMA of at least 32%), with Fab only 1 of 18 patients receiving single injections became positive, although after multiple injections, the incidence increased sharply.[103] For imaging or for multiple administrations for therapeutic purposes, the development of HAMA is detrimental.

If RIS is to find routine serial use as a screening agent for recurrent disease, approaches to deal with the development of HAMA will be necessary. An exception to the development of HAMA has been patients with CLL who are immunodeficient and cannot develop an immune response.[102] In other patient populations, strategies for dealing with the problem of HAMA must be developed. One can attempt to prevent the production of HAMA via the use of immunosuppressants or by alterations in the immunoglobulin structure. Alternatively, one can attempt to reduce the levels of HAMA once they have formed by either plasmapheresis, affinity columns, or preloading with unlabeled antibody.

V. SPECIFICITY OF UPTAKE

It is known that antibodies may bind to cells via their Fc segment.[107] It has also been shown that tumors have expanded extracellular and extravascular volumes and can accumulate radiolabeled proteins nonspecifically.[108] There are several ways to directly determine the specific and nonspecific deposition of antibodies in tumor. Several groups have compared the ratio of tumor to normal tissue uptake. Although this is of some utility, the ratios may vary significantly depending upon which normal tissues are obtained, due in part to the fact that tissues can have different partition coefficients for molecules of various size. Most groups have reported tumor to normal tissue ratios of less than nine to one;[31,33,54,88,109] in our experience, ^{131}I-labeled B72.3 has given some of the highest ratios reported to date.[61] A more representative measure of the specificity of targeting is obtained by coinjections of specific and nonspecific antibody labeled with different isotopes (^{131}I and ^{125}I) that can be discriminated in a gamma counter, permitting comparison of their ratios of uptake on biopsied tumor and normal tissue. Table 7 shows some of the ratios reported to date. These data clearly indicate the specificity of targeting with radiolabeled antibodies. As shown in Table 8, the absolute amounts deposited in the tumor unfortunately are relatively small. The tumor uptake seen with ^{111}In-labeled T101 (0.01 to 0.03% of the injected dose per gram) has been among the highest consistently seen with this technique. A comparison with corresponding work in animal models shows that significantly lower uptake and smaller specificity ratios are obtained in patients (Table 8). In the case of most xenografted tumors, the potential to target radiolabeled MoAb is at its best — there is no cross-reacting antigen, it is a murine antibody in a mouse, the mouse has a small body relative to the size of the tumor, and there are high levels of antigen expression of the tumor.

Ways to improve tumor uptake in patients are under investigation and include targeting malignancies with more accessible antigens (leukemias and selected lymphomas), delivery via alternate routes — intralymphatic, subcutaneous, intraperitoneal, or intraarterial; therapeutic interventions that could improve capillary permeability and tumor blood flow; the use of cocktails; the effect of larger doses of antibody and utilizing antibody fragments.

VI. SUBTRACTION TECHNIQUES

A common problem with many of the studies performed to date has been the low concentration of radiolabeled antibodies in tumor tissue. In addition, relatively low tumor to non-tumor uptake ratios (Table 7) result in poor quality images which are difficult to interpret. This has necessitated the use of methods to enhance tumor-to-nontumor contrast. The most common image-enhancement method has been the blood pool subtraction technique introduced by Goldenberg[31] and Deland.[113] In this method, Tc-99m labeled human serum albumin, which mimics the "nonspecific" distribution of the radiolabeled antibody, is injected intravenously. Utilizing the ability of the gamma camera to differentiate between ^{131}I and ^{99m}Tc, sequential images of each isotope can be obtained and stored on a computer. The "nonspecific" blood pool distribution can then be subtracted from the ^{131}I-labeled antibody distribution which should result in visualization of antigen-specific binding sites. Unfortunately, there are many technical difficulties encountered with this technique:[114]

Table 7
TUMOR ANTIBODY UPTAKE

Antibody	Percent injected dose gram	Tumor to non-tumor ratio	Specific to nonspecific ratio	Ref.
Goat Anti-CEA IgG		2.5:1		31
Goat anti-CEA IgG	0.002—0.005 Mean 0.003	1.8 to 3.5:1 mean 3.8:1	4 to 5:1	10
Murine MoAb 17-1A IgG2a		3.6 to 6.3:1 mean 4.6:1	2.8 to 7 mean 4.5:1	49
Murine MoAb 791T/36 IgG2b	0.005	1.1 to 5.8:1 mean 2.8:1		54
Murine MoAb 17-1A 19-9 IgG			2.1 to 3.1:1	50
Murine MoAb LICR-LON-M8 IgG1		<11.7:1 mean 6.2:1		109
Murine MoAb IgG, 96.5 (anti-p97)	0.006—0.01	4.1 and 7.4:1	1.8 and 2:1	66
Murine MoAb Fab 96.5 and 8.2 (anti-p97)	mean 0.001	Mean 2.3:1	3.4 to 3.7:1	11
Murine MoAb Fab 48.7 (anti-HMWA)	0.0001	Mean 4.1:1	1.2 to 5.9:1 mean 3.6:1	67
Murine MoAb T101 IgG2a	0.01—0.033			99
Murine MoAb B72.3 anti-TAG 72 IgG1	<0.01	2.1 to 38.1:1		61
Murine MoAb IgG, 96.5	0.002	10:1		70
Murine MoAb 228.25S IgG2a & $F(ab')_2$	IgG2a 0.0007—0.007 mean 0.0037 $F(ab')_2$ 0.0009 and 0.0025	IgG2a 0.25 to 3.6:1 mean 2.3:1 $F(ab')_2$ 1.39 and 3.5:1 mean 2.4:1		74

1. The in vivo biological behavior of the isotopes is different.
2. The attenuation characteristics of the gamma rays from ^{131}I and ^{99m}Tc are different.
3. The subtraction procedure introduces additional statistical fluctations, decreasing the signal to noise ratio.

In short, image artifacts are often introduced.[33,44]

In an effort to eliminate the need for blood pool subtraction by accelerating the clearance of nontumor-bound antibody into the reticuloendothelial system, Begent et al. utilized an ^{131}I-labeled goat anti-CEA (specific) polyclonal antibody followed by an injection of a

Table 8
TUMOR UPTAKE AND SPECIFICITY (HUMAN VS. ANIMAL MODEL)

	Percent injected dose per gram		Specific to Nonspecific		
Antibody	**Human**	**Animal**	**Human**	**Animal**	**Ref.**
Goat Anti-CEA	0.002—0.005	9.1	4 to 5:1	3.4 to 6.8:1	33, 110
Murine MoAb 96.5 IgG	<0.01	8.9			66, 3
Murine MoAb 791T/36 IgG2b	0.005	13			54, 6
Murine MoAb Fab 8.2	0.001	1.5 to 3.5	3.4 to 3.7:1	25:1	11, 111
Fab 96.5	0.001	2	3.4 to 3.71:1	20:1	
Murine MoAb B72.3 IgG1	<0.01	26.8			61, 112

liposomally entrapped second antibody (LESA) directed against the goat anti-CEA.[39] By this technique, they demonstrated enhanced blood pool clearance of ^{131}I goat anti-CEA in four of five patients with improvement in tumor-to-nontumor ratios. Later work by the same group demonstrated that direct administration of the second antibody gave similar results without the need for liposome entrapment.[115]

Unfortunately, all these methods are cumbersome and do not address some of the basic problems causing low tumor-to-nontumor ratios. These are more related to:

1. The antibody — for example, crossreactivity with normal tissue, poor immunoreactivity after labeling, and/or rapid deiodination
2. Delivery at the tumor level because of problems with vascularity, capillary permeability or antigen heterogeneity
3. To limitations imposed by the gamma camera due to its limited spatial resolution[116]

VII. ALTERNATIVE RADIOISOTOPES

Several isotopes that can be used for labeling antibodies for imaging applications are listed in Chapter 6. The choice of radiolabel depends to a large extent on the time required for the antibody or its fragments to equilibrate in tissue and to obtain maximum target to background concentration ratios. Until recently, the radiolabeling of antibodies was limited to iodine isotopes, mainly via the chloramine T[117] and iodogen[118] methods, because of the well-known chemistry of radiohalogenation. Iodine isotopes suffer several limitations and are not ideal for imaging: Iodine-131 has a high energy gamma ray of 364 keV which requires thick lead septa collimation reducing the sensitivity and resolution of the gamma camera. The associated beta radiation and the long half life result in a relatively high radiation absorbed dose to the patient. In addition, dehalogenation occurs in vivo as demonstrated by several groups.[4,11,44] Although ^{123}I has been utilized successfully[86-88,90] with the advantage that its energy characteristics are more suitable (159 keV and no beta radiation), it has the limitation of a short half-life of 13 hr. This is likely to require the associated use of antibody fragments, although some studies with intact IgG have shown tumor targeting as early as 3 min post injection.[87]

Halpern et al. performed comparative studies demonstrating in vivo dehalogenation of radioiodinated antibodies and improved targeting and stability of ^{111}In-labeled MoAb which distributed similarly to endogenously labeled ^{75}Se-methionine MoAb.[4] In addition to a higher concentration of radioactivity in tumor, ^{111}In has more favorable characteristics than ^{131}I for imaging with gamma energies of 173 and 247 keV, which are well suited for the gamma camera, a higher photon abundance and a half-life of 2.83 days. The technical details of ^{111}In labeling methodologies are covered in Chapter 6.

The results of studies comparing ^{111}In and ^{131}In labeled antibodies indicate a greater sensitivity of tumor detection with ^{111}In. Fairweather et al.,[41] in a direct comparison in five patients, demonstrated 13 of 15 lesions with ^{111}In anti-CEA vs. 8 of 15 with ^{131}I. Not only was the ^{111}In more sensitive, but also the lesions were better delineated. In a group of patients with breast metastases, ^{111}In-labeled anti-HMFG was able to localize bone metastases, but for unknown reasons was unsuccessful in localizing soft tissue metastases. In contrast, neither ^{131}In or ^{123}I localized in any site.[109]

The advantage of ^{111}In is related to improved count rates and longer retention by tumors. This is probably related to its properties as a trivalent metal and, thus, its ability to bind to intracellular elements and remain locally deposited,[101] while ^{131}I, when separated from the antibody, will be rapidly excreted.

Although improved images have been obtained with ^{111}In-labeled MoAb, some drawbacks have been observed. Frequently, a high degree of liver uptake is seen.[41,70,71,73] In tumors with a high incidence of metastases to the liver, this precludes adequate evaluation of the liver. The mechanism of liver uptake has not been completely elucidated, but appears to be multifactorial with some antibodies crossreacting with the normal liver (anti-p97) and other causing clearance of tagged cells into the liver (T101). There is some instability of ^{111}In chelates in vivo which may lead to the translocation of ^{111}In to transferrin and other metal binding proteins. Other factors such as liver catabolism and Fc binding may also have a role in the liver concentration of ^{111}In. Another problem has been excretion (or binding) of radioactivity into the gut which may interfere with visualization of abdominal disease. The mechanism of gastrointestinal uptake is unknown.

The ideal isotope for gamma camera imaging is ^{99m}Tc, because its energy not only is optimal for imaging, but also it results in a low radiation absorbed dose to the patient. Technetium chemistry is difficult, however methods for producing stable ^{99m}Tc-labeled antibody conjugates are being developed. The 6 hr half-life of ^{99m}Tc may be a disadvantage when utilizing the whole immunoglobulin since most studies suggest that optimal images are obtained beyond 24 hr post infusion. This may require using ^{99m}Tc in conjunction with antibody fragments which localize faster or delivering the MoAb via alternate routes-intra-lymphatic, s.c., or intracavitary — where targeting occurs very rapidly. Currently, experience using ^{99m}Tc labeled antibodies for imaging is extremely limited and has involved direct labeling,[79] a method which in general has been considered to produce unstable labeled antibodies.[119]

The use of positron emitters as labels for antibodies has received little attention. These isotopes have the potential of permitting quantitation of uptake as well as improved contrast though the use of positron emission tomography. Many of these isotopes are short lived and would be of questionable utility. There are several longer lived nuclides such as zirconium-89 and possibly some arsenic isotopes which could be of clinical utility, but no in vivo data is currently available.

VIII. FRAGMENTS

The vast majority of experience in RIS has been with the use of whole immunoglobulin. As discussed in earlier sections, several problems exist with the use of whole IgG. Many studies have found prolonged plasma and whole body retention of the intact IgG. The relatively large size of the IgG molecule may result in decreased capillary permeability and contribute to the difficulty in delivery through the tumor capillary bed. These factors combine to cause relatively low tumor-to-nontumor uptake ratios. An additional problem with the use of IgG is the high incidence of HAMA which may be reduced by the use of fragments. A limited number of trials have appeared in the literature evaluating the use of fragments. In the case of anti-melanoma antibodies, Larson et al. have utilized Fab fragments successfully and have shown that their kinetics are dramatically different from the IgG, with more rapid plasma and whole body clearance and earlier localization in tumor which resulted in improved tumor to nontumor ratios.[11,67] With the exception of several animal studies, no other significant comparison of the distribution of Fab fragments vs. IgG has been performed. In order to obtain some of the benefit of faster kinetics while maintaining bivalent binding with a resultant higher affinity, several studies utilizing $F(ab')_2$ fragments have been performed.[13,49,50,79] The kinetics of plasma and whole body clearance, as expected, has been intermediate between the IgG and the Fab. The available studies comparing $F(ab')_2$ with IgG[49,50,74] suggest an improvement in imaging with $F(ab')_2$ albeit the difference is not tremendous. Further systematic comparisons of IgG, $F(ab')_2$, and Fab with larger numbers of patients are warranted.

IX. SINGLE PHOTON EMISSION TOMOGRAPHY (SPECT)

In an attempt to improve the sensitivity of lesion detection, several groups have evaluated imaging with SPECT, a technique which offers improved contrast resolution.[120] Berche et al. employed ^{131}I-labeled anti-CEA MoAb in patients with medullary thyroid carcinoma and gastrointestinal cancer; a sensitivity of 44% was obtained with conventional imaging while 94% of the lesions were detected by SPECT with improved concordance between observers.[36] This can be compared to the 50% (14 of 25) detection rate reported by Mach et al.[33] utilizing the same antibody and blood pool subtraction techniques. Several groups have found SPECT imaging helpful in delineating tumor from surrounding vasculature and in evaluating the three-dimensional nature of antibody distribution (Figure 7). Although improved contrast has been obtained, reconstruction artifacts may be seen secondary to low count rates.[33] The experience to date is encouraging and further studies will be required to assess its ultimate role.[36,87] Because of the more rigorous requirements for SPECT imaging, its implementation may require the use of ^{123}I, ^{99m}Tc, or ^{111}In and an approach more directed towards the investigation of areas of high risk for metastases.

X. CONCLUSIONS

The field of RIS has evolved from the initial work targeting antigens with little specificity for tumors to targeting better-characterized tumor-associated antigens. The use of polyclonal antibodies has been largely supplanted by MoAb. MoAb have the advantages that they can be produced in unlimited amounts with little variability between lots, a prerequisite for carrying out large clinical trials. The lack of variability between lots ensures reproducibility and permits intercomparison of data. Although the limited trials that have been performed directly comparing polyclonal and MoAb have not shown dramatic differences in sensitivity of tumor localization, the imaging reported with MoAb has been greatly improved. Most studies with polyclonal antibodies have required blood pool subtraction resulting in poor quality images with questionable abnormalities, while several studies with MoAb have reported good imaging without the need for blood pool subtraction.

While this technique is very promising, many technical problems still persist and will require systematic evaluation before clinical use of RIS becomes widespread. Promising

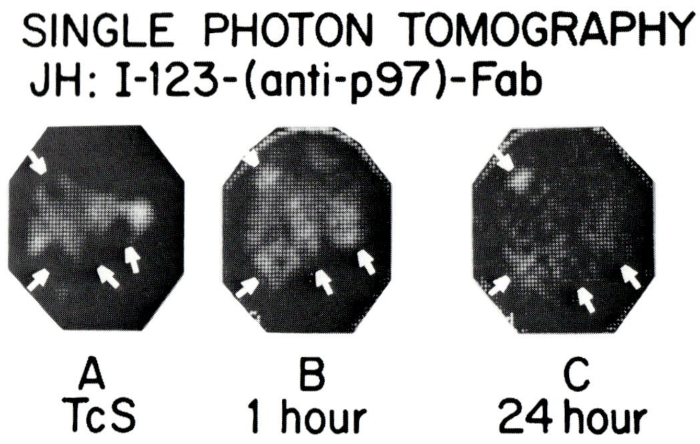

FIGURE 7. A 56-year-old man had biopsy-proved melanoma metastatic to the liver. Panel A is a coronal section through the liver after administration of technetium-99m sulfur colloid. There are several ''cold'' defects corresponding to metastatic deposits (arrows). Panel B is the corresponding coronal section obtained 1 hr after i.v. injection of ^{123}I-(anti-p97) Fab. There is rapid accumulation of the radiolabeled antibody in tumor (arrows). Some radioactivity is seen in the blood contained in the heart (arrowhead) and in the normal liver. By 24 hr after infusion, residual activity is seen in the tumor-bearing areas in the liver (arrows) and the radioactive antibody has been cleared from the blood and normal liver (panel C). This study represents the first successful SPECT study of I-123-labeled antitumor monoclonal antibodies in humans. (From *J.A.M.A*, Feb. 11, 1983, Vol. 249, No. 6, pages 811-812.)

work is being done to overcome the difficulties of decreased sensitivity for lesion detection, immunogenicity, and targeting. Improvements in the future are likely to come as a result of the utilization of better MoAb, cocktails of MoAb, fragments, better isotopes (^{99m}Tc, ^{123}I, and ^{111}In), improved labeling methods, and SPECT.

REFERENCES

1. **DeLand, F. H. and Goldenberg, D. M.,** In vivo cancer diagnosis by radioimmunodetection, in *Radioimmunoimaging and Radioimmunotherapy,* Burchiel, S. W., Rhodes, B. A., Eds., Elsevier Science, New York, 1983, 329.
2. **Colcher, D., Zalutsky, M., Kaplan, W., Kufe, D., Austin, F., and Schlom, J.,** Radiolocalization of human mammary tumors in athymic mice by a monoclonal antibody, *Cancer Res.,* 43, 736, 1983.
3. **Matzku, S., Mahem, J., Georgi, P., and Hellstrom, I.,** Radioimmunolocalization of melanomas with monoclonal antibodies directed against a p97 marker. Model experiments in vitro and in nude mice bearing transplanted human melanomas, Radioactive Isotope, in *Klinik und Forschung,* Vol. 5(1), 1982, 295.
4. **Halpern, S. E., Hagan, P. L., Garver, P. R., Koziol, J. A., Chen, A. W. N., Frincke, J. M., Bartholomew, R. M., Davis, G. S., and Adams, T. H.,** Stability, characterization, and kinetics of ^{111}In-labeled monoclonal antitumor antibodies in normal animals and nude mouse-human tumor models, *Cancer Res.,* 43, 5347, 1983.
5. **Moshakis, V., McIlhinney, R. A. J., Raghavan, D., and Neville, A. M.,** Localization of human tumor xenografts after I.V. administration of radiolabeled monoclonal antibodies, *Br. J. Cancer,* 44, 91, 1981.
6. **Pimm, M. V., Embleton, M. J., Perkins, A. C., Price, M. R., Robins, R. A., Robinson, G. R., and Baldwin, R. W.,** In vivo localization of anti-osteogenic sarcoma 79IT monoclonal antibody in osteogenic sarcoma xenografts, *Int. J. Cancer,* 30, 75, 1982.

7. **Herlyn, D., Powe, J., Alava, A., Mattis, J. A., Herlyn, M., Ernst, C., Vaum, R., and Koprowski, H.,** Radioimmunodetection of human tumor xenografts by monoclonal antibodies, *Cancer Res.,* 43, 2731, 1983.
8. **Epenetos, A. A., Nimmon, C. C., Arklie, J., Elliott, A. T., Hawkins, L. A., Knowles, R. W., Britton, K. E., and Bodmer, W. F.,** Radioimmunodiagnosis of human cancer in an animal model using labeled tumor associated monoclonal antibody, *Br. J. Cancer,* 46, 1, 1982.
9. **Ghose, T., Ferrone, S., Imai, K., Norvell, S. T., Luner, S. J., Martin, R. H., and Blair, A. H.,** Imaging of human melanoma xenografts in nude mice with a radiolabeled monoclonal antibody, *J. Natl. Cancer Inst.,* 69(4), 823, 1982.
10. **Mach, J. P., Carrell, S., Forni, M., Ritschard, J., Donath, A., and Alberto, P.,** Tumor locationization of radiolabeled antibodies against carcinoembryonic antigen in patients with carcinoma, *New Engl. J. Med.,* 5, 303, 1980.
11. **Larson, S. M., Carrasquillo, J. A., Krohn, K. A., Brown, J. P., McGuffin, R. W., Ferens, J. M., Graham, M. M., Hill, L. D., Beaumier, P. L., Hellstrom, K. E., and Hellstrom, I.,** Localization of I-131 labeled p97 specific FAB fragments in human melanoma as a basis for radiotherapy, *J. Clin. Invest.,* 72, 2101, 1983.
12. **Mach, J. P., Chatal, J. F., Lumbroso, J. D., Buchegger, F., Forni, M., Ritchard, J., Berche, C., Douillard, J. Y., Carrel, S., Herlyn, M., Steplewski, Z., and Koprowski, H.,** Tumor localization in patients by radiolabeled monoclonal antibodies against colon carcinoma, *Cancer Res.,* 43, 5593, 1983.
13. **Moldofsky, P. J., Powe, J., Mulhern, C. B., Hammond, N., Sears, H. F., Gatenby, R. A., Steplewski, Z., and Koprowski, H.,** Metastatic colon carcinoma detection with radiolabeled $F(ab')_2$ monoclonal antibody fragments, *Radiology,* 149, 549, 1983.
14. **DeLand, F. H., Kim, E. E., and Goldenberg, D. M.,** Lymphoscintigraphy with radionuclide-labeled antibodies to carcinoembryonic antigen, *Cancer Res.,* 40, 2997, 1980.
15. **Thompson, C. H., Lichtenstein, M., Stacker, S. A., Leyden, M. J., Salehi, N., Andrews, J. T. and McKenzie, I. F.,** Immunoscintigraphy for detection of lymph node metastases from breast cancer, *Lancet,* 2, 1245, 1984.
16. **Keenan, A. M., Weinstein, J. N., Carrasquillo, J. A., Reynolds, J. C., Perentesis, P., Foon, K. A., Mulshine, J. L., Bunn, P. A., and Larson, S. M.,** Immunolymphoscintigraphy with Indium-111 labeled T101 monoclonal antibody, *J. Nucl. Med.,* 26, 56, 1985.
17. Hammersmith Oncology Group and the Imperial Cancer Research Fund, Antibody-guided irradiation of malignant lesions: three cases illustrating a new method of treatment, *Lancet,* 1, 1441, 1984.
18. **Pressman, D. and Korngold, L.,** The in vivo localization of anti-Wagner osteogenic sarcoma antibodies, *Cancer,* 6, 7619, 1953.
19. **Pressman, D., Day, E. D., and Blau, M.,** The use of paired labeling in the determination of tumor localizing antibodies, *Cancer Res.,* 17, 845, 1957.
20. **Bale, W. F., Spar, I. L., Goodland, R. L., and Wolfe, D. E.,** In vivo and in vitro studies of labeled antibodies against rat kidney and Walker carcinoma, *Proc. Soc. Exp. Biol. Med.,* 89, 564, 1955.
21. **Day, E. D., Planinsek, J. A., and Pressman, D.,** Localization of radioiodinated rat fibrinogen in transplanted rat tumors, *Natl. Cancer Inst.,* 23, 799, 1959.
22. **Rygaard, J. and Pollsen, C. O.,** Heterotransplantation of a human malignant tumor to the mouse mutant "nude", *Acta Pathol. Microbiol. Scand.,* 77, 758, 1969.
23. **Spar, I. L., Bale, W. F., Marrack, D., Dewey, W. C., McCardle, R. J., and Harper, P. V.,** I-131 labeled antibodies to human fibrinogen. Diagnostic studies and therapeutic trials, *Cancer,* 20, 865870, 1967.
24. **Kohler, G. and Milstein, C.,** Continuous culture of fused cells secreting antibody of predefined specificity, *Nature (London),* 256, 495, 1975.
25. **Gold, P. and Freedman, S. E.,** Demonstration of tumor specific antigen in human colonic carcinomata by immunological tolerance and absorption techniques, *J. Exp. Med.,* 121, 439, 1965.
26. **Koo, S. K., Warner, N. L., Lie, J. T., and Mckay, I. R.,** Carcinoembryonic antigenic activity of tissue extracts: a quantitative study of malignant and benign neoplasms, cirrhotic liver, normal adult and fetal organs, *Int. J. Cancer,* 11, 681, 1973.
27. **Hansen, J. H., Snyder, J., Miller, E., Vandervoorde, J. P., Miller, O. N., Hines, L. R., and Burns, J. J.,** Carcinoembryonic antigen (CEA) assay: a laboratory adjunct in the diagnosis and management of cancer, *Hum. Pathol.,* 5, 139, 1974.
28. **Martin, E. W., Jr., James, K. K., Hurtubise, P. E., Catalano, P., and Minton, J. P.,** The use of CEA as an early indicator for gastrointestinal tumor recurrence and secondlook procedures, *Cancer,* 39, 440, 1977.
29. **Martin, E. W., Cooperman, M., King, G., Rinker, L., Carey, C., and Minton, J. P.,** A retrospective and prospective study of serial CEA determinations in the early detection of recurrent colon cancer, *Am. J. Surg.,* 137, 167, 1979.

30. **Zamcheck, N.**, The present status of CEA in diagnosis, prognosis, and evaluation of therapy, *Cancer*, 36, 2460, 1975.
31. **Goldenberg, D. M., DeLand, F. H., Kim, E., Bennett, S., Primus, F. J., Van Nagell, J. R., Estes, N., DeSinome, P., and Rayburn, P.**, Use of radiolabeled antibodies to carcinoembryonic antigen for the detection and localization of diverse cancers by external photoscanning, *N. Engl. J. Med.*, 298, 1384, 1978.
32. **Goldenberg, D. M., Kim, E. E., Bennett, S. J., Nelson, M. O., and Deland, F. H.**, CEA radioimmunodetection in the evaluation of colorectal cancer and in the detection of occult neoplasma, *Gastroenterology*, 84, 524, 1983.
33. **Mach, J. P., Buchegger, F., Forni, M., Ritschard, J., Berche, C., Lumbroso, J.-D., Schreyer, M., Girardet, C., Accolla, R. S., and Carrell, S.**, Use of radiolabeled monoclonal anti-CEA antibodies for the detection of human carcinomas by external photoscanning and tomoscintigraphy, *Immunol. Today*, 2, 239, 1981.
34. **Hine, K. R., Bradwell, A. R., Reeder, T. A., Drolc, Z., and Dykes, P. W.**, Radioimmunodetection of gastrointestinal neoplasms with antibodies to carcinoembryonic antigen, *Cancer Res.*, 40, 2993, 1980.
35. **Ishii, N., Nakata, K., Muro, T., Furukawa, R., Kono, K., Kusumoto, Y., Munehisa, T., Koji, T., Nagataki, S., Nishi, S., Tsukada, Y., and Hirai, H.**, Radioimmunodetection of cancer using antibodies to alpha-fetoprotein and carcinoembryonic antigen, *Ann. N.Y. Acad. Sci.*, 417, 270, 1983.
36. **Berche, C., Mach, J. P., Lumbroso, J. D., Langlais, C., Aubry, F., Buchegger, F., and Carrel, S., Rougier, P., Parmentier, C., and Tubiana, M.**, Tomoscintigraphy for detecting gastrointestinal and medullary thyroid cancers: first clinical results using radiolabeled monoclonal antibodies against carcinoembryonic antigen, *Br. Med. J.*, 285, 1447, 1982.
37. **Smedley, H. M., Finan, P., Lennox, E. S., Ritson, A., Takei, F., Wraight, P., Sikora, K.**, Localization of metastatic carcinoma by a radiolabeled monoclonal antibody, *Br. J. Cancer*, 47, 253, 1983.
38. **Searle, F., Bagshawe, K. D., Begent, R. H. J., Jewkes, R. F., Jones, B. E., Keep, P. A., Lewis, J., and Vernon, P.**, Radioimmunolocalization of tumours by external scintigraphy after administration of ^{131}I antibody to carcinoembryonic antigen, *Nucl. Med. Commun.*, 1, 131, 1980.
39. **Begent, R. H. J., Keep, P. A., Green, A. J., Searle, F., Bagshawe, K. D., Jewkes, R. F., Jones, B. E., Barratt, G. M., and Ryman, B. E.**, Liposomally entrapped antibody improves tumour imaging with radiolabelled (first) antitumour antibody, *Lancet*, 2, 739, 1982.
40. **Ott, R. J., Grey, L. J., Zivanovic, M. A., Flower, M. A., Trott, N. G., Moshakis, V., Coombes, R. C., Neville, A. M., Ormerod, M. G., Westwood, J. H., and McCready, V. R.**, The limitations of the dual radionuclide subtraction technique for the external detection of tumours by radioiodine-labelled antibodies, *Br. J. Radiol.*, 56, 101, 1983.
41. **Fairweather, D. S., Bradwell, A. R., Dykes, P. W., Vaughan, A. T., Watson-James, S. F., and Chandler, S.**, Improved tumour localisation using indium-111 labelled antibodies, *Br. Med. J.*, 287, 167, 1983.
42. **Tranter, R. M., Fairweather, D. S., Bardwell, A. R., Dykes, P. W., Watson-James, S., and Chandler, S.**, The detection of squamous cell tumours of the head and neck using radio-labeled antibodies, *J. Laryngol. Otol.*, 98, 71, 1984.
43. **Dillman, R. O., Beauregard, J. C., Sobol, R. E., Royston, I., Bartholomew, R., Hagan, P., and Halpern, S.**, Lack of radioimmunodetection and complications associated with monoclonal anti-carcinoembryonic antigen anti-body cross reactivity with an antigen on circulating cells, *Cancer Res.*, 44, 2213, 1984.
44. **Sullivan, D. C., Silva, J. S., Cox, C. E., Haagensen, D. E., Harris, C. C., Biner, W. H., and Wells, S. A.**, Localization of I-131 labeled goat and primate anti-carcinoembryonic antigen (CEA) antibodies in patients with cancer, *Invest. Radiol.*, 17, 350, 1982.
45. **Warenius, H. M., Galfre, D., Bleehen, N. M., Milstein, C.**, Attempted targeting of a monoclonal antibody in a human tumor xenograft system, *Eur. J. Cancer Clin. Oncol.*, 17, 1009, 1981.
46. **Hagan, P. L., Halpern, S. E., and Chen, A.**, Effect of tumor size, carcinoembryonic antigen (CEA) production and secretion on the distribution of ^{111}In and ^{125}I monoclonal anti-tumor antibodies (MoAb) in animal models, *J. Nucl. Med.*, 24, 77, 1983.
47. **Herlyn, M., Steplewski, Z., Herlyn, D., and Koprowski, H.**, Colorectal carcinoma-specific antigen: detection by means of monoclonal antibodies, *Proc. Natl. Acad. Sci. U.S.A.*, 76, 1438, 1979.
48. **Sears, H. F., Atkinson, B., Mattis, J., Herlyn, D., Hayry, P., Atkinson, B., Ernst, E., Steplewski, Z., and Koprowski, H.**, Phase-1 clinical trials of monoclonal antibody in treatment of gastrointestinal tumors, *Lancet*, 1, 762, 1982.
49. **Mach, J. P., Chatal, J. F., Lumbroso, J. D., Buchegger, F., Forni, M., Ritschard, J., Berche, C., Douillard, J. Y., Carrel, S., Herlyn, M., Steplewski, Z., and Koprowski, H.**, Tumor localization in patients by radiolabeled monoclonal antibodies against colon carcinoma, *Cancer Res.*, 43, 5593, 1983.
50. **Chatal, J. F., Saccavini, J. C., Fumoleau, P., Douillard, J. Y., Curtet, C., Kremer, M., Le Mevel, B., and Koprowski, H.**, Immunoscintigraphy of colon carcinoma, *J. Nucl. Med.*, 25, 307, 1984.

51. **Magnani, J. L., Brockaus, M., Smith, D. F., Ginsburg, V., Blaszcyk, M., Mitchell, K., Steplewski, Z., and Koprowski, H.,** A monosialoganglioside is a monoclonal antibody-defined antigen of colon carcinoma, *Science*, 212, 55, 1981.
52. **Embleton, M. J., Gunn, B., Byers, V. S., and Baldwin, R. W.,** Anti-tumor reactions of monoclonal antibody against a human osteogenic sarcoma cell line, *Br. J. Cancer*, 43, 582, 1981.
53. **Nuti, M., Teramoto, Y. A., Mariani-Costanti, R., Horan Hand, P., Colcher, D., and Schlom, J.,** A monoclonal antibody (B72.3) defines patterns of distribution of a novel tumor-associated antigen in human mammary carcinoma cell populations, *Int. J. Cancer*, 29, 539, 1982.
54. **Farrands, P. A., Perkins, A. C., Pimm, M. V., Hardy, J. D., Embleton, M. J., Baldwin, R. W., and Hardcastle, J. D.,** Radioimmunodetection of human colorectal cancers by an anti-tumor monoclonal antibody, *Lancet*, 2, 397400, 1982.
55. **Farrands, P. A., Perkins, A. C., Sully, L., Hopkins, J. S., Pimm, M. V., Baldwin, R. W., and Hardcastle, J. D.,** Localisation of human osteosarcoma by antitumor monoclonal antibody, *J. Bone Joint Surg.*, 65-B, 638, 1983.
56. **Symonds, E. M., Perkins, A. C., Pimm, M. V., Baldwin, R. W., Hardy, J. G., and Williams, D. A.,** Clinical implications for immunoscintigraphy in patients with ovarian malignancy, *Br. J. Obstet. Gynae.*, 92, 270276, 1985.
57. **Armitage, N. C., Perkins, A. C., Pimm, M. V., Farrands, P. A., Baldwin, R. W., and Hardcastle, J. D.,** The localization of an antitumor monoclonal antibody (791T/36) in gastrointestinal tumors, *Br. J. Surg.*, 71, 407, 1984.
58. **Pimm, M. V., Perkins, A. C., Armitage, N. C., and Baldwin, R. W.,** The characteristics of blood-borne radiolabels and the effect of anti-mouse IgG antibodies on localization of radiolabeled monoclonal antibody in cancer patients, *J. Nucl. Med.*, 26, 1011, 1985.
59. **Colcher, D., Horan Hand, P., Nuti, M., and Schlom, J.,** Differential binding to human mammary and non-mammary tumors of monoclonal antibodies reactive with carcinoembryonic antigen, *Cancer Invest.*, 1, 127, 1983.
60. **Carrasquillo, J. A., Colcher, D., Sugarbaker, P., Reynolds, J. R., Keenan, A. M., Simpson, S., Bryant, G., Thor, A., Perentesis, P., Esteban, J., Horowitz, M., Schlom, J., and Larson, S. M.,** Radiolocalization of colon cancer with I-131 B72.3 monoclonal antibody, *J. Nucl. Med.*, 16, 15, 1985.
61. **Colcher, D., Carrasquillo, J., Sugarbaker, P., Reynolds, J. C., Bryant, G., Larson, S. M., and Schlom, J.,** Quantitative analyses of selective radiolabeled monoclonal antibody localization in metastatic lesions of colorectal cancer patients, *Cancer Res.*, 47, 1185, 1987.
62. **Hnatowich, D. J., Griffin, T. W., Kosciuczyk, C., Rusckowski, M., Childs, R. L., Mattis, J. A., Shealy, D., and Doherty, P. W.,** Pharmacokinetics of an indium-111-labeled monoclonal antibody in cancer patients, *J. Nucl. Med.*, 26 (8), 849, 1985.
63. **Brown, J. P., Woodbury, R. G., Hart. C. S. Hellstrom, I., and Hellstrom, K. E.,** Quantitative analysis of melanoma associated antigen p97 in normal and neoplastic tissues, *Proc. Natl. Acad. Sci. U.S.A.*, 78, 539, 1981.
64. **Brown, J. P., Hewick, R. M., Hellstrom, I., Hellstrom, K. E., Doolittle, R. F., and Dreyer, W. J.,** Human melanoma associated antigen p97 is structurally and functionally related to transferrin, *Nature (London)*, 296, 171, 1982.
65. **Hellstrom, I., Garrigues, H. J., Cabasco, L., Moseley, L. T., Brown, J. P., and Hellstrom, K. E.,** Studies of a high molecular weight human melanoma associated antigen, *J. Immunol.*, 130, 1467, 1983.
66. **Larson, S. M., Brown, J. P., Carrasquillo, J. A., Wright, P. W., Hellstrom, I., and Hellstrom, K. E.,** Imaging of melanoma with ^{131}I-labeled antibodies, *J. Nucl. Med.*, 24, 123, 1983.
67. **Larson, S. M., Carrasquillo, J. A., McGuffin, R. W., Krohn, K. A., Ferens, J. M., Hill, I. D., Beaumier, P. L., Reynolds, J. C., Hellstrom, K. E., and Hellstrom, I.,** Preliminary clinical experience using an I-131 labeled, murine Fab against a high molecular weight antigen of human melanoma, *Radiology*, 155, 487, 1985.
68. **Carrasquillo, J. A., Krohn, K. A., Beaumier, P., McGuffin, R. W., Brown, J. P., Hellstrom, K. E., Hellstrom, I., and Larson, S. M.,** Diagnosis of and therapy for solid tumors with radiolabeled antibodies and immune fragments, *Cancer Treat. Rep.*, 68, 317, 1984.
69. **Ferens, L., Krohn, K. A., Beaumier, P. L., Brown, J. P., Hellstrom, I., Hellstrom, K. E., Carrasquillo, J. A., and Larson, S. M.,** High level iodination of monoclonal antibody fragments for radiotherapy, *J. Nucl. Med.*, 25, 367, 1984.
70. **Halpern, S. E., Dillman, R. O., Witztum, K. F., Shega, J. F., Hagan, P. L., Burrows, W. M., Dillman, J. B., Clutter, M. L., Sobol, R. E., Fincke, J. M., Bartholomew, R. M., David, G. S., and Carlo, D.,** Radioimmunodetection of melanoma utilizing ^{111}In-96.5 monoclonal antibody: a preliminary report, *Radiology*, 155(2), 493, 1985.

71. **Murray, J. L., Rosenblum, M. G., Sobol, R. E., Bartholomew, R. M., Phager, C., Haynie, T. P., Jahns, M. F., Glen, H., Lamki, L., Benjamin, R. E., Papdopoulus, N., Bodie, A. W., Fringcke, J. F., David, G. S., Carlo, D. J., and Hirsh, E. M.,** Radioimmunoimaging in malignant melanoma with 111 In-labeled monoclonal antibody 96.5, *Cancer Res.*, 45(5), 2376, 1985.
72. **Rosenblum, M. G., Murray, J. L., Haynie, T. P., Glenn, H. J., Jahns, M. F., Benjamin, R. S., Frincke, J. M., Carlo, D. J., and Hirsh, E. M.,** Pharmacokinetics of ^{111}In-labeled anti-p97 monoclonal antibody in patients with metastatic malignant melanoma, *Cancer Res.*, 45(5), 2382, 1985.
73. **Carrasquillo, J. A., Abrams, P. G., Schroff, R. W., Reynolds, J. C., Woodhouse, C. S., Morgan, A. C., Keenan, A. M., Foon, K. A., Perentesis, P., Marshall, S., Horowitz, M., Szymendera, J., Englert, J., Oldham, R. K., and Larson, S. M.,** Effect of antibody dose on the imaging and biodistribution of ^{111}In 9.2.27 anti-melanoma monoclonal antibody, *J. Nucl. Med.*, 29, 39, 1988.
74. **Buraggi, G. L., Callegaro, L., Mariani, G., Turrin, A., Cascinelli, N., Attili, A., Bombardieri, E., Terno, G., Plassio, G., Dovis, M., Mazzuca, N., Natali, P. G., Scassellati, G. A., Rosa, U., and Ferrone, S.,** Imaging with ^{131}I-labeled monoclonal antibodies to a high-molecular-weight melanoma-associated antigen in patients with melanoma: efficacy of whole immunoglobulin and its F(ab')2 fragments, *Cancer Res.*, 45(7), 3378, 1985.
75. **Oldham, R. K., Foon, K. A., Morgan, A. C., Jr., Woodhouse, C. A., Schroff, R. W., Abrams, P. G., Fer, M. F., Schoenberger, C. S., Farrell, M. M., Kimball, E. S., and Sherwin, S. A.,** Monoclonal antibody therapy of malignant melanoma: *in vivo* localization in cutaneous metastasis after intravenous administration, *J. Clin. Oncol.*, 2(11), 1235, 1984.
76. **Lee, L. H.,** The biosynthesis of hormone by nonendocrine tumours-a review, *J. Endocrinol.*, 67, 143, 1975.
77. **McManus, L. M., Naughton, M. A., and Martinez-Herandez, A.,** Human chorionic gonadotropin in human neoplastic cells, *Cancer Res.*, 36, 3476, 1976.
78. **Goldenberg, D. M., Kim, E. E., and DeLand, F. H.,** Human chorionic gonadotrophin radioantibodies in the radioimmunodetection of cancer and for disclosure of occult metastases, *Proc. Natl. Acad. Sci. U.S.A.*, 78, 7754, 1981.
79. **Morrison, R. T., Lyster, D. M., Alcorn, L., Rhodes, B. A., Breslow, K., and Burchiel, S. W.,** Radioimmunoimaging with ^{99m}Tc monoclonal antibodies: clinical studies, *Int. J. Nucl. Med. Biol.*, 11(2), 1984, 1984.
80. **Goldenberg, D. M., Kim, E. E., DeLand, F. H., van Nagell, J. R., Jr., and Javadpour, N.,** Radioimmunodetection of cancer using radioactive antibodies to human chorionic gonadotropin, *Science*, 208, 1284, 1980.
81. **Abelev, G. L.,** Alpha-fetoprotein in oncogenesis and its association with malignant tumors, *Adv. Cancer Res.*, 14, 295, 1971.
82. **Goldenberg, D. M., Kim, E. E., DeLand, F., Spremulli, E., Nelson, M. O., Gockerman, J. P., Primus, F. J., Corgan, R. L., and Alpert, E.,** Clinical studies on the radioimmunodetection of tumors containing alpha-fetoprotein, *Cancer*, 45, 2500, 1980.
83. **Halsall, A. K., Fairweather, D. S., Bradwell, A. R., Blackburn, J. C., Dykes, P. W., Howell, A., Reeder, A., and Hine, K. R.,** Localization of malignant germ-cell tumors by external scanning injection of radiolabelled anti-alphafetoprotein, *Br. Med. J.*, 283, 942, 1981.
84. **Katz, M. E., Schwartz, P. E., Kopp, D. S., and Luikait, S.,** Epithelial carcinoma of the ovaries: current strategies, *Ann. Intern. Med.*, 95, 98, 1981.
85. **Taylor-Papadimitriou, J., Peterson, J. A., Arklie, J., Burchell, J., Ceriani, R. L., and Bodmer, W. F.,** Monoclonal antibodies to epithelium-specific components of the human milk fat globule membrane. Production and reaction with cells in culture, *Int. J. Cancer*, 28, 17, 1981.
86. **Epenetos, A. A., Shepherd, J., Britton, K. E., Hawkins, L., Nimmon, C. C., Taylor-Papadimitriou, J., Durbin, H., Malpas, J. S., Mather, S., Granowska, M., Duke, D., and Bodmer, W. F.,** Radioimmunodiagnosis of ovarian cancer using ^{123}I-labelled, tumor-associated monoclonal antibodies, *Cancer Detection Prev.*, 7, 45, 1984.
87. **Epenetos, A. A., Shepherd, J., Britton, K. E., Mather, S., Taylor-Papadimitriou, J., Granowska, M., Durbin, H., Nimmon, C. C., Hawkins, L., Malpas, J., and Bodmer, W. F.,** ^{123}I radioiodinated antibody imaging of occult ovarian cancer, *Cancer*, 55(5), 984, 1985.
88. **Pateisky, N., Philipp, K., Skooler, W. D., Ckerweuka, K., Hamilton, G., and Burchel, J.,** Radioimmunodetection in patients with suspected ovarian cancer, *J. Nucl. Med.*, 26, 1369, 1985.
89. **Epenetos, A. A., Snook, D., Hooker, G., Begent, R., Durbin, H., Oliver, R. T. D., Bodmer, W. F., and Lavender, J. P.,** Indium-111 labelled monoclonal antibody to placental alkaline phosphatase in the detection of neoplasms of testis, ovary, and cervix, *Lancet*, 2(8451), 350, 1985.
90. **Davies, J. O., Davies, E. R., Howe, K., Jackson, P. C., Pitcher, E. M., Sadowski, C. S., and Sunderland, C. A.,** Radionuclide imaging of ovarian tumors with ^{123}I-labelled monolonal antibody (NDOG2) directed against placental alkaline phosphatase, *Br. J. Obstet. Gynaecol.*, 92(3), 277, 1985.

91. **Goldenberg, D. M., DeLand, F. H., Bennett, S. J., Primus, F. J., Nelson, M. O., Flanigan, R. C., McRoberts, J. W., Bruce, A. W., and Mahan, D. E.,** Radioimmunodetection of prostatic cancer: in vivo use of radioactive antibodies against prostatic acid phosphatase for diagnosis and detection of prostatic cancer by nuclear imaging, *J.A.M.A.*, 250 (5), 630, 1983.
92. **Order, S. E.,** The history and progress of serologic immunotherapy and radiodiagnosis. Radiodiagnosis, *Radiology,* 118, 219, 1976.
93. **Shepherd, P. S., Lazarus, C. R., Mistry, R. D., and Maisey, M. N.,** Detection of thyroid tumor using a monoclonal ^{123}I anti-human thyroglobulin antibody, *Eur. J. Nucl. Med.*, 10(7—8), 291, 1985.
94. **Ettinger, D. S., Order, S. E., Wharam, M. D., Parker, M. K., Klein, J. L., and Leichner, P. K.,** Phase-II study of isotopic immunoglobulin therapy for primary liver cancer, *Cancer Treat. Rep.*, 66, 289, 1982.
95. **Schroff, R. W., Klein, R. A., Farrell, M. M., and Stevenson, H. C.,** Enhancing effects of monocytes on modulation of a lymphocyte membrane antigen, *J. Immunol.*, 133(4), 1641, 1984.
96. **Shawler, D. L., Miceli, M. C., Wormsley, S. B., Royston, I., and Dillman, R. O.,** Interaction of in vitro and in vivo antigenic modulation by the anti-human T-cell monoclonal antibody T101, *Cancer Res.*, 44, 5921, 1984.
97. **Royston, I., Majda, J. A., Baird, S. M., Bland, M., and Griffiths, J. C.,** Human T-cell antigens degined by monoclonal antibodies: the 65,000-dalton antigen of T cells (T65) is also found on chronic lymphocytic leukemia cells bearing surface immunoglobulin, *J. Immunol.*, 125, 725, 1980.
98. **Dillman, R. O., Beauregard, J. C., Lea, J. W., Green, M. R., Sobol, R. E., and Royston, I.,** Chronic lymphocytic leukemia and other chronic lymphoid proliferation surface marker phenotypes and clinical correlations, *J. Clin. Oncol.*, 1, 190, 1983.
99. **Bunn, P. A., Jr., Carrasquillo, J. A., Keenan, A. M., Schroff, R. W., Foon, K. A., Hsu, S. M., Gazdar, A. F., Reynolds, J. C., Perentesis, P., and Larson, S. M.,** Imaging of T-cell lymphoma by radiolabeled monoclonal antibody, *Lancet,* 2, 1211, 1984.
100. **Carrasquillo, J. A., Bunn, P. A., Keenan, A. M., Reynolds, J. C., Schroff, R. W., Foon, K. A., Ming-Hsu, S., Gazdar, A. F., Mulshine, J. M., Perentesis, P., Horowitz, M., and Larson, S. M.,** Radioimmunodetection of cutaneous T-cell lymphoma with ^{111}In-T101 monoclonal antibody, *N. Engl. J. Med.*, 315, 673, 1980.
101. **Thakur, M., Segal, A. W., Louis, W. L., Welch, M., Hopkins, J., and Peters, T.,** In-111 labeled cellular blood components: mechanism of labeling and intracellular location in human neutrophils, *J. Nucl. Med.*, 18, 1022, 1977.
102. **Schroff, R. W., Foon, K. A., Beatty, S. M., Oldham, R. K., and Morgan, A. C.,** Human anti-murine immunoglobulin responses in patients receiving monoclonal antibody therapy, *Cancer Res.*, 45, 879, 1985.
103. **Reynolds, J. C., Carrasquillo, J. A., and Larson, S. M.,** Human anti-murine response following administration of radiolabeled monoclonal antibodies, *J. Nucl. Med.*, 26, 55, 1985.
104. **Sears, H. F., Herlyn, D., Steplewski, Z., and Koprowski, H.,** Effects of monoclonal antibody immunotherapy on patients with gastrointestinal adenocarcinoma, *J. Biol. Resp. Modifiers,* 3, 138, 1984.
105. **Miller, R. A., Oseroff, A. R., Stratte, P. T., and Levy, R.,** Monoclonal antibody therapeutic trials in seven patients with T-cell lymphoma, *Blood,* 62, 988, 1983.
106. **Pimm, M. V., Perkins, A. C., Armitage, N. C., and Baldwin, R. W.,** The characteristics of blood-borne radiolabels and the effect of anti-mouse IgG antibodies on localization of radiolabeled monoclonal antibody in cancer patients, *J. Nucl. Med.*, 26, 1011, 1985.
107. **McNabb, T., Koh, T. Y., Dorrington K. J., and Painter, R. J.,** Structure and function of immunoglobulin domains. V. Binding of immunoglobulin G and fragments to placental membrane preparations, *Immunology,* 117, 882, 1976.
108. **Bale, W. F., Contreras, M. A., and Grady, E. D.,** Factors influencing localization of labeled antibodies in tumors, *Cancer Res.*, 20, 1488, 1980.
109. **Rainsbury, R. M., Westwood, J. H., Coombes, R. C., Neville, A. M., Ott, R., Kalirai, T. S., McCready, V. R., and Gazet, J. C.,** Location of metastatic breast carcinoma by a monoclonal antibody chelate labeled with indium-111, *Lancet,* 2, 934, 1983.
110. **Mach, J.-P., Carrel, S., Merenda, C., Sordat, B., and Cerrottini, J. C.,** In vivo localization of radiolabeled antibodies to carcinoembryonic antigen in human colon carcinoma grafted in the nude mouse, *Nature (London),* 248, 704, 1974.
111. **Beaumier, P. L., Larson, S. M., Krohn, K. A., Ferens, J. M., Nelp, W. B., and Brown, J. P.,** Effects of iodination of p97 antigen-specific binding and in vivo tumor localization using monoclonal antibody fragments, *J. Nucl. Med.*, 24, 116, 1983.
112. **Keenan, A. M., Colcher, D., Larson, S. M., and Schlom, J.,** Radioimmunoscintigraphy of human colon cancer xenografts in mice with radioiodinated monoclonal antibody B72.3, *J. Nucl. Med.*, 25, 1197, 1984.
113. **DeLand, F. H., Kim, E. E., and Simmons, G.,** Imaging approach in radioimmunodetection, *Cancer Res.*, 40, 3046, 1980.

114. **Bradwell, A. R., Fairweather, D. S., Dykes, P. W., Keeling, A., Vaughan, A., and Taylor, J.,** Limiting factors in the localization of tumours with radiolabeled antibodies, *Immunol. Today*, 6, 163, 1985.
115. **Chester, K. A., Begent, R. H. J., Pedley, B., Keep, P. A., Boden, J. A., Searle, F., and Bagshawe, K. D.,** The use of second antibody to improve selective localization of tumours: animal model studies, *Br. J. Cancer*, 50, 556, 1984.
116. **Rockoff, S. D., Goodenough, D. S., and McIntire, K. R.,** Theoretical limitations in the immunodiagnostic imaging of cancer with computer tomography and nuclear scanning, *Cancer Res.*, 40, 3054, 1980.
117. **McConahey, P. J. and Dixon, F. J.,** A method of trace iodination of proteins for immunologic studies, *Int. Arch. Aller. Appl. Immunol.*, 29, 185, 1966.
118. **Fraker, P. J. and Speck, J. C., Jr.,** Protein and cell membrane iodinations with a sparingly soluble chloroamide, 1,3,4,6-tetrachloro-3a,6a-diphenylglycoluril, *Biochem. Biophys. Res. Commun.*, 80, 849, 1978.
119. **Paik, C. H., Phan, L. N., Hong, J. J., Herman, D. E., Eckelman, W. C., and Reba, R. C.,** The labeling of high affinity sites of antibodies with ^{99m}Tc, *Int. J. Nucl. Med. Biol.*, 12(1), 3, 1985.
120. **Ell, P. J. and Khan, O.,** Emission computerized tomography: clinical applications, *Semin. Nucl. Med.*, 11, 50, 1981.
121. **Carrasquillo, J. A., Mulshine, J. L., Bunn, P. A., Jr., Reynolds, J. C., Foon, K. A., Schroff, R. W., Perentesis, P., Steis, R. G., Keenan, A. M., Horowitz, M., and Larson, S. M.,** Indium-111 T101 monoclonal antibody is superior to iodine-131 T101 in imaging of cutaneous T-cell lymphoma, *J. Nucl. Med.*, 28, 281, 1987.

Chapter 10

ANTIBODY RADIOTHERAPY: CURRENT STATUS

Shalom Kalnicki and William D. Bloomer

TABLE OF CONTENTS

I. INTRODUCTION

Shortly after the turn of the century, Paul Ehrlich et al.[1] recognized the therapeutic potential of anti-tumor antibodies as carriers of toxic substances that could be selectively targeted to tumor cells. Although the concept of specific antibodies reacting with specific antigens on the surface of tumor cells, but not normal cells, is easily appreciated, its realization is not without problems.[2] Antibodies to tumor-associated antigens have proved to be valuable research tools and have moved rapidly from the laboratory into the clinic as diagnostic and imaging tools. Their role as a major therapeutic modality is in an embryonic stage. The next few years will be critical as interest broadens and ongoing studies come to fruition.

Successful targeting of radiolabeled antibodies to tumor cells requires not only carrier specificity but also radionuclides with appropriate decay characteristics. More than 25 years ago the pioneering French radiotherapists Claude Regaud and Antoine Lacassagne[3] envisioned localizing within tumor cells radionuclides whose range of action would be limited just to tumor cells and not the surrounding normal tissues.

II. TUMOR-ASSOCIATED ANTIGENS

Tumor-associated antigens were recognized as early as 1929 when Witebsky[4] developed a rabbit antiserum against a uterine carcinoma that did not cross react with normal tissues. In the same year, Hirszfeld et al.[5] reported similar results with anaplastic tumors. However, it was not until the mid-1960s, when Gold and Freedman[6] reported that many human colon cancers contain a carcinoembryonic antigen (CEA), that a major thrust was made to exploit tumor immunology for clinical diagnosis and therapy. CEA, which is shed by tumor cells into the general circulation, can be detected by radioimmunoassay of patients' sera. Anti-CEA antibodies have also been used scintigraphically to localize tumors.[7] CEA and alpha-fetoprotein[8] are two of the best known tumor-associated antigens. These and other so-called tumor-specific antigens are more properly called tumor-associated antigens. In general, they represent dedifferentiation products of gene expression, and because they are often found normally in the fetus, they are sometimes referred to as oncofetal antigens. Because they are products of cellular dedifferentiation, oncofetal antigens can be expressed by a variety of tumor cell types. Some oncofetal antigens such as CEA may be expressed in the adult in certain nonmalignant inflammatory conditions. Despite their lack of specificity, tumor-associated antigens are of great value in assessing the response to therapy in patients with known malignancies and elevated titers of these tumor markers.

III. RADIOIMMUNOTHERAPY: HISTORICAL PERSPECTIVES

In 1895, Hericourt and Richet[9] reported the use of antisera against osteogenic sarcoma and observed responses in treating a fibrosarcoma and gastric carcinoma. Subsequent experiences were inconsistent and limited by the lack of antiserum specificity and cross reactivity with normal tissues.

Pressman and Keighley[10] were among the first to use radiolabeled antibodies successfully. They demonstrated that ^{131}I-labeled antiserum to rat kidney localized in rat kidney without significant alteration of the antiserum specificity. Pressman and Korngold[11] subsequently developed the double labeling technique using two different iodine isotopes, ^{125}I and ^{131}I. This has become the standard methodology for documenting specific immune uptake while allowing correction for passive localization of foreign protein within the extracellular space. A specificity ratio can be calculated when the uptakes of immune and nonimmune antisera are compared. In early studies,[12] this ratio was about 2:1. Later work by Bale et al.[13] improved the specificity ratio to almost 8:1. It soon became apparent that the observed localization was the result of antibodies directed against fibrin or fibrinogen associated with rapidly growing tumors rather than against tumor cell surface antigens.[14] Fibrin accumulation in rapidly growing tumors is secondary to an inflammatory response associated with local tumor invasion. Nonetheless, radiolabeled anti-fibrinogen antibodies proved to be very successful in imaging a whole host of tumors.[15]

Ferritin is another tumor-associated product that is the subject of much current laboratory and clinical investigation. It has been isolated from Hodgkins Disease, hepatoma, lung cancer, neuroblastoma, acute myelogenous leukemia, as well as carcinomas of the breast and pancreas.[16-21] As opposed to fibrinogen, which accumulates secondary to blood vessel invasion, ferritin is synthesized and secreted by tumor cells.[22-25]

IV. HYBRIDOMA TECHNOLOGY

Köhler and Milstein[26] revolutionized the field of immunology when they reported the development of mouse spleen-myeloma hybridomas in 1975. Hybridoma technology has greatly facilitated the production and isolation of large quantities of identically formulated antibody to a defined antigenic determinant. The technique is simplistically elegant. Mice, immunized against an antigen of interest, are sacrificed and a suspension of spleen cells harvested and then fused with mouse myeloma cells lacking a necessary replication enzyme. Since the hybridoma cells contain the necessary enzyme, they survive in media conditioned to kill enzyme-deficient unfused myeloma cells. Because unfused spleen cells lack the capacity for sustained replication, they will die. The surviving hybridoma cells are then cloned in microtiter dishes to isolate individual clones of antibody-producing cells. These clones can then be screened for specific antibody production using the immunizing antigen. Desired clones can then be grown in tissue culture or as ascites tumors to produce large amounts of monoclonal antibody.

Successful hybridoma production is not without some difficulties.[27] The yield of specific monoclonal antibody-producing clones is usually very low. The efficiency of viral or polyethylene glycol fusion techniques has been low, but may be improved using receptor-mediated electrically induced cell fusion.[28] The use of nonimmunoglobulin-producing myeloma cells has eliminated the potential problem of nonantibody-myeloma immunoglobulin production.[29] On the other hand, weak immunogens result in hybridomas that are poor producers of the desired antibody and such hybridomas are often unstable with respect to antibody production.

Conventionally produced antiserum usually contains antibodies against a wide spectrum of antigenic determinants that include both tumor and normal tissue antigens. Absorption techniques using a variety of normal tissue cell homogenates or fractions can be used to remove cross-reacting antibodies. However, absorption techniques cannot be used to remove cross-reacting antibodies when hybridomas are used to produce the antibody. In this circumstance, cross reactivities can only be removed by further purification of the immunizing antigen.

Because adverse allergic reactions may occur in humans after multiple applications of foreign proteins, the development of monoclonal antibodies of human origin is a top priority. It is now possible to construct chimeric antibodies in which the antigen-recognizing variable regions of mouse antibodies are joined with the constant regions of human antibodies.[30-32] It remains to be seen whether or not such chimeric antibodies are less likely to produce an immune response in humans.

Another interesting approach to antibody radiotherapy involves the use of bispecific antibodies as carriers of radioactivity. Bispecific antibodies are hybrid immunoglobulins with two different antigen-binding sites. Milstein and Cuello[33] have recently described the preparation of bispecific monoclonal antibodies by the fusion of different antibody-producing cells. Another approach involves the chemical recombination of monoclonal immunoglobulin-G_1 fragments, a procedure that generates the desired bispecific reagent in high yield as the sole reaction product.[34]

V. CHOICE OF RADIONUCLIDE

Although therapeutic strategies abound for using radiolabeled monoclonal or polyclonal antibodies, optimal characteristics for such a radionuclide are unclear.[35] Clearly, radionuclides appropriate for immunoscintigraphy may not be appropriate for antibody radiotherapy. Gamma emitters of a defined energy range are useful for diagnostic purposes, but lack a sufficient differential in absorbed dose between target and normal tissues to be useful for therapy.

Beta emitters are the classic radionuclides used for therapy and have a well-established role in the treatment of hyperthyroidism and thyroid malignancy. Because thyroid tissue concentrates radioiodide to a level at least 25 times greater than the level in plasma,[36] there is no need for a carrier. Unfortunately, the ability of thyroid tissue to concentrate iodide to such a high level represents a unique circumstance in nature. Nonspecific beta-emitting radiocolloids have been used to treat malignant ascites and pleural effusions for palliation. They also provide an attractive alternative to surgical synovectomy for the treatment of chronic synovitis involving specific joints.[37] However, the role of beta-emitting radiocolloids is much less established when compared with the role of radioiodine for treatment of thyroid disorders.[38]

Alpha particles from astatine-211 have been used successfully for therapy of experimental malignant ascites.[39] Furthermore, monoclonal antibodies have been labeled with this radionuclide and antigenic specificity preserved.[40,41] Because of their mass and charge, alpha particles are densely ionizing and have short path lengths relative to both beta and gamma emitters. On the other hand, astatine-211 has such a short physical half-life (7.2 hr) that a high extraction coefficient from the general circulation is necessary to minimize normal tissue irradiation.

Depending upon what biological assumptions are used, theoretical models of antibody radiotherapy will make certain radionuclides appear more attractive than others. For example, iodine-125 is a low energy beta emitter and is exquisitely radiotoxic when disintegration occurs in close proximity to nuclear structures.[42] Unfortunately, there is no reason to think that radiolabeled antibodies undergo nuclear sequestration. Among the beta emitters that do not require nuclear localization for cytotoxicity are iodine-131, yttrium-90, rhenium-186, copper-67, and palladium-109.

Beta emitters appear to be the most attractive radionuclides for antibody radiotherapy at the present time. Physical characteristics to be considered in selecting such a radionuclide include, but are not restricted to, physical half-life, beta particle energy, associated gamma radiation, stability of daughter decay products, mode of production, and availability. The important chemical parameters to be considered include innate reactivity, ability to form a stable chelate or direct chemical bond with antibody, stability of the radiolabeled antibody at physiological pH and in biological fluids, and the specific activity of labeled antibody, i.e., the number of radionuclides per antibody molecule. From a biological standpoint, tumor cell retention time and fate of catabolized radiolabel will influence selection of radionuclide and may limit ultimate applicability and therapeutic efficacy.

Probably the most extensively studied beta emitter for antibody radiotherapy is iodine-131. Its physical half-life of 8.05 days and stable decay products make it suitable for both immunoscintigraphy and antibody radiotherapy. Investigations using 64 hr half-life yttrium-90 labeled antibody are currently underway in several centers. Its in vivo metabolism is not clearly understood, but bone sequestration of free isotope may limit applicability.

VI. SOME BIOLOGICAL CONSIDERATIONS

The biological half-life of radiolabeled antibody is a function of immunological specificity, tumor cell expression of antigenic determinants, the presence of circulating antigen, and antibody catabolism. Most radiolabeling techniques degrade, at least to some extent, the immunological specificity of native antibody by slight chemical alterations and/or steric hindrance introduced by the addition of a foreign element.

Morphological heterogeneity, as well as differences within tumors with respect to cell surface receptors, metastatic potential, growth rate, and response to specific therapies, are well-known variables.[43,44] Using heterologous antisera and monoclonal antibodies, antigenic heterogeneity within tumors is also well established.[45-47] However, with the use of monoclonal antibodies for therapy, it has been observed that the binding of antibody to antigens on the surface of tumor cells can result in the disappearance of target antigens from the cell surface.[48,49] This process is called antigenic modulation. In one experience,[48] 5 of 11 leukemia patients showed evidence of an immune reaction to mouse monoclonal antibodies used for therapy. Antigenic modulation usually requires bivalent antibody binding. The use of monovalent monoclonal antibodies, prepared by limited proteolysis, may prevent antigenic modulation and actually enhance tumor cell lysis in the presence of complement.[50]

Despite morphological disparities, it has generally been assumed that tumors arise from a single genetic clone. However, a recent study of B-cell lymphomas suggests that as many as 10% of such tumors are actually biclonal.[51] Fortunately, antigenic modulation is usually temporary and more often associated with hematopoietic tumors rather than solid tumors. Nonetheless, because it can decrease the efficacy of repeated antibody administrations, some investigators advocate the use of heterologous antiserum or a battery of monoclonal antibodies for tumor therapy. Another complicating factor to be considered in the future is that natural somatic mutations within B-cell lymphomas lead to lability of idiotype expression and define a mechanism by which such tumors may become unresponsive to anti-idiotype antibody therapy.[52]

The presence of circulating tumor antigens that can bind with antibody in the blood stream will adversely affect not only diagnostic studies but also therapy by interfering with the targeting of antibody to tumor cells.[53] In the presence of antigens such as CEA, some patients show a transient decrease in antigen level after infusion of antibody.[54]

Sequestration of infused monoclonal antibody is influenced by tumor weight, larger tumors being visualized earlier and more easily than small tumors.[55] Nonspecific immunoglobulin localizes in tumors much more and for longer periods of time than it does in normal tissues,[56] suggesting that newly formed tumor blood vessels may be more permeable than capillaries of normal tissues. An equally plausible explanation, however, is that antibody sequestration by tumors is the result of decreased antibody clearance. Evidence abounds that many tumors grow at such a rate that they outstrip their ability to induce an adequate blood supply. In fact, autoradiographs of tumors after administration of radiolabeled antisera demonstrate large amounts of perivascular antibody deposition with much smaller amounts in necrotic areas.[57] Thus, whereas the extraction coefficient of radiolabeled antibody from the general circulation varies according to tumor size and the number of newly formed capillaries, detection and therapy may be more dependent on antibody clearance from a poorly perfused environment.

VII. IMMUNOSCINTIGRAPHY

Current antibody radiotherapy studies are a natural outgrowth of the burgeoning experience using radiolabeled antibodies for tumor detection. Immunoscintigraphy began in earnest after it was shown that anti-CEA antibody could be used to image diverse tumors successfully.[58]

Computer-assisted image enhancement and subtraction, as well as absorption techniques, improve sensitivity.[59,60] Nonetheless, the use of whole antiserum rarely detects lesions not otherwise readily apparent by more conventional radiographic techniques. Monoclonal antibody and enzyme prepared fragments thereof are the subject of much current investigation. Although there appears to be some controversy over the merits of monoclonal antibody vs. conventional antiserum, the more rapid rate of clearance of monoclonal antibody from the circulation should be more advantageous.[61] On the other hand, the localizing efficiency of monoclonal antibodies may be limited if a difference in epitope expression exists between the primary tumor used to produce the monoclonal and subsequent metastases. Of particular interest is the recent report showing that $F(ab')_2$ fragments of monoclonal antibody can detect metastic tumor deposits not detectable by other radiographic techniques including computed tomography.[62]

VIII. THE BASIS FOR ANTIBODY RADIOTHERAPY

The encouraging results of radiolabeled antibody for the detection of tumors led investigators to consider antibodies for therapy. Although ^{131}I labeled antibodies had been used as early as 1957 to treat malignant melanoma,[63] the development of monoclonal antibodies spurred many groups into active studies. Radiolabeled monoclonals have been used to detect human tumor xenografts in animal systems.[64-66] Nonradioactive monoclonal antibodies have inhibited the growth of solid tumor xenografts in animal models[67-68] as well as leukemia.[69,70] Moreover, they have also been used to treat cutaneous T-cell lymphoma and leukemia.[71-73] Other studies have investigated chemotherapeutic agents and toxins attached to monoclonal antibodies.[74-77] Immunomicrospheres have also been suggested as therapeutic agents. Such microspheres would have antibodies chemically bound to their surface and these antibody-coated microspheres would react in a highly specific manner with target cells.[78]

Much investigational work needs to be done before conclusions can be made regarding optimal radionuclides for antibody-mediated radiotherapy. As opposed to external beam irradiation where a wide spectrum of options are available, compromises may be necessary in the case of a therapeutic radionuclide. Controversies also exist regarding the merits of monoclonal antibody, polyclonal antibodies, or heterologous antisera. Theoretically, monoclonal antibodies allow one to choose a specific IgG subclass and epitope to be targeted, maximize antigen-antibody affinity, eliminate cross reactivity with normal tissues, and prepare immune antibody fragments such as $F(ab')_2$ that have optimal pharmacokinetics.

IX. ANTIFERRITIN ANTIBODY STUDIES

Iodine-131 labeled antiferritin polyclonal antibody has been the subject of extensive investigation by Order and colleagues.[79,80] Phase I studies in patients with hepatocellular carcinoma provided an opportunity to perform dosimetric analyses. The tumor effective half-life was 3 to 4 days and the radiation dose rate low. Using a combination of computed tomography and immunoscintigraphy, it was determined that the tumor uptake of antibody was linearly related to tumor volume when tumor volumes were less than 1700 cm^3. In addition, the mean tumor-to-liver ratio (per gram tissue) was almost five to one. On the other hand, there was no correlation between tumor uptake of antibody and tumor volume when tumors exceeded 2300 cm^3; moreover, the mean tumor-to-liver ratio was less than two to one. This finding can be attributed to a combination of tumor necrosis and poor vascularization. Normal liver uptake was linearly related to volume. On the basis of these dosimetric analyses as well as normal tissue toxicity studies, a treatment regimen of 30 mCi ^{131}I-antiferritin polyclonal antibody on day zero followed by a second dose of 20 mCi on day five was considered to be optimal per cycle of therapy. The results of this protocol have recently been reported for patients with Hodgkin's disease and hepatocellular carcinoma.

In Hodgkin's disease, 37 patients with advanced disease, refractory to at least two potentially curative combination chemotherapy programs, were studied with ^{131}I-antiferritin antibody of rabbit, pig, or monkey origin.[81] Objective partial responses of measurable disease were recorded in 40% of patients, and one complete response was observed. Of the 22 patients with B-cell symptoms referable to their Hodgkin's disease, 77% showed improvement or complete clearing. Toxicity was mild. No patient developed a skin rash or anaphylactic reaction. The major toxicity was hematological, thrombocytopenia being most prominent. Fifty percent of patients showed depression of their platelet counts to less than 100,000 per dℓ. Platelet transfusions were required in four patients whose counts fell below 20,000 per dℓ.

The lack of allergic reactions to repeated cycles of antibody therapy is presumed to be the result of changing species of origin with each cycle, e.g., rabbit antibody for the first cycle, pig for the second cycle, and monkey for the third cycle. The interval between cycles was 8 weeks. Of those patients achieving a partial remission after the first cycle of therapy, only two showed continued improvement with a second cycle. Fourteen patients remained stable, while six progressed after the second and subsequent cycles of treatment.

Further studies of yttrium-90 labeled antiferritin antibody are planned. Because of its decay characteristics, ^{90}Y-antiferritin antibody may deliver a higher tumor dose without adding to the total body dose. Equally important, outpatient administration may be possible because ^{90}Y is a pure beta emitter.

While uncommon in the United States, hepatocellular carcinoma is a serious medical problem in Asia and sub-Saharan Africa. In a large series of patients reported from Japan,[82] the median survival of medically treated patients was 1.6 months and ranged between 0.7 and 8.3 months depending on stage. The median survival of patients undergoing hepatic resection was 26 months for Stage I and 12 months for Stage II patients. The major cause of death was locally uncontrolled disease rather than distant metastases.

A total of 105 patients with hepatoma have been studied in three sequential phase I-II protocols using ^{131}I-antiferritin.[83] Therapy in all three trials included external beam irradiation (2100 rad in 300 rad fractions over 2 weeks) and chemotherapy (15 mg doxorubicin and 500 mg 5-fluorouracil) integrated with 30 mCi ^{131}I-antiferritin on day zero followed by 20 mCi antibody on day five. Alternating cycles of antibody of rabbit, pig, monkey, and bovine origin were used at 8-week intervals.

Responses were obtained in 48% of patients - 7% complete and 41% partial responses. Previously untreated patients without metastases who were alpha-fetoprotein positive had a median survival of 5 months compared to alpha-fetoprotein negative patients whose survival was almost 11 months. Of the four complete responders, one is alive 3.5 years later. The longest partial response lasted 5.7 years.

The variables affecting tumor localization of ^{131}I-antiferritin antibody have been studied in an experimental rat hepatoma model.[84] The in vivo localization of both ^{131}I-antiferritin antibody and, normal ^{131}I-IgG was investigated over a broad range of weights and specific activities. The dose distribution of antiferritin antibody in tumor was three times that of normal IgG without any significant increase in dose to normal tissues. Tumor localization of ^{131}I-antiferritin antibody could be blocked by nonradioactive antibody but not by normal IgG. Normal tissues bound IgG and antiferritin antibody nonspecifically in a linear relationship directly related to weight.

X. HUMAN MELANOMA STUDIES

Malignant melanoma arises from the pigment producing cells that originate embryologically from neural crest derivatives and migrate early in gestation to skin, uveal tract, meninges, and ectodermal mucosa.[85] The melanocytes of skin are found in the basal layer of the epidermis and are responsible for the biosynthesis and transport of the pigment melanin. Melanomas are not rare malignancies. In fact, the rate of increase in their incidence during recent years is second only to lung cancer.[86] Melanomas account for about 1% of all malignancies in the United States and for about the same percentage of cancer deaths. Although only 3% of cutaneous neoplasms are melanomas, melanomas cause 65% of all skin cancer deaths.[87] Deaths from malignant melanoma are always the result of metastases to critical organs such as lung, liver, and brain. This is in sharp contrast to the natural history and biological behavior of heptocellular carcinomas. Melanoma is notoriously resistant to both chemotherapy and external beam radiotherapy[88] and is an ideal tumor in which to study new therapeutic modalities such as antibody radiotherapy.

A melanoma-associated antigen characterized as p97 has been studied extensively as a diagnostic agent and, more recently, as the basis for antibody-mediated radiotherapy. The p97 antigen is a 97,000 mol wt cell surface glycoprotein that can be present in concentrations as high as 400,000 molecules per cell.[89-91] Although it is expressed at very low concentrations in many adult tissues, its concentration in about 50% of melanomas is very high. It can, thus, be called an oncofetal antigen. The amino acid structure shows considerable homology with serotransferrin and lactotransferrin.[92]

Imaging studies using whole anti-p97 IgG demonstrated localization in 88% of tumors measuring greater than 1.5 cm.[93] The major problems identified were prolonged blood pool retention, relatively low target-to-nontarget ratios, and the appearance of human antimouse antibodies. Subsequent imaging studies[94] using Fab fragments rather than whole antibody revealed a higher tumor extraction coefficient for p97-specific Fab than for nonspecific Fab. Moreover, the egress of nonspecific Fab fragments from tumor was greater than p97-specific Fab fragments.

On the basis of these scintigraphic studies, phase I radiotherapy studies were initiated in seven patients.[94] Twelve therapeutic doses of ^{131}I-labeled anti-p97 Fab fragments were given. Despite a broad range of specific activity, excellent tumor localization was obtained and no major normal tissue toxicity was observed. Cumulative doses ranged between 132 and 529 mCi. Allergic reactions were rare and responded to symptomatic treatment. In two patients who developed isotype-specific immunity after multiple injections of Fab (IgG_1) fragments, readministration was possible by changing to a different isotype, e.g., Fab (IgG_{2a}). Dosimetry estimations were performed based upon the distribution obtained from scintigraphic analyses. For every 100 mCi administered, the tumor received 1040 rad, liver 325 rad and bone marrow 30 rad. No tumor responses were reported when ^{131}I-Fab fragments were used. Whole antibody without an attached radionuclide also has not produced objective tumor regressions or histological changes in biopsy specimens.[95]

On the basis of these observations, Larson et al.[96] have identified specific areas for investigation that will apply to both diagnostic studies and therapy. These include antigen distribution on tumor cells, antigen-antibody affinity, the mass amount of antibody administered, radiolabeling technique, specific activity, quality control, and whether or not to use whole antibody or fragments thereof.

XI. PRECLINICAL STUDIES

Studies of antibody-mediated radiotherapy systems are not as plentiful as one might have expected. This probably reflects the relative lack of good animal tumor models and the major effort necessary to define tumor antigens and develop appropriate antibodies.

Monoclonal antibodies against the Thy 1.1 T-cell differentiation antigen by themselves are ineffective in treating AKR T-cell lymphoma in mice once palpable tumor has developed.[98,99] However, ^{131}I-labeled anti-Thy 1.1 antibodies not only localized within subcutaneous tumor nodules, but also caused significant tumor regression.[100] Doses of 500 μCi led to tumor regression in 44% of animals, prolonged survival, and resulted in locally cured tumor nodules in two of five cases. In contrast, therapy with ^{131}I-labeled nonspecific antibody, even in doses of 1 mCi, had no therapeutic efficacy.

Total tumor uptake of both specific anti-Thy 1.1 and nonspecific antibody increased with increasing tumor size. Antigen-antibody affinity was preserved as long as each anti-Thy 1.1 molecule was labeled with less than two iodine atoms. Bone marrow toxicity developed with anti-Thy 1.1 doses in excess of 1 mCi. A dose of 1 mCi anti-Thy 1.1 antibody was estimated to deliver about 3300 rad tumor dose.

By comparison, studies of ^{131}I-labeled monoclonal immunoglobulin against Rauscher murine erythroleukemia showed no therapeutic advantage for specific vs. nonspecific antibody.[69,101,102] Rather, radioimmunotherapy in this system was totally nonspecific, regardless of radionuclide carrier — tumor-specific monoclonal antibody, nonspecific antibody, $F(ab')_2$ fragments, polyclonal gamma globulin, and serum albumin. Dose-response curves using reduction in splenomegaly as the therapeutic endpoint showed that about 90% reduction in spleen size occurred with 80 μCi injected dose, irrespective of carrier. Therapeutic efficacy was influenced by size of the radionuclide carrier, serum half-life of the carrier, and serum concentration of circulating antigen.

XII. CONCLUSION

Despite technical refinements and integrated administration, a quantum leap forward in cancer therapy using conventional modalities appears most unlikely. However, newer strategies based upon the use of radionuclides attached to anti-tumor antibodies offer the potential of making this great next step forward. Although easily conceptualized, the actual formulation of such "magic bullets" presents a number of technical and biological options that will require careful investigation. The necessary data for radiation treatment planning can be obtained from tracer studies and supplemented with tomographic scanning and sophisticated dynamic mathematical modeling of physiological parameters.[97] Compromises may be necessary in the choice of radionuclide. Extraction coefficient, tumor cell retention time, and fate of catabolized radionuclide will influence applicability. Nonetheless, most investigators are optimistic that the immune system and tumor milieu can be exploited to produce the necessary distribution and therapeutic efficacy.

REFERENCES

1. **Ehrlich, P., Herta, C. A., and Shiga, K.,** Über einige Verwendungen der Naphtochinosulfosaure, *Z. Physiol. Cheum.*, 61, 379, 1904.
2. **Bloomer, W. D., Lipsztein, R., and Dalton, J. F.,** Antibody mediated radiotherapy, *Cancer*, 55, 2229, 1985.
3. **Regaud, C. and Lacassagne, A.,** La radiosensibilife cellulaire dans ses manifestations générales, *Radiophysiol. Radiother.*, 104, 1927.
4. **Witebsky, E.,** Disponibilität und Spezifität alkohölloslicher Strukturen von Organen und bösartigen Geschwulsten, *Z. Immunitaetsforsch.*, 62, 35, 1929.
5. **Hirszfeld, L., Halber, W., and Laskowski, J.,** Untersuchungen uber die serologischen Eigenschaften der Gewebe; über serologische Eigenschaften der Neubildungen, *Z. Immunitaetsforsch*, 64, 81, 1929.
6. **Gold, P. and Freedman, S. O.,** Demonstration of tumor specific antigens in human colonic carcinomata by immunological tolerance and absorption techniques, *J. Exp. Med.*, 121, 439, 1965.
7. **Mach, J. P., Carrel, S., Merenda, C., Sordad, B., and Cerottini, J. C.,** In vivo localization of radiolabeled antibodies to carcinoembryonic antigen in human colon carcinoma grafted into nude mice, *Nature (London)*, 248, 704, 1974.

8. **Abelev, G. I.,** Alpha-fetoprotein in oncogenesis and its association with malignant tumors, *Adv. Cancer Res.,* 14, 295, 1971.
9. **Hericourt, J., Richet, C.,** Traitment d'un cas de sarcome par la serotherapie. *C. R. Acad. Sci.,* 120, 948, 1895.
10. **Pressman, D. and Keighley, G.,** The zone of activity of antibodies as determined by the use of radioactive tracers: the zone of activity of nephrotoxic antikidney serum, *J. Immunol.,* 59, 141, 1948.
11. **Pressman, D. and Korngold, L.,** The in vivo localization of anti-Wagner osteogenic sarcoma antibodies, *Cancer,* 6, 7619, 1953.
12. **Pressman, D., Day, E. D., and Blau, M.,** The use of paired labeling in the determination of tumor localizing antibodies, *Cancer Res.,* 17, 845, 1957.
13. **Bale, W. F., Spar, I. L., Goodland, R. L., and Wolfe, D. E.,** In vivo and in vitro studies of labeled antibodies against rat kidney and Walker carcinoma, *Proc. Soc. Exp. Biol. Med.,* 89, 564, 1955.
14. **Day, E. D., Planisek, J. A., and Pressman, D.,** Localization of radioiodinated rat fibrinogen in transplanted rat tumors, *J. Natl. Cancer Inst.,* 23, 799, 1959.
15. **Spar, I. L., Bale, W. F., Marrack, D., Dewey, W. C., McCarole, R. J., and Harper, P. V.,** ^{131}I-Labeled antibodies to human fibrinogen: diagnostic studies and therapeutic trials, *Cancer,* 20, 865, 1967.
16. **Order, S. E., Porter, M., and Hellman, S.,** Hodgkin's disease: evidence for a tumor-associated antigen, *New Engl. J. Med.,* 285, 471, 1974.
17. **Marcus, D. M. and Zinberg, N.,** Isolation of ferritin from human mammary and pancreatic carcinomas by means of antibody immunoabsorbents, *Arch. Biochem. Biophys.,* 162, 495, 1974.
18. **Hann, H. L., Stahlhut, M. W., and Millman, I.,** Human ferritins present in the sera of nude mice transplanted with human neuroblastoma or hepatocellular carcinoma, *Cancer Res.,* 44, 3898, 1984.
19. **White, G. P., Worwood, M., Parry, D. H., and Jacobs, A.,** Ferritin synthesis in normal and leukemic lymphocytes, *Nature (London),* 250, 584, 1974.
20. **Gropp, C., Havemann, K., and Lehmann, F. G.,** Carcinoembryonic antigen and ferritin in patients with lung cancer before and during therapy, *Cancer,* 42, 2802, 1978.
21. **Kew, M. C., Vorrance, J. D., Derman, D., Simon, M., Macnab, G. M., Charlton, R. W., and Bothwell, T. H.,** Serum tumor ferritins in primary liver cancer, *Gut,* 19, 294, 1978.
22. **Richter, G. W.,** Comparison of ferritins from neoplastic and non-neoplastic human cells, *Nature (London),* 207, 616, 1965.
23. **McGuire, R. A., Pretlow, T. G., Wareing, T. H., and Bradley, E. D.,** Hodgkin's cells and attached lymphocytes, *Cancer,* 44, 183, 1979.
24. **Sarcione, E. J., Smalley, J. R., Lema, M. J., and Stutzman, L.,** Increased ferritin synthesis and release by Hodgkin's disease peripheral blood lymphocytes, *Int. J. Cancer,* 70, 339, 1977.
25. **Eshhar, Z., Order, S. E., and Katz, D. H.,** Ferritin, a Hodgkin's disease associated antigen, *Proc. Natl. Acad. Sci. U.S.A.,* 71, 3956, 1974.
26. **Köhler, G. and Milstein, C.,** Continuous culture of fused cells secreting antibody of proven defined specificity, *Nature (London),* 256, 495, 1975.
27. **Diamond, B. A., Yelton, D. E., and Scharff, M. D.,** Monoclonal antibodies: a new technology for producing serologic reagents, *N. Engl. J. Med.,* 304, 1344, 1981.
28. **Lo, M. M. S., Tsong, T. Y., Conrad, M. K., Strittmatter, S. M., Hester, L. D., and Snyder, S. H.,** Monoclonal antibody production by receptor-mediated electrically induced cell fusion, *Nature (London),* 310, 792, 1984.
29. **Shulman, M., Wolde, C. D., and Köhler, G.,** A better cell line for making hybridoma secreting specific antibodies, *Nature (London),* 276, 269, 1978.
30. **Boulianne, G. L., Hozumi, N., and Shulman, M. J.,** Production of function chimaeric mouse/human antibody, *Nature (London),* 312, 643, 1984.
31. **Morrison, S. L., Johnson, M. J., and Herzenberg, L. A.,** Chimeric human antibody molecules: mouse antigen binding domains with human constant region domains, *Proc. Natl. Acad. Sci. U.S.A.,* 81, 6851, 1984.
32. **Neuberger, M. S., Williams, G. T., and Fox, R. O.,** Recombinant antibodies possessing novel effector functions, *Nature (London),* 312, 604, 1984.
33. **Milstein, C. and Cuello, A. C.,** Hybrid hybridomas and their use in immunohistochemistry, *Nature (London),* 305, 537, 1983.
34. **Brennan, M., Davison, P. F., and Paulus, F.,** Preparation of biospecific antibodies by chemical recombination of monoclonal immunoglobulin G_1 fragments, *Science,* 229, 81, 1985.
35. **O'Brien, H. A.,** Overview of radionuclides useful for radioimmunoimaging, radioimmunotherapy and current status of preparing radiolabeled antibodies, in *Radioimmunoimaging and Radioimmunotherapy,* Burchiel, S. W. and Rhodes, B. A., Eds., Elsevier, Amsterdam, 1983, 161.
36. **Ingbar, S. H. and Woeber, K. A.,** The thyroid gland, in *Textbook of Endocrinology,* 4th ed., Williams, R. H., Ed., W. B. Saunders, Philadelphia, 1968, 105.

37. **Sledge, C. B., Atcher, R. W., Shortkroff, S., Anderson, R. J., Bloomer, W. D., and Hurson, B. J.,** Intra-articular radiation synovectomy, *Clin. Orthop.*, 182, 37, 1984.
38. **Spencer, R. P.,** *Therapy in Nuclear Medicine,* Grune and Stratton, New York, 1978.
39. **Bloomer, W. D., McLaughlin, W. H., Neirinckx, R. D., Adelstein, S. J., Gordon, P. R., Ruth, T. J. and Wolf, A. P.,** Astatine-211-tellurium radiocolloid cures experimental malignant ascites, *Science,* 212, 340, 1981.
40. **Vaughan, A. T. M., Bateman, W. J., Brown, G., and Cowan, J.,** The specific inhibition of cellular clonogenic proliferation using ^{211}At labeled lectins and antibodies, *Int. J. Nucl. Med. Biol.*, 9, 167, 1982.
41. **Vaughan, A. T. M., Bateman, W. J., and Fischer, D. R.,** The in vivo fate of ^{211}At labeled monoclonal antibody with known specificity in a murine system, *Int. J. Radiat. Oncol. Bio. Phys.*, 8, 1943, 1982.
42. **Bloomer, W. D., McLaughlin, W. H., and Adelstein, S. J.,** Therapeutic implications of iodine -125 cytotoxicity, *Int. J. Radiation Oncol. Bio. Phys.*, 8, 1903, 1982.
43. **Foulds, L.,** The experimental study of tumor progression: a review, *Cancer Res.*, 14, 327, 1954.
44. **Hart, I. R., and Fidler, I. J.,** The implications of tumor heterogeneity for studies on the biology and therapy of cancer metastases, *Biochim. Biophys. Acta,* 651, 37, 1981.
45. **Prehn, R. T.,** Analyses of antigenic heterogeneity within individual 3 - methylcholanthrene-induced mouse sarcomas, *J. Natl. Cancer Inst.*, 45, 1039, 1970.
46. **Muller, F. R. and Heppner, G. H.,** Immunologic heterogeneity of tumor cell subpopulations from a single mouse mammary tumor, *J. Natl. Cancer Inst.*, 63, 1457, 1979.
47. **Colcher, D., Horan-Hand, P., Teramoto, Y. A., Wunderlich, D., and Schlom, J.,** Monoclonal antibodies define diversity of mammary tumor viral gene products in virions and mammary tumors of the genus Mus, *Cancer Res.*, 41, 1451, 1981.
48. **Meeker, T. C., Lowder, J., Maloney, D., Miller, R. A., Thielemans, K., Warnke, R., and Levy, R.,** A clinical trial of antiidiotype therapy for B-cell malignancy, *Blood,* 65, 1349, 1985.
49. **Ritz, J., Pesando, J. M., Notis-McConarty, J., and Schlossman, S. F.,** Modulation of human acute lymphoblastic leukemia antigen induced by monoclonal antibody in vitro, *J. Immunol.*, 125, 1506, 1980.
50. **Cobbold, S. P. and Waldmann, H.,** Therapeutic potential of monovalent monoclonal antibodies, *Nature (London),* 308, 460, 1984.
51. **Sklar, J., Cleary, M. L., Thielemans, K., Gralow, J., Warnke, R., and Levy, R.,** Biclonal B-cell lymphoma, *N. Engl. J. Med.*, 311, 20, 1984.
52. **Raffeld, M., Neckers, L., Longo, D. L., and Cossman, J.,** Spontaneous alteration of idiotype in a monoclonal B-cell lymphoma, *N. Engl. J. Med.*, 312, 1653, 1985.
53. **Mach, J. P., Forni, M., Ritchard, J., Buchegger, F., Carrel, S., Widgren, S., Donath, A., and Alberto, P.,** Use and limitations of radiolabeled anti-CEA antibodies and their fragments for photoscanning detection of human colorectal carcinomas, *Oncodev. Biol. Med.*, 1, 49, 1980.
54. **Dillman, R. O., Beauregard, J. C., Sobol, R. E., Royston, I., Bartholomew, R. M., Hagan, P. S., and Halpern, S. E.,** Lack of radioimmunodetection and complications associated with monoclonal anticarcioembryonic antigen antibody cross-reactivity with an antigen in circulating cells, *Cancer Res.*, 44, 2213, 1984.
55. **Mann, B. D., Cohen, M.B., Saxton, R. E., Morton, D. L., Benedict, W. F., Korn, E. L., Spolter, L., Graham, L. S., Chang, C. C., Burk, M. W.,** Imaging of human tumor xenografts in nude mice with radiolabeled monoclonal antibodies: limitations of specificity due to nonspecific uptake of antibody, *Cancer,* 54, 1318, 1984.
56. **Duran-Reynolds, F.,** Studies in the localization of dyes and foreign proteins in normal and malignant tissues, *Am. J. Cancer,* 35, 98, 1939.
57. **Rostock, R. A., Klein, J. L., Leichner, P. K., Order, S. E.,** Distribution of and physiologic factors that affect ^{131}I-antiferritin tumor localization in experimental hepatoma, *Int. J. Radiat. Oncol. Biol. Phys.*, 10, 1135, 1984.
58. **Goldenberg, D. M., DeLand, F., Kim, E.,** Use of radiolabeled antibodies to carcinoembryonic antigen for the detection and localization of diverse cancers by external photoscanning, *N. Engl. J. Med.*, 298, 1384, 1978.
59. **DeLand, F. H., Kim, E. E., and Simmons, G.,** Imaging approach in radioimmunodetection, *Cancer Res.*, 40, 3046, 1980.
60. **Primus, F. F. and Goldenberg, D. M.,** Immunological considerations in the use of goat antibodies to carcinoembryonic antigen for the radioimmunodetection of cancer, *Cancer Res.*, 40, 2979, 1983.
61. **Ghose, T., Ferrone, S., Iniai, K., Norvell, S. T., Luner, S. J., and Martin, R. H.,** Imaging of human melanoma xenografts in nude mice with a radiolabeled monoclonal antibody, *J. Natl. Cancer Inst.*, 69, 823, 1982.
62. **Moldofsky, P. J., Sears, H. F., Mulhern, C. B., Jr., Hammond, N. D., Powe, J., Gatenby, R. A., Steplewski, Z., and Koprowski, H.,** Detection of metastatic tumor in normal-sized retroperitoneal lymph nodes by monoclonal antibody imaging, *N. Engl. J. Med.*, 311, 106, 1984.

63. **Vial, A. B. and Callahan, W.**, The effect of some tagged antibodies in human melanoblastoma, *Cancer*, 10, 999, 1957.
64. **Colcher, D., Zalutsky, M., Kaplan, W., Kufe, D., Austin, F., and Sclom, J.**, Radiolocalization of human mammary tumors in athymic mice by a monoclonal antibody, *Cancer Res.*, 43, 736, 1983.
65. **Moshakis, V., McIlhinney, R. A. J., Raghaven, D., and Neville, A. M.**, Localization of human tumor xenografts after intravenous administration of radiolabeled monoclonal antibodies, *Br. J. Cancer.*, 44, 91, 1981.
66. **Houston, L. L., Nowinski, R. C., and Bernstein, I. D.**, Specific in vivo localization of monoclonal antibodies directed against the Thy 1.1 antigen, *Immunology*, 125, 837, 1980.
67. **Herlyn, D. M., Steplewski, Z., Herlyn, M. F., and Koprowski, H.**, Inhibition of growth of colorectal carcinoma in nude mice by monoclonal antibody, *Cancer Res.*, 40, 717, 1980.
68. **Herlyn, D. M., Steplewski, Z., Herlyn, M. F., and Koprowski, H.**, Monoclonal antibodies in cell-mediated cytotoxicity against human melanoma and colorectal carcinoma, *Eur. J. Immunol.*, 9, 657, 1979.
69. **Scheinberg, D. A. and Strand, M.**, Leukemic cell targeting and therapy by monoclonal antibody in a mouse model system, *Cancer Res.*, 42, 44, 1982.
70. **Bernstein, I. D., Tam, M. R., and Nowinski, R. C.**, Mouse leukemia: therapy with monoclonal antibodies against a thymus differentiation antigen, *Science*, 207, 68, 1980.
71. **Miller, R. A. and Levy, R.**, Response of cutaneous T-cell lymphoma to therapy with hybridoma monoclonal antibody, *Lancet*, 2, 226, 1981.
72. **Miller, R. A., Maloney, D. G., McKellop, J., and Levy, R.**, *In vivo* effects of murine hybridoma monoclonal antibody in a patient with T-cell leukemia, *Blood*, 58, 78, 1981.
73. **Ritz, J., Pesando, J. M., Sallan, S. E., Clavell, L. A., and Notis-McConarty, J.**, Serotherapy of acute lymphoblastic leukemia with monoclonal antibody, *Blood*, 58, 141, 1981.
74. **Casellas, P., Brown, J. P., Gros, P., Hellstrom, I., Jansen, F. K., and Ponert, P. S.**, Human melanoma cells can be killed *in vitro* by an immunotoxin specific for melanoma associated antigen p97, *Int. J. Cancer*, 30, 437, 1982.
75. **Ghose, T., Norvell, S. T., Gucla, A., Cameron, D., Bodurtha, A., and McDonald, A. S.**, Immunochemotherapy of cancer with chlorambucil-carrying antibody, *Br. Med. J.*, 3, 495, 1972.
76. **Tsukada, Y., Hurwitz, E., Kashi, R., Sela, M., Hibi, N., Hara, A., and Hirai, H.**, Chemotherapy by intravenous administration of conjugates of daunomycin with monoclonal and conventional antirat alpha-feto-protein antibodies, *Proc. Natl. Acad. Sci. U.S.A.*, 79, 7896, 1982.
77. **Vitetta, E. S., Krolick, K. A., Miyama-Inaba, M., Cushley, W., and Uhr, J. W.**, Immunotoxins: a new approach to cancer therapy, *Science*, 219, 644, 1983.
78. **Rembaum, A., Dreyer, W. J.**, Immunomicrospheres: reagents for call labeling and separation, *Science*, 208, 364, 1980.
79. **Leichner, P. K., Klein, J. L., Garrison, S. B., Jenkins, R. E., Nickloff, E. L., Ettinger, D. S., and Order, S. E.**, Dosimetry of ^{131}I-labeled antiferritin in hepatoma: a model for radioimmunoglobulin dosimetry, *Int. J. Radiat. Oncol. Bio. Phys.*, 7, 323, 1981.
80. **Ettinger, D. S., Order, S. E., Wharan, M. D., Parker, M. K., Klein, J. L., Leichner, P. K.**, Phase 1-11 study of isotopic immunoglobulin therapy for primary liver carcinoma, *Cancer Treat. Rep.*, 66, 289, 1982.
81. **Lenhard, R. E., Order, S. E., Spunberg, J. J., Asbell, S. O., and Leibel, S. A.**, Isotopic immunoglobulin: a new systemic therapy for advanced Hodgkin's Disease, *J. Clin. Oncol.*, 3, 1296, 1985.
82. **Okuda, K., Oktsuki, T., Obata, H., Tomimatsu, M., Okasaki, N., Hasegawa, H., Nakajima, V., and Ohnishi, K.**, Natural history of hepatocellular carcinoma and prognosis in relation to treatment. Study of 850 patients, *Cancer*, 56, 918, 1985.
83. **Order, S. E., Stillwagon, G. B., Klein, J. L., Leichner, P. K., Siegelman, S. S., Fishman, E. K., Ettinger, D. S., Haulk, T., Kopher, K., Finney, K., Surdyke, M., Seir, S., and Leibel, S.**, Iodine-^{131} antiferritin, a new treatment modality in hepatoma: a Radiation Therapy Oncology Group Study, *J. Clin. Oncol.*, 3, 1573, 1985.
84. **Rostock, R. A., Klein, J. L., Kopher, K. A., and Order, S. E.**, Variables affecting the tumor localization of ^{131}I-antiferritin in experimental hepatoma, *Am. J. Clin. Oncol. (CCT)*, 6, 9, 1984.
85. **Rawles, M. E.**, Origin of the mammalian pigment cell and its role in the pigmentation of hair, in *Pigment Cell Growth*, Gordon, M., Ed., Academic Press, Orlando, 1953, 1.
86. **Elwood, J. M., Lee, J. A. H.**, Recent data on the epidemiology of malignant melanoma, *Semin. Oncol.*, 2, 149, 1975.
87. **Cutler, S. J. and Young, J. L., Jr.**, *Third National Cancer Survey: Incidence Data, Natl. Cancer Inst. Monogr.*, 41, 20, 1975.
88. **Mastrangelo, M. J., Rosenberg, S. A., Baker, A. R., Katz, H. R.**, Cutaneous melanoma, in *Cancer: Principles and Practice of Oncology*, DeVita, V. J., Jr., Hellman, S., and Rosenberg, S. A., Eds., Lippincott, Philadelphia, 1982, 1124.

89. **Brown, J. P., Nishiyamau, K., Hellstrom, I., and Hellstrom, K. E.,** Structural characterization of human melanoma-associated antigen p97 using monoclonal antibodies, *J. Immunol.*, 127, 539, 1981.
90. **Brown, J. P., Woodbury, R. G., Hart, C. E., Hellstrom, I., and Hellstrom, K. E.,** Quantitative analysis of melanoma-associated antigen p97 in normal and neoplastic tissues, *Proc. Natl. Acad. Sci. U.S.A.*, 78, 539, 1981.
91. **Woodbury, R. J., Brown, J. P., Yeh, M. Y., Hellstrom, I., and Hellstrom, K. E.,** Identification of cell surface protein, p97, in human melanomas and certain other neoplasms. *Proc. Natl. Acad. U.S.A.*, 77, 2183, 1980.
92. **Brown, J. P., Hewick, R. M., Hellstrom, I., Hellstrom, K. E., Doolittle, R. F., Dreyer, W. J.,** Human melanoma-associated antigen is structurally and functionally related to transferrin, *Nature (London)*, 296, 171, 1982.
93. **Larson, S. M., Brown, J. P., Wright, P. W., Carrasquillo, J. A., Hellstrom, I., and Hellstrom, K. E.,** Imaging of melanoma with ^{131}I-labeled monoclonal antibodies, *J. Nucl. Med.*, 24, 123, 1983.
94. **Larson, S. M., Carrasquillo, J. A., Korhn, K. A., Brown, J. P., McGuffin, R. W., Ferens, J. M., Graham, M. M., Hill, L. D., Beumier, P. L., Hellstrom, K. E., and Hellstrom, I.,** Localization of ^{131}I-labeled p97-specific Fab fragments in human melanoma as a basis for radiotherapy, *J. Clin. Invest.*, 72, 2101, 1983.
95. **Goodman, G. E., Baumier, P., Hellstrom, I., Fernyhough, B., and Hellstrom, K. E.,** Pilot trial of murine monoclonal antibodies in patients with advanced melanoma. *J. Clin. Oncol.*, 3, 340, 1985.
96. **Larson, S. M., Carrasquillo, J. A., and Reynolds, J. C.,** Radioimmunodetection and radioimmunotherapy, *Cancer Invest.*, 2, 363, 1984.
97. **DeNardo, G. L., Raventos, A., Hines, H. H., Scheibe, P. O., Maley, D. J., Hays, M. T., and DeNardo, S. J.,** Requirements for a treatment planning system for radioimmunotherapy, *Int. J. Radiat. Oncol. Biol. Phys.*, 11, 335, 1985.
98. **Badger, C. C. and Bernstein, I. D.,** Monoclonal antibody therapy of murine leukemia. *J. Exp. Med.*, 157, 828, 1983.
99. **Bernstein, I. D., Tam, M. C., and Nowinski, R. C.,** Mouse leukemia: therapy with monoclonal antibodies against a thymus differentiation antigen, *Science*, 207, 68, 1980.
100. **Badger, C. C., Krohn, K. A., Peterson, A. V., Shulman, H., and Bernstein, I. D.,** Experimental radiotherapy of murine lymphoma with ^{131}I-labeled anti-Thy 1.1 monoclonal antibody, *Cancer Res.*, 45, 1536, 1985.
101. **Scheinberg, D. A. and Strand, M.,** Kinetic and catabolic considerations of monoclonal antibody targeting in erythroleukemic mice, *Cancer Res.*, 43, 265, 1983.
102. **Redwood, W. R., Tom, T. D., and Strand, M.,** Specificity, efficacy and toxicity of radioimmunotherapy in erythroleukemic mice, *Cancer Res.*, 44, 5681, 1984.

Chapter 11

ANTIBODY-MEDIATED RADIOTHERAPY: FUTURE PROSPECTS

Michael R. Zalutsky

TABLE OF CONTENTS

I. INTRODUCTION

Although the development of monoclonal antibodies may result in major advances in the diagnosis of cancer, it is anticipated that their major impact will be on the treatment of human malignancies. A particularly attractive approach to cancer therapy is to employ antibodies directed against tumor-associated antigens as carriers for the selective delivery of toxic doses of radiation to tumor cells. Since isotopes are available which emit radiation with different ranges of action, an advantage of radioimmunotherapy is the potential for choosing the type of radiation with a range which is most compatible with a particular tumor type, size, and anatomic location. This is in contrast to the use of immunotoxins, an approach in which the therapeutic effect is always dependent upon internalization of the toxin-antibody conjugate by each individual target cell.[1,2]

While the idea of selectively destroying tumors by combining a cytotoxic agent with a tumor-directed antibody was first recognized more than 80 years ago,[3] it was not until 1960 that Bale and co-workers[4] demonstrated that an antibody could be used to carry a therapeutic dose of radioactivity to a tumor. The isotope used in this study was iodine-131, which has an 8-day half-life and decays by the emission of beta particles which have a maximum range of 2.1 mm in tissue. It is worth noting that the vast majority of radioimmunotherapeutic trials reported since this initial study have continued to use iodine-131 as the isotope.

Although iodine-131 is probably an adequate label for some radioimmunotherapeutic applications, it also has several characteristics which limit its utility, principally because they can cause significant irradiation of normal tissues. These properties include

1. Dehalogenation in vivo
2. Emission of medium-energy gamma rays
3. Relatively long half-life
4. Maximum beta range of about 200 cell diameters

In this chapter, the potential utility of isotopes other than iodine-131 is explored. Factors influencing the selection of an isotope for antibody-mediated radiotherapy including dosimetric considerations are discussed, not only for other beta emitters, but also for isotopes decaying by the emission of alpha particles and short-range electrons. The evaluation of radioimmunotherapeutic agents both in vitro and in animal models is also described. Finally, several stratagies are presented for improving the therapeutic index of radiolabeled antibodies.

II. DOSIMETRIC CONSIDERATIONS

The systematic evaluation of the efficacy of radioimmunotherapy requires the development of techniques for calculating the radiation absorbed dose to both the tumor and surrounding normal tissues. In nuclear medicine, the conventional approach is to use the procedures developed by the Medical Internal Radiation Dose Committee (MIRD).[5,6] In this formalism, the average dose rate to an organ or tissue is given by:

$$D = \frac{2.13A}{m} \sum_i n_i E_i \phi_i \text{ rad}$$

where A is the cumulated activity in μCi hours, m is the mass of the tissue in grams, n_i is the fractional abundance of the radiative event, E_i is the average energy in MeV, and ϕ_i is the absorbed fraction for the organ volume.

In the standard MIRD approach, certain assumptions are made which in some cases may not be appropriate for antibody radiotherapy dosimetry calculations. It is assumed, for example, that the isotope and resultant radiation dose are distributed homogeneously throughout each organ. Kwok et al.[7] have recently used a modified MIRD approach to calculate the dose received by a 1 gm target and surrounding normal tissue from three types of target activity distributions: uniform, diffusion limited into target, and limited by diffusion and including time dependent redistribution of the isotope into peripheral regions of the target volume. This methodology will be helpful in evaluating the effects of poorly perfused necrotic areas and antigen shedding on the heterogeneity of absorbed doses received by different regions in a tumor.

Since the binding of antibody to antigen occurs in cellular dimensions, it will often be more relevant to consider the dose received by the target cells at a cellular level. Indeed, since most radiobiological studies have demonstrated that the cell nucleus, in particular the DNA, is the most radiosensitive cellular component, distribution of radiation dose at a subcellular level will sometimes be required. The need for microdosimetric approaches will, of course, depend upon the range of the radiation employed and upon the uniformity of its distribution relative to the dimensions of a particular tumor target.

The inadequacy of MIRD dosimetry calculations for predicting radiation effects occurring at the cellular level has been illustrated in several recent studies. These experiments employed isotopes decaying by the emission of electrons of cellular range that had been localized intracellularly. Kassis et al.[8] have compared the in vitro cytotoxicity of Tl-201, which decays in part by the emission of electrons of subcellular range, to that of three beta emitters. Contrary to what would have been predicted by macroscopic dosimetry calculations, the lower energy electrons were more toxic than the higher energy beta particles of K-42, K-43 and Rb-86. In addition, the radiotoxicity of Tl-201 could be inhibited by ouabain, suggesting that intracellular localization was a prerequisite for the toxic effect of this isotope. The same group has also measured the in vitro cytotoxicity of Cr-51 and reported that the dose received by cells taking up this isotope is more than 100 times greater than would have been predicted from a MIRD-type calculation.[9] Similar differences have been observed in vivo. Rao et al.[10] have reported that Tl-201 was more effective in reducing sperm heads in mice than the higher energy beta emitter Tl-204.

The need for microdosimetric approaches is most evident for isotopes decaying by emission of low energy electrons and/or alpha particles. Sastry and Rao[11] have recently considered several dosimetric approaches for use with electrons of subcellular range. An approach for calculating the microdosimetry of monoclonal antibodies labeled with alpha emitters has also been reported.[12] A general review of microdosimetry can be found in Reference 13.

III. SELECTION OF THE RADIONUCLIDE

The goal of radioimmunotherapy is to exploit the potential tumor specificity of monoclonal antibodies to selectively destroy cancer cells. Strategies must be devised which will permit the delivery of cytotoxic doses of radiation to the tumor while minimizing the irradiation of surrounding normal tissues. The selection of an appropriate isotope for antibody radiotherapy will depend upon a multitude of factors many of which must also be considered for diagnostic applications. These include the chemical aspects of antibody labeling, the stability of the bond between the radionuclide and antibody in vivo, the density of antigenic sites on the tumor cell (and on normal tissues), and the pharmacokinetics of antibody uptake and retention in both target and nontarget tissues. These issues are addressed in detail in other chapters in this volume.

Several groups have performed calculations in an attempt to evaluate the potential utility of various isotopes for use in radioimmunotherapy. Wessels and Rogus[14] used standard MIRD formalism to compare the efficacy of treating a 500 gm tumor located in the liver with an antibody labeled with several different isotopes. Animal biodistribution data from

Table 1
DISTANCES IN CELL DIAMETERS[a] FOR DEPOSITION OF 50% AND 90% OF THE ENERGY FROM A POINT SOURCE OF SELECTED ISOTOPES

	Cell diameters	
Isotope	**50% Deposition**	**90% Deposition**
^{67}Cu	18	57
^{97}Ru	12	61
^{100}Pd	2.6	5.7
^{101m}Rh	0.5	77
^{119}Sb	0.4	0.6
^{123}I	8.3	25
^{131}I	26	71
^{197}Hg	3.1	5.5

[a] Assuming cell diameter of 10 μm.

Adapted from Jungerman, J. A., Yu, K-H. P., and Zanelli, C. I., *Int. J. Appl. Radiat. Isotop.*, 35, 883, 1984.

the literature were used to estimate tumor-to-normal-tissue ratios. Based on these assumptions, the beta emitters Re-186 and Y-90 were predicted to be valuable isotopes for use in antibody radiotherapy.

Jungerman and co-workers[15] have calculated the dose distribution in cellular dimensions for seven potential electron-emitting radionuclides. In Table 1, their data have been adapted to compare the range in cell diameters required for 50% and 90% energy deposition. Beta emitters such as Cu-67 and I-131 deposit most of their energy over a range of greater than 50 cells while some of the conversion and Auger electron emitters deposit their energy in a volume approximating that of a single cell.

Of critical importance to the success of radioimmunotherapy is the selection of a radionuclide that de-excites by emission of radiation of a range which is most appropriate for each individual therapeutic application. The ideal isotope for treating a stage III hepatoma of 500 gm is likely to be different from either the one selected for treating a micrometastases of a few hundred cells or a tumor of the circulatory system such as a lymphoma. The degree of heterogeneity of antigen expression among the cells in the tumor will also dictate the relative efficacy of using radiation of cellular or macro range. In addition, the proximity of the tumor to highly radiosensitive cell populations must also be considered.

Isotopes of potential utility for antibody radiotherapy are available which emit radiation of subcellular to multicellular range. Beta emitters with ranges of several millimeters are probably the isotopes of choice for treating larger tumors whose anatomic location precludes surgery. Isotopes decaying by alpha or, in some cases, low energy electron emission might be employed for micrometastatic disease. If the antibody is internalized into the tumor cell, it may be possible to exploit the exquisite radiotoxicity and subcellular range of certain Auger and Coster-Kronig electron emitters. The details of these approaches will be discussed in the sections which follow.

IV. BETA EMITTERS

The clinical application of nuclides for radiotherapy has been confined to the use of beta-

Table 2
SOME BETA-EMITTING ISOTOPES OF POTENTIAL UTILITY FOR ANTIBODY RADIOTHERAPY

Isotope	Half-life	E_{max}(keV)	Yield per 100 decays
^{47}Sc	3.42 days	450	74
		610	26
^{67}Cu	2.58 days	395	45
		484	35
		577	20
^{90}Y	6.41 hr	2288	100
^{109}Pd	13.4 hr	1028	100
^{131}I	8.08 days	336	13
		606	86
^{186}Re	90.6 hr	934	22
		1072	70
^{188}Re	16.9 hr	1973	24
		2128	74
^{212}Bi	60.6 min	1550	6
		2270	40

emitting isotopes. With the exception of a recent report describing the use of ^{90}Y-labeled antiferritin in patients,[16] radioimmunotherapeutic trials have been limited to the use of iodine-131. Although some of the responses obtained following treatment with ^{131}I-labeled antibodies have been encouraging, it is clear that for some applications, a higher therapeutic index could be obtained by labeling the antibody with a different isotope.

Several beta-emitting nuclides of potential utility for antibody radiotherapy are listed in Table 2. Use of these isotopes could offer the following advantages:

1. Decreased loss of label from the antibody in vivo due to improved chemical stability
2. A beta particle range which is more compatible with the dimensions of the tumor
3. A shorter half-life which could minimize irradiation of normal tissues due to loss of label from the antibody over time

A. Rhenium-188

Rhenium-188 has a half-life of 16.9 hr and a maximum beta energy of 2.128 MeV. This isotope is particularly attractive because it could be supplied conveniently from a radionuclide generator system using 69.4-day ^{188}W as the parent. Tungsten-188 can be produced in a nuclear reactor by irradiation of ^{186}W via double neutron capture.[17] Generator systems for the separation of ^{188}Re from ^{188}W which utilize columns of anion exchange resin,[18] alumina,[19] and zirconium oxide[17,20] have all been reported. With zirconium oxide columns, elution yields of about 85% could be obtained with breakthrough of the ^{188}W parent of less than 10^{-4}%.

Since the chemistry of rhenium is similar to that of technetium, it may be possible to adapt some of the methodologies which have been developed for ^{99m}Tc, the most commonly used isotope in nuclear medicine, to the labeling of antibodies with ^{188}Re (and ^{186}Re). It should be expected, however, that the synthesis of rhenium complexes will be considerably more difficult because rhenium is more kinetically inert than technetium. Fritzberg and coworkers[21] have been investigating the possibility of labeling antibodies with rhenium isotopes through the formation of rhenium complexes with diamine dimercaptide ligands because technetium readily forms complexes of this type. One such complex, Re-CO_2DADS, could be prepared by an exchange reaction between $ReO_2(en)_2Cl$ and the N_2S_2 ligand at slightly alkaline pH.

B. Yttrium-90

There is considerable interest in using ^{90}Y-labeled antibodies for radiotherapeutic applications. Properties of this isotope which might be suitable for this application include its 64 hr half-life, lack of gamma emissions, and chemical properties which may permit the labeling of antibodies via bifunctional chelates. Unfortunately, use of DTPA chelates originally developed for labeling antibodies with ^{111}In does not appear to produce a ^{90}Y-labeled protein which is stable in vivo. For example, when an anti-CEA antibody was labeled with ^{90}Y using DTPA anhydride and injected into mice, a significant fraction of the injected dose was recovered in the liver.[22] Hnatowich et al.[23] have used the cyclic anhydride of DTPA to label human IgG and the $F(ab')_2$ fragment of antibody 19-9 with ^{90}Y. Incubation of the labeled proteins with human serum at 37°C followed by analysis by antitransferrin and CA 19-9 affinity chromatography was used to demonstrate a loss of 13% of the ^{90}Y from the antibody per day. The availability of ^{90}Y-labeled antibodies with adequate stability in vivo will probably require the development of chelates which are more specifically designed for use with ^{90}Y.

C. Copper-67

One of the most attractive radionuclides for use in antibody-mediated radiotherapy is ^{67}Cu. As shown in Table 2, this isotope has a half-life of 2.58 days and decays by the emission of beta particles with maximum energies of 395 to 577 keV. Calculations based on the data of Jungerman et al.[15] indicate that a point source of ^{67}Cu would deposit 90% of its energy over a range of about 60 cell diameters (see Table 1). Copper-67 also emits several gamma rays of 91 to 185 keV which are of appropriate energy for imaging. Quantitative images of the distribution of ^{67}Cu in patients undergoing therapy could provide valuable data for the calculation of the radiation absorbed dose received by both normal tissues and possibly tumor.

Antibodies have been labeled with ^{67}Cu using several DTPA and EDTA bifunctional chelates. Chelates which have been employed include isothiocyanobenzyl-EDTA[24] and the cyclic anhydride of DTPA.[25] The stability of ^{67}Cu-labeled proteins prepared using EDTA and DTPA chelates has not been satisfactory. DeNardo et al.[26] have compared the stability of several DTPA and EDTA chelates of both ^{111}In and ^{67}Cu in the presence of serum by high-performance liquid chromatography (HPLC) analysis. In contrast to the results obtained with the ^{111}In chelates, the ^{67}Cu complexes rapidly dissociated in serum. The differential stability which was observed was attributed to the fact that copper forms strong complexes with proteins such as albumin.[27]

In an effort to produce ^{67}Cu monoclonal antibodies with improved stability, several groups have been investigating alternative chelate systems. Franz et al.[28] have synthesized a cyclam analogue tetradentate macrocyclic amine for use with ^{67}Cu. Although no exchange of copper activity to EDTA was observed over 3 days, stability studies in the presence of serum were not reported. N-benzyl porphyrin chelating agents are also being investigated for use with ^{67}Cu.[29]

Perhaps the most promising results obtained to date have involved the use of a new macrocycle, TETA, which was specifically designed for use with copper.[27] A bifunctional chelate, 6(p-bromoacetamidobenzyl)-TETA was then used to label antibodies with ^{67}Cu. Loss of ^{67}Cu activity from the protein in the presence of serum was only about 1%/day.

D. Palladium-109

Fawwaz and co-workers[30] have been investigating the feasibility of labeling antibodies with the 13.4-hr half-life beta emitter ^{109}Pd. An antimelanoma monoclonal antibody was labeled in about 10% yield with ^{109}Pd using the cyclic anhydride of DTPA. The ^{109}Pd-labeled antibody bound specifically to human melanoma but not to lymphoma cells in vitro. Uptake

Table 3
SOME ISOTOPES EMITTING RADIATION WITH RANGES LESS THAN TEN CELL DIAMETERS

Isotope	Half-life	Type	E(KeV)	Yield per 100 decays
^{211}At	7.2 hr	Alpha	5866	42
		Alpha	7450	58
^{212}Bi	60.6 min	Alpha	6051	25
		Alpha	6090	10
^{100}Pd	3.64 days	Conv. elec. (L)	71-81	6
		Conv. elec. (K)	52-61	47
^{197}Hg	2.71 days	Auger (K)	52	4
		Conv. elec. (L)	64	65
		Conv. elec. (M)	74	15

of ^{109}Pd activity in human melanoma xenografts implanted in nude mice was more than 18%/g from 13 to 48 hr after injection of labeled antibody, while activity in the blood was at least an order of magnitude lower.

V. ALPHA EMITTERS

One of the principal drawbacks to using beta-emitting isotopes for antibody-directed radiotherapy is that significant irradiation of normal tissue can occur due to the relatively long range (greater than 1 cm for ^{90}Y, for example) of their radiation. With the caveat that the problem of tumor-cell heterogeneity can be addressed through the use of mixtures of monoclonal antibodies, an attractive alternative for radioimmunotherapy would be to combine the potential tumor cell specificity of these antibodies with a nuclide decaying by the emission of radiation more approximating cellular dimensions.

Alpha-particle-emitting isotopes could be ideal for this purpose for several reasons. First, the range of 5 to 8 MeV alpha particles in tissue equivalent medium is only about 4 to 6 cell diameters. Second, their cytotoxic effects appear to be relatively oxygen independent. Alpha particles are a type of radiation of high linear energy transfer, about 100 to 125 keV/μm. Because of their short range and high linear energy transfer, alpha particles have a higher probability of causing double DNA strand breaks than beta particles. Thus, the considerable cytotoxicity of alpha particles is not unexpected. Indeed, both in-beam and radionuclide studies have shown that only 2 to 16 alpha traversals per cell are required to achieve cell killing.[31-33]

Among the alpha emitters, few nuclides can both be produced in reasonable yield and possess half-lives which are appropriate for use in antibody radiotherapy. Two alpha-emitting isotopes which might be suitable for some applications are ^{212}Bi and ^{211}At. Pertinent decay properties of these isotopes are listed in Table 3.

A. Astatine-211

Among the alpha-emitting nuclides, ^{211}At appears to be a promising candidate for use in radioimmunotherapy. The decay scheme of ^{211}At is shown in Figure 1. This nuclide has a half-life of 7.2 hr and the emission of an alpha particle is associated with every decay of ^{211}At. The plonium X-rays which are also emitted facilitate the measurement of ^{211}At activity levels during the course of chemical and biological investigations. Although astatine possesses some metallic characteristics, it has some chemical similarities to iodine, an element whose isotopes are readily incorporated into proteins.

Astatine-211 can be produced in a cyclotron by the irradiation of a natural bismuth target

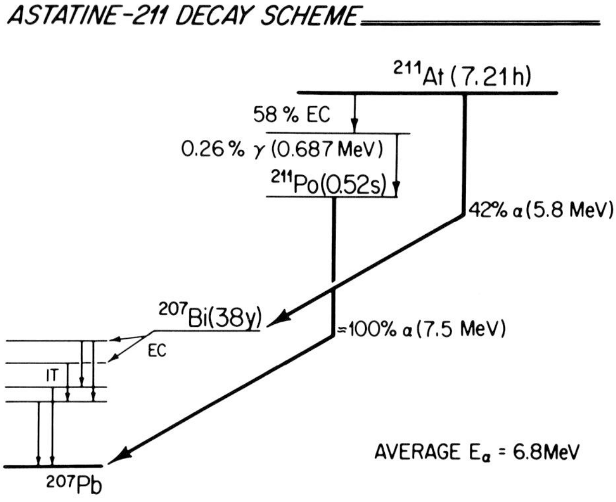

FIGURE 1. Decay scheme of astatine-211.

with alpha particles via the ^{209}Bi(α, 2n)^{211}At reaction. Care must be taken to keep the incident alpha energy below 29 MeV, the threshold for ^{210}At production, because this 8.1-hr half-life isotope decays to ^{210}Po, which is a 138-day half-life alpha emitter. Isolation of ^{211}At from the bismuth target can be most conveniently achieved by distillation at 600 to 700°C into a solution of dilute sodium hydroxide and sodium metabisulfite.[34,35] A recent modification of this procedure is the distillation of ^{211}At onto a small column of silica, permitting the subsequent isolation of astatine in a variety of solvent systems.[36]

Attempts to label proteins using the standard methods for protein iodination have not produced an astatinated protein that is stable either in vitro or in vivo.[34,37] This can probably be attributed to the fact that astatotyrosine has been shown to deastatinate in the presence of oxidants such as those used in electrophilic halogenation.[38] Visser et al.[39] have observed that when astatide was reacted with different proteins in the presence of hydrogen peroxide, only proteins containing free thiol groups could be labeled, suggesting the formation of S–At bonds. Although the rate of deastatination of proteins with free thiols was lower, the stability reported for the ^{211}At-labeled thiolated proteins would not be sufficient for radioimmunotherapeutic applications.

In an effort to produce an astatinated protein which would be more stable in vivo, we developed a two-step procedure which involves the synthesis of an astatinated intermediate followed by the addition of this compound to the protein via an acylation reaction.[35,40] In the first step, illustrated in Figure 2, p-astatobenzoic acid was synthesized in 70 to 90% yield by reacting astatide with the diazonium sulfate salt of p-aminobenzoic acid. Following purification of the product by extraction with diethyl ether, an astatinated mixed anhydride was formed by reaction with tributylamine and isobutylchloroformate. The labeled anhydride was then reacted with several model proteins including bovine serum albumin.

Following purification by size-exclusion chromatography, 10 to 15% of the ^{211}At activity could be isolated in the protein fraction. Comparison of the tissue distribution in mice of ^{211}At-labeled BSA to that of astatide and astatobenzoic acid suggested that the astatinated protein was stable in vivo. In addition, haemagglutination inhibition assays and immunodiffusion measurements were used to demonstrate that the labeling procedure did not significantly alter the antigenic properties of BSA.

One of the difficulties with this approach is that the specific activity of the astatinated protein is low, only about 200 μCi/mg. As shown in Figure 3, with a large excess of diazonium salt, in addition to the synthesis of astatobenzoic acid, several competitory re-

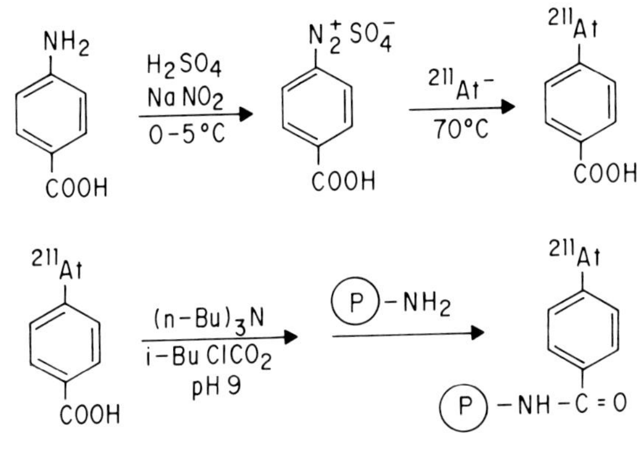

FIGURE 2. The astatobenzoic acid method for labeling proteins with astatine. First step: synthesis of p-astatobenzoic acid from corresponding diazonium salt. Second step: conjugation to protein using a mixed anhydride.

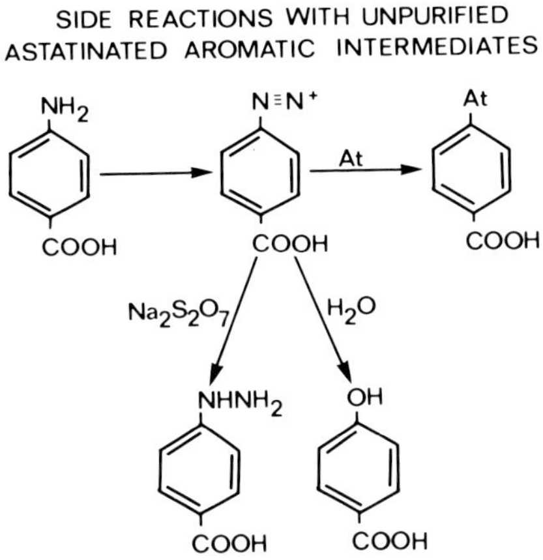

FIGURE 3. Side reactions possible with diazonium salt.

actions are possible including hydrolysis to a phenol and reduction by sodium metabisulfite (present in the solution used to trap the ^{211}At in the target distillation) to carboxyphenylhydrazine. These impurities could create two types of problems as shown in Figures 4 and 5. First, it is possible that other compounds containing free amino groups will be able to compete with the protein for astatobenzoic acid. And second, other mixed anhydrides can be formed by reaction with carboxylated impurities which can then compete with the astatinated anhydride for the amine sites on the protein.

Several groups have attempted to improve the specific activity of proteins labeled using the astatobenzoic acid method. In an attempt to avoid some of the side reactions described above, Vaughan[41] has removed the metabisulfite from the catcher solution used in the target distillation step and has used a large molar excess of iodide in the diazotization reaction. Harrison and Royle[42] have used ion-pair, reverse-phase high pressure liquid chromatography to separate p-astatobenzoic acid from unlabeled impurities such as p-hydroxybenzoic acid. While both groups reported that the overall yield for protein astatination could be increased to 30 to 40%, less than 0.05% of the protein molecules could be labeled with ^{211}At.

Our group has been investigating alternative approaches for the synthesis of astatobenzoic acids and other potential astatinated acylation reagents. Reports of the regiospecific iodination

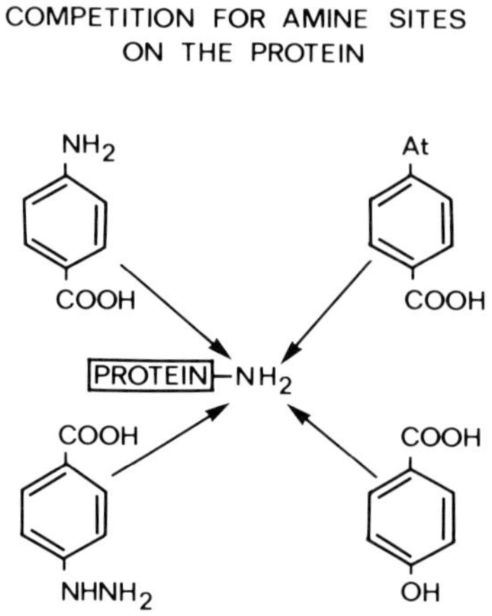

FIGURE 4. Competition of carboxylated impurities with astatobenzoic acid for amine sites on protein.

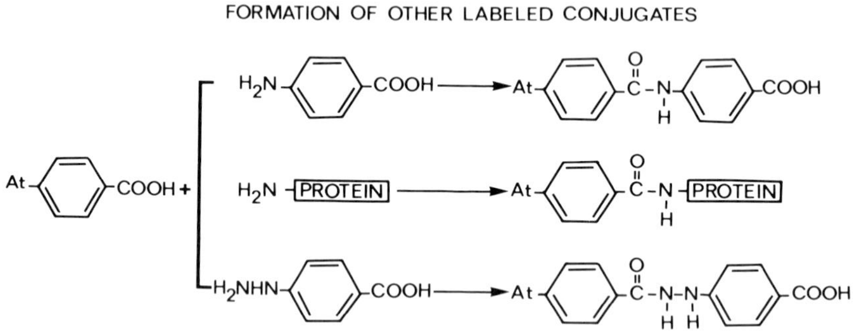

FIGURE 5. Formation of astatinated conjugate impurities.

of several compounds using aryl trialkylstannanes[43,44] encouraged us to explore the synthesis of astatobenzoic acids using this route.[45] The isomers of tri-*n*-butylstannylbenzoic acid oxazalone were synthesized in three steps from the corresponding bromobenzoic acids. Astatinations of the stannyl derivatives were performed in pH 5.5 tetrahydrofuran/ammonium acetate buffer by addition of Na ^{211}At and hydrogen peroxide. The reaction was quenched by the addition of sodium bisulfite and the astatobenzoic acids were generated by rapid sequential treatment of the labeled oxazolines with HCl and NaOH at 100°C. A rapid purification technique for the astatobenzoic acids was developed using a reverse-phase Sep-Pak® cartridge. Radiochemical yields of 10%, 82%, and 84% were obtained for o-, m-, and p-astatobenzoic acid, respectively.

The in vitro stability of the three astatobenzoic acids synthesized via the stannyl derivatives was measured in both phosphate buffered saline (PBS) and 50% fetal calf serum and compared to that of p-astatobenzoic acid which had been prepared from the diazonium salt intermediate.[46] As shown in Figure 6, the four astatobenzoic acid preparations were all stable in PBS with less than 1% deastatination observed over 37 hr for the m- and stannyl-derived p-isomers. The m- and stannyl derived p-isomers were also the most stable in the presence of serum (Figure 7). In both PBS and serum, the deastatination of p-astatobenzoic acid was much greater when the compound was prepared via the diazonium salt. This is presumably due to the formation of astatinated impurities such as azo conjugates which may be more rapidly deastatinated in serum.

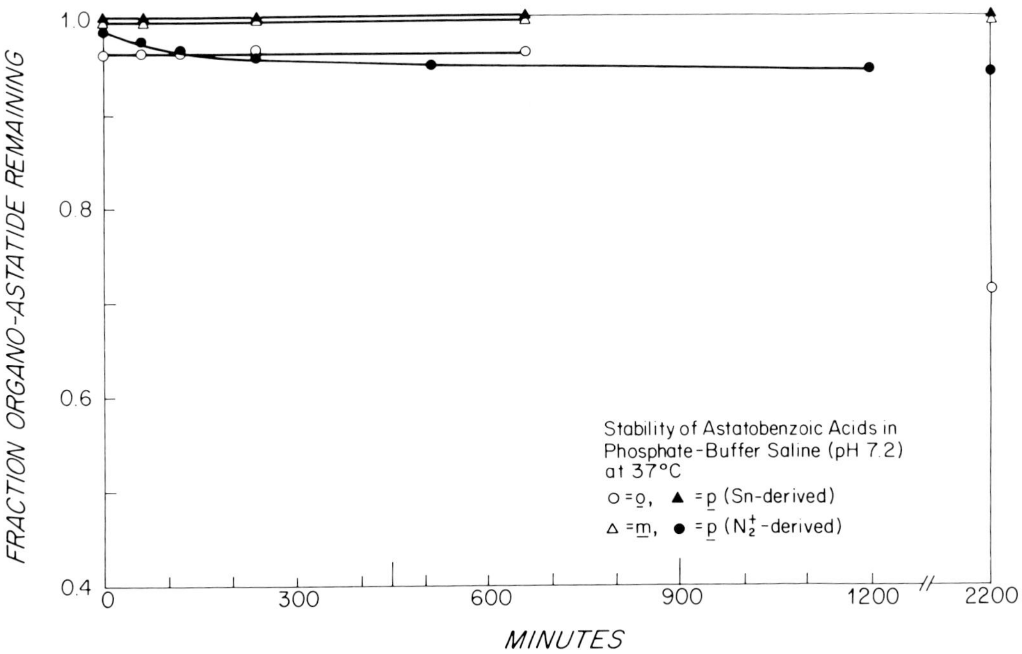

FIGURE 6. Stability of astatobenzoic acids in phosphate buffered saline.

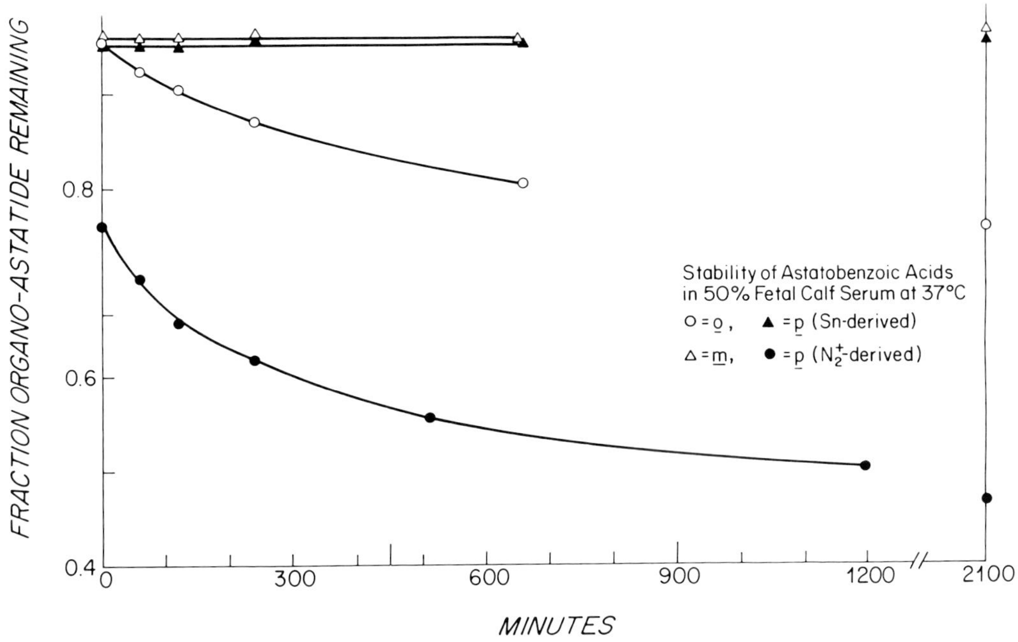

FIGURE 7. Stability of astatobenzoic acids in 50% fetal calf serum.

Vaughn[33,47-49] and co-workers have labeled several proteins including monoclonal antibodies with ^{211}At using the astatobenzoic acid method. Clonogenic assays using ^{211}At-labeled antitransferrin receptor and antihuman leukocyte monoclonal antibodies as well as Concanavalin A were used to demonstrate the exquisite cytotoxicity of cell-associated ^{211}At. Death of 63% of cells (D_{37} value) for various mouse and human cell lines could be achieved with

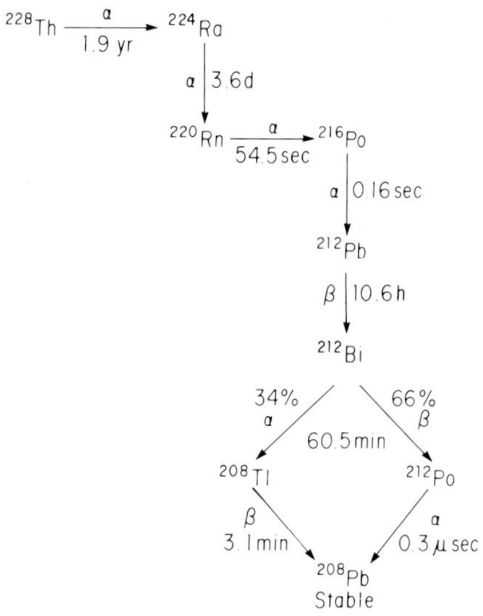

FIGURE 8. Thorium-228 decay series to ^{212}Pb and ^{212}Bi.

only 7 to 26 ^{211}At atoms bound per cell. Interpretation of these results is rendered problematic by the fact that less than 2% of the ^{211}At-labeled antibodies could be bound to antigen-positive cells in vitro and, unfortunately, no data for binding to control cell lines was reported. When the labeled antibody was injected into nude mice bearing HL60 xenografts, the localization index for ^{211}At activity in the tumor, determined by comparison to an ^{125}I-labeled control antibody, was 2 to 3 times that observed in normal tissues.

B. Bismuth-212 and the ^{212}Pb-^{212}Bi Generator

One of the main drawbacks to the use of ^{211}At-labeled monoclonal antibodies in radioimmunotherapy is that a relatively high energy cyclotron is required for the production of ^{211}At. This limits the utilization of ^{211}At to only a few research centers. A more convenient approach would be to use an alpha-emitting isotope which could be provided routinely from a radionuclide generator system with a long-lived parent.

A generator for the production of the alpha-emitting nuclides ^{212}Pb and ^{212}Bi from 1.9-year ^{228}Th was first proposed by Zucchini and Friedman.[50] As shown in Figure 8, ^{228}Th decays after the emission of four alpha particles to 10.6-hr ^{212}Pb. Lead-212 decays by beta emission to 61-min ^{212}Bi which in turn deexcites by two pathways, both of which involve the emission of an alpha and a beta particle.

In the original generator system, ^{228}Th and its ^{224}Ra daughter were absorbed on a column of sodium titanate. The gaseous ^{220}Rn daughter was eluted from the column with distilled water, and allowed to decay to ^{212}Pb which was then absorbed on a cation exchange column. Removal of ^{212}Pb and ^{212}Bi from the column was accomplished in approximately 80 to 90% yield by elution with 2*N* HCl. Addition of an anion exchange column in series with the cation column reduced the breakthrough of ^{228}Th and ^{224}Ra to less than 0.001%.

Recently, a new generator has been developed for the production of ^{212}Pb and ^{212}Bi which utilizes ^{224}Ra as the parent.[51] This approach eliminates the potential radiation hazard of using the long-lived parent, ^{228}Th in a hospital environment. The ^{224}Ra was separated from ^{228}Th by isolating the latter on an anion exchange column in nitric acid. The ^{224}Ra activity in dilute HCl was added to a 300 $\mu\ell$ cation exchange column and could be isolated in approximately 50% yield using either 0.15 *N* HI or 0.5 *N* HCl as the eluant.

Although the 10.6-hr half-life of ^{212}Pb would appear to make it a more suitable isotope than ^{212}Bi for use in radioimmunotherapy, there are two problems associated with the use of ^{212}Pb in applications requiring radiation of cellular dimensions. The first is the fact that at least one beta particle is also emitted per ^{212}Pb decay resulting in a mixture of short-range, high LET and long-range, low LET radiation. While the equilibrium absorbed dose constant for the beta radiation of ^{212}Pb is almost an order of magnitude less than that for its alpha radiation, it is actually greater than that for ^{32}P, a beta emitter commonly used in radiotherapy. And second, because ^{212}Pb decays via multiple sequential nuclear transformations, disruption of the chemical bond between the subsequent daughter products and the antibody is a strong possibility.

Monoclonal antibodies have been labeled with ^{212}Bi using several bifunctional chelates containing DTPA. In a study evaluating the relative utility of the cyclic anhydride of DTPA and 1-(p-thiocyanatobenzyl)DTPA for labeling antibodies with bismuth, it was reported that proteins labeled using the latter chelate were considerably more stable both in vitro and in vivo.[52] Recently, a monoclonal antibody directed against the human interleukin 2 (IL-2) receptor has been labeled with ^{212}Bi using the isobutylcarboxycarbonic anhydride of DTPA.[53] Cytotoxicity of the ^{212}Bi-labeled anti-Tac antibody for IL-2 receptor-positive T-cell leukemia cells was demonstrated using assays of both clonogenic survival and inhibition of protein synthesis. At a dose of 24 rad/mℓ, the survival fraction of the leukemia cells was only 1 in 1000, while the growing potential of receptor-negative cells was only reduced by 50%. Control experiments including pretreatment with cold anti-Tac and the use of a labeled irrelevant antibody support the specificity of the cytotoxic response. Although these results are encouraging, the 61-min half-life of ^{212}Bi may limit the utility of this isotope to those applications such as T-cell leukemia where rapid delivery of the labeled antibody to the tumor may be possible.

VI. LOW ENERGY ELECTRON EMITTERS

Low energy electrons are considered to be those with ranges in tissue of cellular or subcellular dimensions. The three types of electrons which can fall within these categories are conversion electrons, Auger electrons, and Coster-Kronig electrons. The two nuclear decay processes which can lead to the production of these electrons are internal conversion and electron capture.

Internal conversion results from an electromagnetic interaction between the nucleus and the atomic electrons and is an alternative decay route to gamma emission. Instead, conversion electrons are created with an energy equal to the difference between the energy of the gamma ray and the binding energy of the atomic electron. In some cases, this energy difference is only 10 to 80 keV which yields conversion electrons with ranges of about 1 to 10 cell diameters. Several examples of isotopes which emit conversion electrons in this range with half-lives which could be appropriate for antibody radiotherapy are listed in Tables 3 and 4. One can use the relationship developed by Cole[54] to estimate the range of low energy electrons in tissue:

$$R = 0.0431\,(E + 0.367)^{1.77} - 0.007$$

where R is the range in microns and E is the energy of the electron in keV.

Both internal conversion and electron capture create vacancies in the inner atomic shells of the daughter atom which are transferred by a series of rearrangements to outer atomic shells. The energy difference between the binding energies of the inner and outer shell electrons may be transferred to other outer shell electrons which are ejected from the atom. These ejected electrons are classified as Auger electrons if they arise from higher shells and as Coster-Kronig electrons if they originate from higher subshells. Each nuclear decay can

Table 4
SOME ISOTOPES EMITTING RADIATION OF SUBCELLULAR AND UNICELLULAR RANGE

Isotope	Half-life	Type	E(keV)	Yield per 100 decays
^{123}I	13.0 hr	Auger (L)	3.2	95
		Auger (K)	22.7	12
^{77}Br	57.0 hr	Auger (L)	1.3	113
		Coster-Kronig (LM)	0.04—0.08	357
^{100}Pd	3.64 days	Auger (L)	2.2	91
		Auger (K)	16.8—19.5	19
^{119}Sb	1.58 days	Auger (L)	4.0	88
		Conv. elec. (L)	19.1	86
		Auger (K)	21.0	14
^{101m}Rh	4.34 days	Auger (L)	2.2	92
		Auger (K)	16.4—18.8	19
^{197}Hg	2.71 days	Auger (L)	12	50
^{97}Ru	2.88 days	Auger (L)	2.2	96
		Auger (K)	15.5—17.8	21
^{58m}Co	9.2 hr	Conv. elec. (K)	17	66
		Conv. elec. (L,M)	24	34
^{189m}Os	5.7 hr	Conv. elec. (L)	20	77
		Conv. elec. (M)	28	23

result in the creation of a multitude of these electrons, most of which have ranges far less than a single cell diameter. Several isotopes which emit subcellular-range Auger and Coster-Kronig electrons and have half-lives which may be suitable for use in radioimmunotherapy are listed in Table 4.

A. Isotopes Requiring Nuclear Localization

Since there are no reports in the literature to date of the use of low energy electron emitters as labels for antibody radiotherapy, the potential utility of this approach must be gleaned from other radiotherapeutic applications of these isotopes. The isotope most frequently employed in these studies has been iodine-125 which emits a multitude of electrons of subcellular range per decay. The average number of electrons emitted and the electron energy distribution for iodine-125 decay is dependent on the chemical environment of the atom.[55,56]

When discussing the radiotoxicity of radiation of subcellular or cellular range (the majority of electrons emitted by iodine-125 have ranges less than 0.1 μm), it is important to bear in mind that conventional MIRD-type dosimetry is not applicable because of its macro, whole tissue perspective. Most radiobiological studies have shown that the cell nucleus is by far the most radiosensitive structure in a cell. Damage to DNA structure occurring at the molecular level such as multiple strand breakage[57] and ring fragmentation[58] can be correlated with radiotoxicity. Indeed, following irradiation, the cellular survival fraction will be proportional to the total number of chromosomal alterations which occur per cell.[59]

The extremely focal nature of the radiotoxicity associated with iodine-125 has been demonstrated by both theoretical calculation and by experiment. Sastry and Rao[11] have calculated that the dose received by the genome from iodine-125 homogeneously distributed in a sphere approximating the volume of the DNA helix would be at least an order of magnitude greater than if the isotope were distributed throughout a typical cellular volume. Martin and Hazeltine[57] used DNA fragments labeled with both iodine-125 and phosphorous-32 to demonstrate that most of the DNA strand breaks occur within only five nucleotides of the site of iodine-125 decay.

As would be expected, the radiotoxicity of isotopes like iodine-125 are critically dependent upon their localization in close proximity to the cell nucleus. This has been demonstrated in several studies using halogenated analogues of thymidine which are rapidly incorporated into the DNA of proliferating cells. Several groups have demonstrated in multiple cell lines that ^{125}I-iododeoxyuridine (^{125}IUdR) is highly cytotoxic.[59,60-62] In contrast, iodine-125 located extracellularly or on the cell membrane is much less radiotoxic,[63,64] supporting the fact that iodine-125 toxicity is dependent on uptake by the nucleus. It is also interesting to note that when IUdR is labeled with the beta emitter ^{131}I, it is considerably less cytotoxic than when labeled with ^{125}I despite the fact that the equilibrium dose constant for ^{125}I is about ten times lower than that of ^{131}I.[65] This difference demonstrates the inadequacy of MIRD formalism for calculating the radiation absorbed dose from short-range radiation.

Iodine-125 IUdR has also been shown to be therapeutically efficacious against a peritoneally implanted ascites tumor in the mouse.[66,67] Although these results demonstating the cytotoxicity of ^{125}I both in vitro and in vivo are encouraging, the 60-day half-life of iodine-125 could preclude its use at therapeutic doses in humans. It may be possible to label an antibody with a shorter half-life isotope which emits low-energy electrons such as those listed in Table 4. Bromine-77, for example, emits a multitude of Auger and Coster-Kronig electrons with ranges of less than 0.1 μm.[68] McElvany et al.[69] have synthesized ^{77}Br labeled deoxyuridine and the radiotoxicity of ^{77}BrUdR has been shown to be comparable to that of the ^{125}I labeled analogue.[68] The potentially lower rate of dehalogenation and the relatively low thyroid accumulation of bromide are two additional advantages of ^{77}Br relative to ^{125}I.

If radiotherapy using antibodies labeled with isotopes emitting electrons of subcellular range is to be feasible, it will be necessary to demonstrate that a significant fraction of the radioactivity can be translocated to the nucleus following antibody binding to the tumor cell membrane. Although this has yet to be demonstrated for an antibody, the potential of this type of approach has been shown using ^{125}I-labeled tamoxifen. This compound binds to cell-surface estrogen receptors forming a complex which is translocated to the nucleus.[70] Bloomer et al.[71,72] have shown that ^{125}I-labeled tamoxifen is cytotoxic to cells bearing estrogen receptors and significantly less toxic to control lines which lack membrane receptor.

The attractiveness of this approach is that if cytotoxicity is dependent upon internalization, it may be possible to treat tumors while minimizing irradiation of surrounding normal tissues. It will be critical, therefore, to identify antibodies that rapidly internalize into malignant, but not normal, cell populations. We have recently investigated the internalization of antibody F77-129 which is directed against an antigen present on human prostate tumors.[73,74] The half time for internalization measured by fluorescence was only about 30 min in vitro. However, the subcellular distribution of the antibody has not been measured.

Because of the potential for rapid degradation of antibodies within the cell, it will be important to develop labeling strategies which will maximize retention of radioactivity within the cell by inhibiting catabolism of the labeled antibody. One approach reported by Pittman et al.[75] is the use of cellobiose spacers between an iodinated tyramine and the protein. When proteins labeled by this procedure were introduced into cells, the retention of iodine-125 was considerably greater than that observed with proteins labeled by conventional methods.

B. Isotopes Localized Outside the Cell Nucleus

Selective irradiation of cells from isotopes localized outside the cell nucleus could also be achieved by using isotopes which emit conversion electrons and Auger electrons of appropriate range. The ideal electron energy for maximizing energy deposition in the cell nucleus will depend on a number of factors including the dimensions of the cell, the relative volume of the nucleus and the cytoplasm, and whether the isotope is affixed to the cell membrane or distributed throughout the cytoplasm. Kassis et al.[76] have calculated the average energy absorbed by the nucleus from electrons of varying energies located in different cellular compartments. The V79 Chinese hamster fibroblast with an average radius of 5.2 μm and a nuclear radius of 4.0 μm was used as the cell model for these calculations. For electron emitters distributed uniformly throughout the cytoplasm, the maximum deposition of energy in the nucleus, 2.9 keV, could be achieved with 16 keV electrons. We have extended these calculations to electrons located on the cell membrane; in this case, optimal irradiation of the cell nucleus requires electrons of about 17 keV. The energy deposited in the nucleus per decay decreases rapidly as a function of electron energy. Less than 1 keV per decay would be deposited in the cell nucleus by electrons with an energy of more than 50 keV located either on the cell membrane or in the cytoplasm. Some of the conversion and Auger electron-emitting isotopes that could be considered as potential labels for radioimmunotherapeutic applications involving the irradiation of micrometastatic foci are listed in Tables 3 and 4.

VII. EVALUATION OF RADIOLABELED ANTIBODIES AS THERAPEUTIC AGENTS

A. In Vitro Assessment

The most commonly used technique for evaluating the cytotoxic effects of radiation in vitro is the clonogenic assay.[77] Cell death is defined in terms of the loss of reproductive capacity as reflected by the inability to form clones or colonies of cells after exposure to radiation. Results are expressed in terms of D_o, the dose required to reduce the number of clones formed to 37% of their control value. Several examples of cell survival curves can be found in References 59 to 67. The shape of the survival curve is indicative of the relative biological effectiveness of the radiation employed. With high linear energy transfer radiation, such as alpha particles and intracellularly localized Auger electron emitters, a plot of the logarithm of the surviving fraction vs. radiation absorbed dose is a straight line. However, with sparsely ionizing radiation, a shoulder which is related to the oxygen enhancing effect[78] is generally observed at low radiation doses.

An alternative measurement of cytotoxicity is the determination of the effect of potential toxins on the ability of cells to synthesize protein.[79] In this procedure, cells are treated with varying doses of radioactivity and the ability of the cells to incorporate a labeled amino acid such as ^{3}H-leucine is measured.

With both types of cytotoxicity assays, radiation can be expressed either as activity per milliliter incubation volume or as radioactivity bound per cell. The latter method is preferable for use with labeled antibodies, particularly when using isotopes decaying by emission of short range radiation. Cell-bound radioactivity can be measured conveniently using a rapid method developed by Kassis and Adelstein.[80] When isotopes emitting radiation of subcellular range are used, a determination of the distribution of activity among the various cellular compartments may also be required.

In addition, meaningful evaluation of the in vitro cytotoxicity of radiolabeled antibodies will be dependent upon obtaining data for the appropriate controls. These include measuring the radiotoxicity of the radiolabeled tumor-reactive antibody in an antigen-negative cell line and the toxicity of an isotype-matched, tumor-unreactive antibody in the target cell line.

B. In Vivo Assessment

Several approaches have been reported for evaluating the therapeutic efficacy of radiolabeled antibodies in animal models. To date, these studies have been limited to antibodies labeled with iodine-131. One method which has been used as a preliminary indicator is the measurement of tumor growth in vivo following an in vitro incubation of tumor cells with labeled antibody. Zalcberg and co-workers[81] were able to show significant and specific decreases in tumor growth in a human colon carcinoma mouse xenograft model following in vitro incubation with iodine-131 specific but not control antibody. This type of study, as the authors suggest, is only the first step in demonstrating therapeutic utility in vivo.

Changes in tumor size and prolongation in median survival are the endpoints which have been used in most radioimmunotherapeutic trails in animal models. While all studies indicate that iodine-131 labeled antibodies have a therapeutic effect against a variety of tumors, the specificity of this effect has not been uniformly demonstrated.

Zalcberg et al.[81] reported that iodine-131 labeled 250-30.6 monoclonal antibody was effective in retarding tumor growth in two different animal models, but that in the murine thymoma, unlabeled control antibody was also effective. Similarly, dose-dependent reduction in splenomegaly and survival were observed in erythroleukemic mice following administration of both tumor-specific and control antibodies labeled with ^{131}I.[82] Goldenberg et al.[83] were able to demonstrate preferential treatment of human colonic tumor implants in the hamster with labeled specific antibody at doses of 1 mCi per animal. However, at both higher and lower doses, no significant advantage of tumor-directed antibody compared to normal goat IgG was observed. An additional study in a neuroblastoma xenograft model is difficult to interpret because no data for labeled control antibody was reported.[84]

Badger et al.[85] have demonstrated that an iodine-131 labeled monoclonal antibody directed against the Thy 1.1 differentiation antigen could be used to treat a murine lymphoma. Doses of 500 to 1500 μCi of iodine-131 labeled anti-Thy 1.1 resulted in significant regression of an established lymphoma while labeled control antibody had no effect except at the highest dose. Histopathological studies of mice treated with the higher doses of labeled antibody indicated severe bone marrow hypoplasia 2 weeks after antibody administration with recovery noted 1 week later.

Based on these studies, a number of factors emerge which must be considered in the design of radioimmunotherapeutic trials in animals. First, the importance of performing adequate controls cannot be overemphasized. These should include a labeled nonspecific antibody and unlabeled tumor-associated antibody. It is also important to study multiple doses of labeled antibody so that the width of the "therapeutic window" can be established. Therapeutic efficacy for a given dose of labeled antibody will also depend upon the interval between tumor inoculation and labeled antibody administration. The rate of tumor cell doubling relative to the pharmacokinetics of antibody uptake and washout in vivo must also be considered. Finally, the problem of calculating the radiation dose to a tumor whose size changes rapidly during the course of the experiment must be solved.

A significant problem in assessing the efficacy of antibody-mediated radiotherapy is the lack of a realistic animal model. Because of the size of the nude mouse relative to the range of the beta particles of ^{131}I (maximum range 2.2 mm), toxicity to normal tissues proximal to organs which concentrate radioactivity may be greater than would be encountered clinically. The magnitude of this effect would, of course, be greatest for high energy beta particles and least for low energy electron emitters. In addition, toxicity to normal tissue adjacent to tumor cannot be measured in the nude mouse model.

One approach to developing a more useful model is to place the tumor in a more clinically relevant anatomic site. For example, Bullard et al.[86] have developed an intracranially implanted human glioma xenograft model in the rat. The radiotherapeutic efficacy of iodine-131 labeled 81C6, an antibody directed against a glioma associated antigen, was evaluated in this model.[87] Iodine-131 labeled 81C6 was found to be significantly more effective in prolonging survival compared to unlabeled 81C6, buffer, and iodine-131 labeled isotype-matched control antibody.

VIII. IMPROVING THE THERAPEUTIC INDEX

The success of antibody-mediated radiotherapy is critically dependent upon the ability to maximize the uptake and retention of labeled antibody by the tumor while minimizing the dose received by normal tissues. Although the results obtained with ^{131}I-labeled antibodies have, in general, been less than encouraging, it seems likely that utilization of some of the isotopes described above could help achieve these goals. In addition to radioisotopic considerations, there are several factors of a more pharmacological nature which could also be exploited to increase the therapeutic index for monoclonal antibodies.

One approach to increasing the clearance of radioactivity from normal tissues is the use of $F(ab')_2$ and Fab fragments. With these fragments, higher tumor-to-normal-tissue ratios have been obtained and at earlier time points than with intact IgG.[88,89] Thus, antibody fragments could be of particular utility for use with shorter half-life isotopes. While use of labeled antibody fragments results in a more rapid clearance of radioactivity from the body, particularly from the blood pool, a significant reduction in tumor uptake is, in general, also observed. An exception is a recent report by Harwood and co-workers[90] in which the uptake of an anti-CEA $F(ab')_2$ fragment in human colon tumor xenografts in nude mice was equal to that measured following injection of intact IgG. However, loss of radioactivity from the tumor was more rapid with the $F(ab')_2$ fragment. If sufficient labeled antibody can be delivered to a tumor, then use of $F(ab')_2$ fragments may decrease the radiation absorbed dose received by normal tissues.

Depending upon the location of the tumor, it may be possible to increase both the rate and magnitude of tumor uptake by administering the antibody via a nonintravenous route. For example, ovarian and colorectal cancers which have metastasized within the peritoneal cavity may be treated more effectively by intraperitoneal injection of labeled antibody. Colcher et al.[91] have compared the utility of intravenous (i.v.) and intraperitoneal delivery of ^{131}I-labeled B72.3 monoclonal antibody in patients with peritoneal carcinomatosis. Following intraperitoneal injection, the ratio of radioactivity in the tumor to surrounding normal tissues was 3 to 8 times higher than that obtained by the i.v. route.

We have been investigating the relative ability of delivering radioiodinated monoclonal antibody 81C6 to intracranial glioma xenografts following i.v. and intracarotid injection.[92] A paired injection protocol was used to demonstrate a 20% advantage in integrated tumor uptake when antibody was administered via the carotid artery.

Epenetos and co-workers[93] are studying the efficacy of treating tumors by the direct injection of ^{131}I-labeled HMFG2 antibody into isolated body spaces containing tumor. One patient was injected intrapleurally, another intrapericardially, and a third received antibody via an intraperitoneal injection. Higher tumor-to-normal-tissue ratios than those following i.v. administration were reported. In addition, doses of only 20 mCi of ^{131}I-labeled antibody resulted in some therapeutic benefit to the three patients studied. Epenetos et al.[94] have also reported that arterial infusion of an ^{131}I-labeled antibody against epidermal growth factor receptor resulted in significant regression of tumor in a patient with an advanced glioma. Compared to i.v. delivery, a twofold increased tumor dose was reported following intracarotid delivery.

Several groups have been investigating various approaches which utilize a second antibody reactive with the anti-tumor antibody in order to expedite clearance of activity from normal tissues. Begent et al.[95] have studied the effect of liposome-entrapped second antibody (horse antibody to goat immunoglobulin) on the distribution of ^{131}I-labeled goat anti-CEA in patients. Although the clearance of radioactivity from the blood pool was accelerated by a factor of two- to fourfold after injection of the liposomes, increased accumulation of radioactivity in the liver was also observed for the first 24 hr after liposome administration. Sharkey and co-workers[96] have investigated the utility of a second antibody not encapsulated in liposomes for decreasing blood pool activity following injection of ^{131}I-labeled anti-CEA in hamsters bearing human colonic tumor xenografts. Injection of the second antibody decreased activity levels in the blood by a factors of 4 and 16 at 2 and 24 hr, respectively, without increasing the accumulation of ^{131}I activity in the liver or spleen. Unfortunately, by 24 hr, the absolute percent of injected dose in the tumors of animals receiving second antibody had decreased to about one third of the level observed in animals injected with ^{131}I-labeled anti-CEA alone. Similar observations on the effect of second antibody administration have been reported by the Charing Cross group.[97,98]

An interesting approach to increasing the rate of tumor uptake and normal tissue washout has been reported by Goodwin and co-workers.[99] This method is based on the use of a monoclonal antibody which had been developed which was highly specific for the indium-benzyl-EDTA complex.[100] Rapid tumor uptake and clearance of activity from both the blood pool and the liver was achieved using the following protocol: anti-chelate antibody was injected into tumor-bearing mice. Twenty-four hours later, cold indium chelate covalently linked to a carrier protein was administered, followed 1 hr later by injection of ^{111}In-benzyl-EDTA. Tumor uptake in this study was based on nonspecific processes. However, the development of hybrid antibodies with one arm recognizing the chelate and the other binding to the tumor should permit more effective utilization of this approach.

ACKNOWLEDGMENTS

The personal research described in this chapter was supported in part by National Cancer Institute Grant CA42324 and by a grant from the Preuss Foundation.

REFERENCES

1. **Frankel, A. E., Houston, L. L., Issell, B. F., and Fathman, G.,** Prospects for immunotoxin therapy in cancer, *Annu. Rev. Med.*, 37, 125, 1986.
2. **Frankel, A. E.,** Antibody-toxin hybrids: a clinical review of their use, *J. Biol. Response Mod.*, 4, 437, 1985.
3. **Ehrlich, P., Herta, C. A., and Shiga, K.,** Uber einige Verwendungen der Naphtochinosulfosaure, *Z. Physiol. Cheum.*, 61, 379, 1904.
4. **Bale, W. F., Spar, I. L., and Goodland, R. L.,** Experimental radiation therapy of tumors with ^{131}I-carrying antibodies to fibrin, *Cancer Res.*, 20, 1488, 1960.
5. **Loevinger, R. and Berman, M.,** A schema for calculations for biologically-distributed radionuclides, *J. Nucl. Med., Suppl.*, 1, 7, 1968.
6. **Snyder, W. S., Ford, M. R., Warner, G. G., and Fisher, H. L., Jr.,** Estimates of absorbed fractions for monoenergetic photon sources uniformly distributed in various organs of a heterogeneous phantom, *J. Nucl. Med., Suppl.*, 3, 5, 1969.
7. **Kwok, C. S., Prestwich, W. V., and Wilson, B. C.,** Calculation of radiation doses for nonuniformly distributed β and γ radionuclides in soft tissue, *Med. Phys.*, 12, 405, 1985.
8. **Kassis, A. I., Adelstein, S. J., and Sastry, K. S. R.,** Thallium-201: an experimental and a theoretical radiobiological approach to dosimetry, *J. Nucl. Med.*, 24, 1164, 1983.
9. **Kassis, A. I., Sastry, K. S. R., and Adelstein, S. J.,** Intracellular distribution and radiotoxicity of chromium-51 in mammalian cells: Auger-electron dosimetry, *J. Nucl. Med.*, 26, 59, 1985.
10. **Rao, D. V., Govelitz, G. F., and Sastry, K. S. R.,** Radiotoxicity of thallium-201 in mouse testes. Inadequacy of conventional dosimetry, *J. Nucl. Med.*, 24, 145, 1983.
11. **Sastry, K. S. R. and Rao, D. V.,** Dosimetry of low energy electrons, in *Physics of Nuclear Medicine Recent Advances*, Rao, D. V., Chandra, R., and Graham, M. C., Eds., American Institute of Physics, New York, 1984, 169.
12. **Fisher, D. L.,** The microdosimetry of monoclonal antibodies labeled with alpha emitters, Report BN-SA-2204, Battelle Pacific Northwest Laboratory, 1985.
13. International Commission on Radiation Units and Measurements, *Microdosimetry,* ICRU Report 36, 1983.
14. **Wessels, B. W. and Rogus, R. D.,** Radionuclide selection and model absorbed dose calculations for radiolabeled tumor associated antibodies, *Med. Phsy.*, 11, 638, 1984.
15. **Jungerman, J. A., Yu, K.-H. P., and Zanelli, C. I.,** Radiation absorbed dose estimates at the cellular level for some electron-emitting radionuclides for radioimmunotherapy, *Int. J. Appl. Radiat. Isot.*, 35, 883, 1984.

16. **Order, S. E., Klein, J. L., Leichner, P. K., Frincke, J., Lollo, C., and Carlo, D. J.,** ^{90}Yttrium antiferritin-A new therapeutic radiolabled antibody, *Int. J. Radiat. Oncol. Biol. Phys.*, 12, 277, 1986.
17. **Lewis, R. E. and Eldridge, J. S.,** Production of 70 day tungsten-188 and development of a 17 hour rhenium-188 radioisotope generator, *J. Nucl. Med.*, 7, 804, 1966.
18. **Blanchot, J., Herment, J., and Moussa, A.,** Une generator ^{188}Re parte ^{188}W, *Int. J. Appl. Radiat. Isot.*, 20, 467, 1969.
19. **Misheyev, N. B., Popovits, W. B., Rumer, I. A., Savelyev, G. I., and Volkova, N. L.,** A rhenium-188 generator, *Isotopenpraxis*, 8, 248, 1972.
20. **Malyshev, K. V. and Smirnov, V. V.,** Rhenium-188 generator based on hydrated zirconium oxide, *Radiokhimiya*, 17, 249, 1975.
21. **Fritzberg, A. R., Rao, T. N., Adhikesavlu, D., Camerman, A., and Vanderheyden, J.-L.,** Synthesis and characterization of Re and Tc complexes of N_2S_2 and N_3S ligands, *J. Labelled Cmpd. Radiopharm.*, 23(Abstr.), 1120, 1986.
22. **Vaughan, A. T. M., Keeling, A., and Yankuba, S. C. S.,** The production and biological distribution of yttrium-90 labelled antibodies, *Int. J. Appl. Radiat. Isot.*, 36, 803, 1985.
23. **Hnatowich, D. J., Virzi, F., and Doherty, P. W.,** DTPA-coupled antibodies labeled with yttrium-90, *J. Nucl. Med.*, 26, 503, 1985.
24. **Cole, W., DeNardo, S., Meares, C., DeNardo, G., and O'Brien, H.,** Development of copper 67 chelate conjugated monoclonal antibody, *J. Nucl. Med.*, 24(Abstr.), 30, 1983.
25. **Mirzadeh, S., Mausner, L. F., and Srivastava, S.,** Production of no-carrier added ^{67}Cu, *Int. J. Appl. Radiat. Isot.*, 37, 29, 1986.
26. **DeNardo, S. J., Meares, C. F., Moi, M. K., Cole, W. C., McCall, M. J., DeNardo, G. L., and O'Brien, H. A.,** Comparative serum stability of Cu-67 and In-111 chelates for diagnostic and therapeutic antibody applications, *J. Nucl. Med.*, 26(Abstr.), 119, 1985.
27. **Moi, M. K., Meares, C. F., McCall, M. J., Cole, W. C., and DeNardo, S. J.,** Copper chelates as probes of biological systems, *Anal. Biochem.*, 148, 249, 1985.
28. **Franz, J., Barefield, E. K., Freeman, G. M., Volkert, W. A., and Holmes, R. A.,** Employment of a macrocyclic amine bifunctional chelate to label antibodies, *J. Nucl. Med.*, 26(Abstr.), 129, 1985.
29. **Figard, S. D., Mercer-Smith, J. A., Taylor, W. A., and Lavallee, D. K.,** Labeling antibodies with copper-67, *J. Nucl. Med.*, 27(Abstr.), 1042, 1986.
30. **Fawwaz, R. A., Wang, T. S. T., Srivastava, S. C., Rosen, J. M., Ferrone, S., Hardy, M. A., and Alderson, P. O.,** Potential of palladium-109-labeled antimelanoma monoclonal antibody for tumor therapy, *J. Nucl. Med.*, 25, 796, 1984.
31. **Barendsen, G. W., Beusker, T. L. J., Vergroesen, A. J., and Budke, L.,** Effects of different ionizing radiation on human cells in tissue culture, *Radiat. Res.*, 13, 841, 1960.
32. **Lloyd, E. L., Gammell, M. A., Henning, C. V., Gammell, D. S., and Zabransky, B. J.,** Cell survival following multiple-track alpha particle irradiation, *Int. J. Radiat. Biol.*, 35, 23, 1979.
33. **Vaughan, A. T. M., Bateman, W. J., and Cowan, J.,** The specific inhibition of cellular clonogenic proliferation using ^{211}At labelled lectins and antibodies-I, *Int. J. Nucl. Med. Biol.*, 9, 167, 1982.
34. **Aaij, C., Tschrotts, W. R. J. M., Lindner, L., and Feltkamp, T. E. W.,** The preparation of astatine labeled proteins, *Int. J. Appl. Radiat. Isot.*, 26, 25, 1975.
35. **Friedman, A. M., Zalutsky, M. R., Wung, W., Buckingham, F., Harper, P. V., Sherr, G. H., Wainer, B., Hunter, R. L., Appelman, E. H., Rothberg, R. M., Fitch, F. W., Stuart, F. P., and Simonian, S. J.,** Preparation of a biologically stable and immunogenically competent astatinated protein, *Int. J. Nucl. Med. Biol.*, 4, 219, 1977.
36. **Lambrecht, R. M., and Mirzadeh, S.,** Cyclotron isotopes and radiopharmaceuticals-XXXV, Astatine-211, *Int. J. Appl. Radiat. Isot.*, 36, 443, 1985.
37. **Vaughan, A. T. M. and Fremlin, J. H.,** The preparation of astatine labeled proteins using an electrophilic reaction, *Int. J. Nucl. Med. Biol.*, 5, 229, 1978.
38. **Visser, G. W. M., Diemer, E. L., and Kaspersen, F. M.,** The preparation and stability of astatotyrosine and astatoiodo-tyrosine, *Int. J. Appl. Radiat. Isot.*, 30, 749, 1979.
39. **Visser, G. W. M., Diemer, E. L., and Kaspersen, F. M.,** The nature of the astatine-protein bond, *Int. J. Appl. Radiat. Isot.*, 32, 905, 1981.
40. **Zalutsky, M. R., Friedman, A. M., Buckingham, F., Wung, W., Stuart, F. P., and Simonian, S. J.,** Synthesis of a non-labile astatine-protein conjugate, *J. Labelled Cmpd. Radiopharm.*, 13, 181, 1977.
41. **Vaughan, A. T. M.,** The labeling of proteins with ^{211}At using an acylation reaction, *Int. J. Appl. Radiat. Isot.*, 30, 576, 1979.
42. **Harrison, A. and Royle, L.,** Preparation of a ^{211}At-IgG conjugate which is stable in vivo, *Int. J. Appl. Radiat. Isot.*, 35, 1005, 1984.
43. **Hanson, R. N., Tonnesen, G. L., McLaughlin, W. H., Bloomer, W. H., and Seitz, D. E.,** Electrophilic radiodestannylation as a new radioiodination method, *J. Labelled Cmpd. Radiopharm.*, 18, 128, 1981.

44. **Tonnesen, G. L., Hanson, R. N., and Seitz, D. E.,** Position-specific radioiodination utilizing an aryltributylstannyl intermediate. Synthesis of [^{125}I] iodotamoxifen, *Int. J. Appl. Radiat. Isot.*, 32, 171, 1981.
45. **Milius, R. A., McLaughlin, W. H., Lambrecht, R. M., Carroll, J. J., Adelstein, S. J., and Bloomer, W. H.,** Organoastatine chemistry. Astatination via electrophilic destannylation, *Int. J. Appl. Radiat. Isot.*, 37, 799, 1986.
46. **Milius, R. A., Zalutsky, M. R., Lambrecht, R. M., and Adelstein, S. J.,** The synthesis and in vitro stability of potential protein astatinating agents: astatobenzoic acids, in preparation.
47. **Vaughan, A. T. M., Bateman, W. J., and Cowan, J.,** The preparation and cytotoxic properties of ^{211}At labelled concanavalin A bound to cell membranes, *J. Radioanal. Chem.*, 64, 33, 1981.
48. **Vaughan, A. T. M., Bateman, W. J., and Fisher, D. R.,** The in vivo fate of a ^{211}At labelled monoclonal antibody with known specificity in a murine system, *Int. J. Radiat. Oncol. Biol. Phys.*, 8, 1943, 1982.
49. **Bateman, W. J., Vaughan, A. T. M., and Brown, G.,** Tumour localization of ^{211}At labelled monoclonal antibody to a sub-cutaneous human heterograft in the nude mouse. II. *Int. J. Nucl. Med. Biol.*, 4, 241, 1983.
50. **Zucchini, G. L. and Friedman, A. M.,** Isotopic generator for ^{211}Pb and ^{212}Bi, *Int. J. Nucl. Med. Biol.*, 9, 83, 1982.
51. **Atcher, R. W., Friedman, A. M., and Hines, J. J.,** An improved generator for the production of ^{212}Pb and ^{212}Bi from ^{224}Ra, *Int. J. Appl. Radiat. Isot.*, 39, 283, 1988.
52. **Anderson-Berg, W. T., Strand, M., Brechbiel, M., Atcher, R. W., and Gansow, O. A.,** Bi-212 labeled monoclonal antibodies for use in radioimmunotherapy, *J. Nucl. Med.*, 27(Abstr.), 1040, 1986.
53. **Kozak, R. W., Atcher, R. W., Gansow, O. A., Friedman, A. M., Hines, J. J., and Waldmann, T. A.,** Bismuth-212-labeled anti-Tac monoclonal antibody: α particle-emitting radionuclides as modalities for radioimmunotherapy, *Proc. Natl. Acad. Sci. U.S.A.*, 83, 474, 1986.
54. **Cole, A.,** Absorption of 20-eV to 50,000-eV electron beams in air and plastic, *Radiat. Res.*, 38, 7, 1969.
55. **Charlton, D. E. and Booz, J.,** A Monte Carlo treatment of the decay of ^{125}I, *Radiat. Res.*, 87, 10, 1981.
56. **Carlson, T. A. and White, R. M.,** Formation of fragment ions from $CH_3{}^{125}Te$ following nuclear decays of $CH_3{}^{125}I$ and $C_2H_5{}^{125}I$, *J. Chem. Phys.*, 38, 2930, 1963.
57. **Martin, R. F. and Hazeltine, W. A.,** Range of radiochemical damage to DNA with decay of iodine-125, *Science*, 213, 896, 1981.
58. **Deutzmann, R. and Stocklin, G.,** Chemical effects of iodine-125 decay in aqueous solution of 5-iodouracil. Ring fragmentation as a consequence of the Auger effect, *Radiat. Res.*, 87, 24, 1981.
59. **Chan, P. C., Lisco, E., Lisco, H., and Adelstein, S. J.,** Cell survival and cytogenetic responses to ^{125}I-UdR in cultured mammalian cells, *Curr. Top. Radiat. Res. Q.*, 12, 426, 1977.
60. **Hofer, K. G. and Hughes, W. L.,** Radiotoxicity of intranuclear tritium, ^{125}iodine and ^{131}iodine, *Radiat. Res.*, 47, 94, 1971.
61. **Burki, H. J., Roots, R., Feinendegen, L. E., and Bond, V. P.,** Inactivation of mammalian cells after disintegrations of ^{3}H or ^{125}I in cell DNA at $-196°C$, *Int. J. Radiat. Biol.*, 24, 363, 1973.
62. **Bradley, E. W., Chan, P. C., and Adelstein, S. J.,** The radiotoxicity of iodine-125 in mammalian cells. I. Effects on the survival curve of radioiodine incorporated into DNA, *Radiat. Res.*, 64, 555, 1975.
63. **Hofer, K. G., Harris, C. R., and Smith, J. M.,** Radiotoxicity of intracellular ^{67}Ga, ^{125}I and ^{3}H. Nuclear versus cytoplasmic radiation effects in murine L1210 leukemia, *Int. J. Radiat. Biol.*, 28, 225, 1975.
64. **Warters, R. L., Hofer, K. G., Harris, C. R., and Smith, J. M.,** Radionuclide toxicity in cultured mammalian cells: elucidation of the primary site of radiation damage, *Curr. Top. Radiat. Res. Q.*, 12, 389, 1977.
65. **Dillman, L. T.,** Radionuclide decay schemes and nuclear parameters for use in radiation-dose estimation, *J. Nucl. Med., Suppl.*, 2, 5, 1969.
66. **Bloomer, W. D. and Adelstein, S. J.,** 5-^{125}I-iododeoxyuridine as prototype for radionuclide therapy with Auger emitters, *Nature (London)*, 265, 620, 1977.
67. **Bloomer, W. D. and Adelstein, S. J.,** Antineoplastic effects of iodine-125 labeled iododeoxyuridine, *Int. J. Radiat. Biol.*, 27, 509, 1975.
68. **Kassis, A. I., Adelstein, S. J., Haydock, C., Sastry, S. K. R., McElvany, K. D., and Welch, M. J.,** Lethality of Auger electrons from the decay of bromine-77 in the DNA of mammalian cells, *Radiat. Res.*, 90, 362, 1982.
69. **McElvany, K. D., Welch, M. J., Katzenellenbogen, J. A., Senderoff, S. G., Bentley, G. B., and Grant, P. M.,** Scope and limitations of a rapid radiobromination technique, *Int. J. Appl. Radiat. Isot.*, 32, 411, 1981.
70. **Heel, R. C., Brogden, R. N., Speight, T. M., and Avery, G. S.,** Tamoxifen: a review of its pharmacological properties and therapeutic use in the treatment of breast cancer, *Drugs*, 16, 1, 1978.
71. **Bloomer, W. D., McLaughlin, W. H., Weichselbaum, R. R., Tonnesen, G. L., Hellman, S., Seitz, D. E., Hanson, R. N., Adelstein, S. J., Rosner, A. L., Burstein, N. A., Nove, J. J., and Little, J. B.,** Iodine-125-labelled tamoxifen is differentially cytotoxic to cells containing oestrogen receptors, *Int. J. Radiat. Biol.*, 38, 197, 1980.

72. **Bloomer, W. D., McLaughlin, W. H., Weichselbaum, R. R., Hanson, R. N., Adelstein, S. J., and Seitz, D. E.,** The role of subcellular localization in assessing the cytotoxicity of iodine-125 labeled iododeoxyuridine, iodotamoxifen, and iodoantipyrine, *J. Radioanal. Chem.*, 65, 209, 1981.
73. **Carroll, A. M., Zalutsky, M. R., Schatten, S., Perry, L. L., Sobotka, C., Benacerraf, B., and Greene, M.,** Monoclonal antibodies to tissue specific cell surface antigens I: characterization of an antibody to a prostate tissue antigen, *Clin. Immunol. Immunopathol.*, 33, 268, 1984.
74. **Carroll, A. M., Zalutsky, M. R., Benacerraf, B., and Greene, M. I.,** Monoclonal antibodies to tissue-associated antigens as anti-tumor reagents, *Surv. Synth. Pathol. Res.*, 3, 189, 1984.
75. **Pittman, R. C., Carew, T. E., Glass, C. K., Green, S. E., Taylor, C. A., Jr., and Attie, A. D.,** A radioiodinated intracellularly trapped ligand for determining the sites of plasma protein degradation in vivo, *Biochem. J.*, 212, 791, 1983.
76. **Kassis, A. I., Adelstein, S. J., Haydock, C., and Sastry, K. S. R.,** Radiotoxicity of ^{75}Se and ^{35}S: theory and application to a cellular model, *Radiat. Res.*, 84, 407, 1980.
77. **Hall, E. J.,** *Radiobiology for the Radiologist,* Harper & Row, New York, 1978, 31.
78. **Hall, E. J.,** *Radiobiology for the Radiologist,* Harper & Row, New York, 1978, 181.
79. **Thorpe, P. E., Rose, W. C. J., Cumber, A. J., Hinson, C. A., Edwards, D. C., and Davies, A. J. S.,** Toxicity of diptheria toxin for lymphoblastoid cells is increased by conjugation to antilymphocytic globulin, *Nature (London),* 272, 752, 1978.
80. **Kassis, A. I. and Adelstein, S. J.,** A rapid and reproducible method for the separation of cells from radioactive media, *J. Nucl. Med.*, 21, 88, 1980.
81. **Zalcberg, J. R., Thompson, C. H., Lichtenstein, M., and McKenzie, I. F. C.,** Tumor immunotherapy in the mouse with the use of ^{131}I-labeled monoclonal antibodies, *J. Natl. Cancer Inst.*, 72, 697, 1984.
82. **Redwood, W. R., Tom, T. D., and Strand, M.,** Specificity, efficacy and toxicity of radioimmunotherapy in erythroleukemic mice, *Cancer Res.*, 44, 5681, 1984.
83. **Goldenberg, D. M., Gaffar, S. A., Bennett, S. J., and Beach, J. L.,** Experimental radioimmunotherapy of a xenografted human colonic tumor (GW-39) producing carcinoembryonic antigen, *Cancer Res.*, 41, 4354, 1981.
84. **Jones, D. H., Goldman, A., Gordon, I., Pritchard, J., Gregory, B. J., and Kemshead, J. T.,** Therapeutic application of a radiolabelled monoclonal antibody in nude mice xenografted with human neuroblastoma: tumoricidal effects and distribution studies, *Int. J. Cancer,* 35, 715, 1985.
85. **Badger, C. C., Krohn, K. A., Peterson, A. V., Shulman, H., and Bernstein, I. D.,** Experimental radiotherapy of murine lymphoma with ^{131}I-labeled anti-Thy 1.1 monoclonal antibody, *Cancer Res.*, 45, 1536, 1985.
86. **Bullard, D. E., Adams, C. J., Coleman, R. E., and Bigner, D. D.,** In vivo imaging of intracranial human glioma xenografts comparing specific versus nonspecific radiolabeled monclonal antibodies, *J. Neurosurg.*, 64, 257, 1986.
87. **Lee, Y.-S., Bullard, D. E., Humphrey, P. A., Colapinto, E. V., Friedman, H. S., Zalutsky, M. R., Coleman, R. E., and Bigner, D. D.,** Treatment of intracranial human glioma xenografts with ^{131}I anti-tenascin monoclonal antibody (Mab)81C6, *Cancer Res.*, 48, 2904, 1988.
88. **Zalutsky, M. R., Colcher, D., Kaplan, W. D., Kufe, D. W.,** Radioiodinated B6.2 monoclonal antibody: further characterization of a potential radiopharmaceutical for the identification of breast tumors, *Int. J. Nucl. Med. Biol.*, 12, 227, 1985.
89. **Buchegger, F., Haskell, C. M., Schreyer, M., Scazziga, B. R., Randin, S., Carrel, S., and Mach, J.-P.,** Radiolabeled fragments of monoclonal antibodies against carcinoembryonic antigen for localization of human colon carcinoma grafted into nude mice, *J. Exp. Med.*, 158, 413, 1983.
90. **Harwood, P. J., Boden, J., Pedley, R. B., Rawlings, G., Rodgers, G. T., and Bagshawe, K. D.,** Comparative tumour localization of antibody fragments and intact IgG in nude mice bearing a CEA-producing human colon tumor xenograft, *Eur. J. Cancer Clin. Oncol.*, 21, 1515, 1985.
91. **Colcher, D., Esteban, J., Carrasquillo, J. A., Sugarbaker, P., Reynolds, J. C., Bryant, G., Larson, S. M., and Schlom, J.,** Comparison of route of administration of radiolabeled monoclonal antibodies in patients with colorectal cancer, *J. Nucl. Med.*, 27(Abstr.), 902, 1986.
92. **Lee, Y., Bullard, D. E., Wikstrand, C. J., Zalutsky, M. R., Muhlbaier, L. H., and Bigner, D. D.,** Comparison of monoclonal antibody delivery to intracranial glioma xenografts by intravenous and intracarotid infusion, *Cancer Res.*, 47, 1941, 1987.
93. Hammersmith Oncology Group and the Imperial Cancer Research Fund, Antibody-guided irradiation of malignant lesions: three cases illustrating a new method of treatment, *Lancet,* 1, 1441, 1984.
94. **Epenetos, A. A., Courtenay-Luck, N., Pickering, D., Hooker, G., Durbin, H., Lavender, J. P., and McKenzie, C. G.,** Antibody guided irradiation of brain glioma by arterial infusion of radioactive monoclonal antibody agaisnt epidermal growth factor receptor and blood group A antigen, *Br. Med. J.*, 290, 1463, 1985.

95. **Begent, R. H. J., Keep, P. A., Green, A. J., Searle, F., Bagshawe, K. D., Jewkes, R. F., Jones, B. E., Barratt, G. M., and Ryman, B. E.,** Liposomally entrapped second antibody improves tumour imaging with radiolabelled (first) antitumor antibody, *Lancet,* 2, 739, 1982.
96. **Sharkey, R. M., Primus, F. J., and Goldenberg, D. M.,** Second antibody clearance of radiolabeled antibody in cancer radioimmunodetection, *Proc. Natl. Acad. Sci. U.S.A.,* 81, 2843, 1984.
97. **Chester, K. A., Begent, R. H. J., Pedley, R. B., Keep, P. A., Boden, J. A., Searle, F., and Bagshawe, K. D.,** The use of 2d antibody to improve selective localization of tumors: animal model studies, *Br. J. Cancer,* 50(Abstr.), 556, 1984.
98. **Begent, R. H. J., Bagshawe, K. D., Pedley, R. B., Searle, F., Ledermann, J. A., Green, A., Keep, P. A., Chester, K. A., Glaser, M. G., and Dale, R.,** Use of 2d antibody in radioimmunotherapy, *Cancer Drug Deliv.,* 2(Abstr.), 234, 1985.
99. **Goodwin, D. A., Meares, C. F., McTigue, M., McCall, M. J., and David, G. S.,** Rapid localization of hapten in sites containing previously administered antibody for immunoscintigraphy with short half-life tracers, *J. Nucl. Med.,* 27(Abstr.), 959, 1986.
100. **Reardan, D. T., Meares, C. F., Goodwin, D. A., McTigue, M., David, G. S., Stone, M. R., Leung, J. P., Bartholomew, R. M., and Frincke, J. M.,** Antibodies against metal chelates, *Nature (London),* 316, 265, 1985.

INDEX

U

V

W

Y